TRADITIONAL INDIAN MEDICINE –
with specific reference to Buddhist and Tribal Medicine

TRADITIONAL INDIAN MEDICINE –

with specific reference to Buddhist and Tribal Medicine

AMIT JHA
Department of History
Sri Aurobindo College (Day)
University of Delhi

RESEARCH INDIA PRESS
New Delhi (INDIA)

Cataloging in Publication Data--DK

Courtesy: D. K. Agencies (P) Ltd. <docinfo@dkagencies.com>

Jha, Amit.

Traditional Indian medicine : with specific reference to Buddhist and tribal medicine / Amit Jha. -- 1st ed.

p. cm.

Includes bibliographical references (p.) and index.

ISBN : 9788189131357

1. Traditional medicine--India. 2. Medicine, Tibetan. 3. Buddhist medicine. I. Title.

DDC 610.954 22

ISBN : 978-81-89131-35-7

Price : 1195

First Edition: 2011

Typesetting by
G. R. Sharma
9968281826

Published by :
RESEARCH INDIA PRESS
E-6/34, Sangam Vihar
New Delhi-110062
Phone: 011-26047013, (M) 9818085794
E-mail: researchindiapress@yahoo.com

CONTENTS

ACKNOWLEDGEMENTS

I would like to record my thanks to the members of the library staff of Sri Aurobindo College, Nehru Memorial Museum and Library, Teen Murti House, New Delhi, JNU Library, New Delhi and the Delhi University Library System. I am also thankful to my respected teachers, Prof. Aditya Mukherjee (Deptt. of Contemporary Studies, JNU), Prof. K. T. S. Sarao (Head, Deptt. of Buddhist Studies, D. U.), Dr. S. M. Patnaik, (Reader, Deptt. of Anthropology, D. U.), and Dr. I. N.Singh (Buddhist Studies, D. U.), whose interest in my work and constructive criticism have helped me in improving this work.

I am really thankful to the UGC for providing me financial assistance for this work. I must also, make it clear that financial benefit is not the motive behind the publication of this work. For this, I must thank Research India Press, Delhi for getting this work published at a very subsidised rate. My only purpose, here, is to popularize the concept of Traditional Indian Medicine especially Buddhist Medicine in India. In this regard, first and foremost, with all my humility, I pay my obeisance to His Holiness Dalai Lama. Actually, I am trying to follow the footsteps of contemporary great Buddhist scholars like Lama Tashi Namgyal, Lama Pasang Yongten Arya and Thirangpu Rinpoche. *For me, also, the works of Dr. P.V.*

Sharma, S. S. Begley, J. Holist Nurs and Subhuti Dharmananda proved to be very inspiring

I will always remain thankful to Prof. B. P. Sahu, (Head of Deptt., Deptt. of History, Delhi University) my teacher, for his guidance, constant encouragement and kindness. He has been kind enough to spare some of his precious time to give valuable suggestions regarding this work.

Last but not the least, I must thank Mrs. Leena Jha, who made an immense contribution to this work. She meticulously collected relevant data by consulting variety of primary and secondary sources (both, the printed version as well as online sources) for this work.

INTRODUCTION

In the great teaching of the Vedas, there is no touch of sectarianism. It is of all ages, climes and nationalities and is the royal road for the attainment of the Great Knowledge. Thoreau, American Thinker.

Traditional medical science in India, is to some extent, gradually accumulated practical and systematic knowledge. They are (viz. Ayurveda, Siddha, Unani, etc.) very ancient, deep rooted and codified. They have their origins in the remote past, their systematisation and canonisation gave rise to the elite (the Greater Tradition) medical science.

It is now recognized that western criteria are not the sole benchmark by which other cultural knowledge should be evaluated. While the term 'traditional' sometimes carries the connotation of 'pre-modern' in the sense of 'primitive' or 'outdated', many of the traditional medical technologies were in fact quite advanced even by western standards as well as better adapted to unique local conditions and needs than their later 'modern' substitutes. In countries with ancient cultural traditions, the folk and elite science were taken as part of the same unified legacy, without any hegemonic categorizations. However, modernization has homogenized various solutions, and this loss of ideas is similar to the destruction of biodiversity. Colonizers systematically derogated, exterminated or undermined the local traditional science, technology and crafts of the lands and people they plundered, because of their intellectual arrogance, and also to control and appropriate the economic means of production and the social means of organization. Modern societies created hegemonic categories of science versus magic, technology versus superstitions etc., which were arbitrary and contrived. But many anthropologists who have recently worked with so-called 'primitive' peoples have been surprised to learn of some of their highly evolved and sophisticated medical technologies. Anthropologists thus coined the term 'Traditional Medical System' as a scientific system, which has its own validity, in contradistinction to 'modern' medical science.

Impact of Globalisation

The vast majority of modern medicines patented by western pharmaceutical firms are based on tropical plants. The most common method to select candidates for detailed testing has been for western firms to scout tropical societies, seek out established 'folk' remedies, and to subject these to 'western scientific legitimizing'. In many cases, patents owned by multinationals are largely for isolating the active ingredients in a lab, and going through rigorous protocols of testing and patent filing. While this is an important and expensive task, and deserves credit, these are seldom-independent discoveries from scratch. Never has the society that has truly discovered it through centuries of empirical testing and trial and error received any recognition, much less any share of royalty. India's recent fights in international courts, over western patents of its traditional intellectual property in agriculture and medicine like **neem** (which GOI won in 2005), **rice** (basmati vs. Texas inc.) have brought much needed publicity for this arena.

Today, the multinationals are mercilessly exploiting the herbal and mineral wealth of remote areas, using the same Traditional Indian Medicine. They throw some crumbs to the local people and make millions out of this traditional knowledge. Actually, the world has suffered and continues to suffer from a profound loss of indigenous peoples and rural groups and their knowledge about the natural world constructed from their intimate ties to land and place. This loss has been accompanied by neglect and the marginalization of their practices and beliefs, often figured as inferior forms of knowing to be replaced by universalized knowledge derived from the Western scientific tradition.

While the latter tradition has great beauty, power and utility, attempts to apply it universally without regard for traditional medical systems has in many cases led to failures in sustainable resource use and the erosion of biological diversity. The imposition of scientific management regimes without the participation of local communities has prompted debate on whether the neglect of traditional knowledge violates human rights, civil rights, and indigenous rights.

Research Methodology

The formation of this work has been influenced by the work of such social scientists, historians and scholars like P.C. Roy, D. D. Kosambi, H. H. Nobel Laureate Dalai Lama, Lama Tashi Namgyal, Thirangpu Rinpoche, C Pierce Salguero, Dr. D.P. Agrawala, DR. P.V Sharma George Sarton's 6-Volumes (1927-57) on the Euro-American Scientific thought and Joseph Needham's 16-Volume (1954-95) on science and civilization in China had been in the back of our mind as architects of this project.

This project has been organized around two interrelated themes: (a) to track the development of traditional Indian medicine, in general, like the Ayurveda, tribal medicine, Buddhist medicine, etc.; and (b) then, in particular, trace the evolution of the Tibetan Medicine (Sowa Rigpa), a hybrid Buddhist medicine as a creative combination of Ayurveda, the Himalayan (Tribal) medicine and the Buddhist medicine.

This work attempts to investigate the development of both philosophy and scientific ideas in India in the context of its cultural background. This is envisaged to be a cooperative study in philosophy, science and culture with a hermeneutic approach. Therefore, a study of vast ancient literature and analysis of variety of archaeological data became imperative. However, unconventional sources of history like study of 'popular culture' or 'folk culture' also formed a very significant part of this work. The basic idea of this work was an inter-disciplinary and comprehensive exploration of the Scientific, Philosophical and Cultural Heritage of India. Emphasis has been laid on showing the relevance of the past to the understanding of the present and the future. That India's heritage is not only rich in spiritual and philosophical insight but also has been sustained by the scientific and technological innovations especially in the medical field, has been highlighted in this work.

An Overview

Among all sciences, medicine was the most advanced considering the fact that the Atharva Veda, (about 1500 BC) one of the four ancient scriptures of India, mentions certain herbs with curative powers. Several ancient texts on physiology identified factors as those, which determined good or ill health. The traditional Indian medicine *Ayurveda*, focused on longevity and prescribed several remedies for the same. Gold, silver, mercury, neem, garlic and honey are described as having specific curative powers in the vast treasury of India's pharmacopoeia, medical texts of ancient India. Modern scientists have subsequently credited some of these with the same curative powers.

Yoga stressed the holistic approach to health based on proper diet and physical exercise. Today, even modern scientists accept its efficacy as one of the most efficient ways to stress-free, healthy living.

Charaka, the great Ayurvedic physician of the 1st Century AD, had written Charaka Samhita, the first scientific medical text. Charaka's work consisted of eight chapters devoted to pharmacology, diet, treatment of major diseases like fever, diarrhoea, consumption, leprosy and tumour among others. He also wrote on such specialised subjects as pathology, embryology and anatomy.

In the fourth century, came Sushruta, who is considered the father of surgery. In his treatise Sushruta Samhita, he lists about 125 surgical instruments used by him in his surgeries, details methods of operations among other subjects. In his time he is believed to have performed Caesarean sections, done plastic surgeries and set compound fractures.

Veterinary science was another field, which had been developed, well in ancient times, with hospitals for horses, elephants and cattle. A special branch of Indian medicine was devoted to the treatment of elephants and was called Hastyayurveda.

Besides *Ayurveda*, Buddhist & Jain medicines, Unani & *Siddha*, and tribal medicines have also played a major role in Traditional Medical Science of India

Siddha medicine is the oldest and the foremost of all other medical systems of the world. This system, which has been in practice since 750 A.D. is also based on the

Tridhatu physiology and the Tridosha pathology similar to Ayurveda. Treatment involves use of mineral compounds in preparing medicine. Herbs and medicinal plants are used to a limited extent.

Therefore, we have two ancient system of medicine in India. The Siddha, which flourished in South India and Ayurveda prevalent in North India.

The Siddha system is the science of cell-regeneration, as taught by Lord Siva to the goddess Parvati who taught it to Nandideva who taught it to Agastya rishi (known also as the Tamil rishi). Unfortunately, researchers have discovered thirteen Agastya rishis... The Quest For Forever Siddha healing concerns itself with preventing cell degeneration so as to allow the body an immortality that reflects the immortality of the soul. This stems from the Hindu belief in the two kinds of salvation- Videha mukti i.e. salvation following death, and Jeevan mukti i.e. salvation during life itself. In the latter, the body remains healthy in the face of chronological old age. Siddha medicinal philosophy believes that medicines (kalpa) and meditation (yoga) together make jeevan mukti possible.

The scienctific theory behind this approach rests on the fact of cell repair and cell waste processes that occur simulataneously upto a certain stage, after which the latter overtakes the former. The prevention of the second phase is the focus of Siddha effort. Only natural then that the materials chosen as medicines be imperishable themselves. Metals (including gold and silver) and minerals constitute the bulk of Siddha treatment, and mercury (rasa) and sulphur (gandhaka) are of particular importance.

The Unani medical system flourished in Persia and India. Today, it is strong in India and Pakistan. The Unani system is sometimes called Hikmat or Unani-Tibb. Its medical practitioners are called Hakims. The Unani medicine system was introduced into India in the thirteetnth century by Arab scholars. Originally a Greek achievement based on and confined to pragmatisms, it received its scientific character from Hippocrates (460-377 BC). The system involved four elements, thus differing from the Ayurvedic system of three doshas and the Chinese system of five elements. The original Greek and the resulting Unani systems involve these four elements: earth, air, water, and fire; along with four natures: cold, hot, wet, and dry; and four humors: blood (which is hot/wet), phlegm (cold/wet), yellow bile (hot/dry), and black bile (cold/dry). Unani medicine, like Western medicine (which also arose from the Greek background) owes its origination to Hippocrates (460-377 B.C.) and his numerous followers. Other Greek medical masters, such as Dioscorides and Galen, who we recognize as the forerunners of Western herbal medicine, are also considered founders of Unani medicine. Unani medicine arrived in the Arab world in the eighth century, was further developed by Rhazes (865-925 AD), author of Al Havi Libre Continents, and Zahravi (born 946 AD) author of Al-Tasreef, a comprehensive surgery text that was regarded as irrefutable testimony to the glories of the Unani system, complete with pictures of instruments that Zahravi invented. Many theories of *Ayurveda* (already at a peak) were incorporated into the Unani system prior to the thirteenth century.

All the three traditional systems, namely, Ayurveda, Siddha and Unani are based on common principles of understanding the human body. Diagnosis and treatment are also done on similar grounds - checking the pulse as a part of diagnosis, laying emphasis on diet regulation in treatment, use of herbs and medicinal plants for preparing drugs, etc., all focussing on treating the 'patient' and not the 'disease'.

Buddhist Medicine and Ayurveda

Buddhism and Ayurvedic medicine originated in India and both aim at eliminating suffering. Buddhism primarily concerns with the well-being of the mind and Ayurveda deals with the well-being of the body. While treating one aspect of a person, one cannot neglect the other because both are inseparably linked together. Both systems regard the body and the mind as interdependent and interlinked. This relationship has been illustrated with a picture of a boat and a boatman. Body is the boat, mind is the boatman. The boat cannot go anywhere without direction from the boatman, but the boatman relies on the boat in order to make his journey. Similarly, with body and mind, both are interdependent and rely on each other. Both have healed the ailing mind and body throughout their history and will continue to do so in the future.

Tribal Medicine

However, some of the traditional medicine were passed down orally through generations and also became part of folklore. In this category falls the tribal medicine. We find that the tribals and rural folk in India use plants and herbs for curing common ailments at less cost. The tribal medicine is basically an indigenous system of medicine where the folk recipe for medicine has its own details of method of preparation, dosage, mixture of their herbs or ingredients used. Numerous, hitherto unrecorded uses of plants and herbs gets reflected in the tribal folklore. This has led to the development of Ethno-botany and Ethno-zoology in India.

Over 10,000 wild plants used by tribals for varied uses have been recorded. Of these, 8,000 are used for medicinal purposes, with 2,000 new claims warranting scientific scrutiny. As many as 4,000 plant species are used by the tribals for food, with 800 new findings of edible use.

Studying the tribals' use of animals is ethno zoology. It has been found that more than 100 animals are used for food. Over-hunting is remains a problem as many of these are threatened. Non-tribals also use tribals to hunt the animals. However, with adequate conservation inputs and captive breeding, many of medicinal uses of animals can be continued without causing any significant harm to their populations.

The tribal healer is also the medium through which they know what is happening. Different tribes use their own theories, like the concept of *tijio* among the Santhals of central India, which is similar to the modern day concept of 'bacteria'. Among the Kanis of Kerala, the concept of *visham* explains cause of disease and using steam with medicine expels them.

Tibetan Medicine

Tibetan medicine is a creative combination of Buddhist, Ayurveda and Tribal medicines. Tibetans use an ancient form of medicine known as Gso-wa Rig-pa or Sowa Rigpa based on Buddhism. *Sowa-Rigpa* means 'science of healing' and the practitioners of this medicine are known as *Amchi* (superior to all). It has been practiced in Tibet, the Himalayan regions and central Asia since ancient times. *Sowa-Rigpa* originated from India[1] and it is still practiced in Ladakh and Paddar-Pangay regions of Jammu and Kashmir, Himachal Pradesh, Arunachal Pradesh, Sikkim, Darjeeling-Kalimgpong (WB), etc., In recent times, apart from Asian countries, Tibetan medicine has also become popular in the western world especially in the USA and many European nations. But it's popularity in the Indian mainstream is still awaited. Therefore, in this work, we have tried to discuss Sowa Rigpa, exclusively.

Ayurveda and Sowa Rigpa

The Tibetan medicine system is essentially based on the Buddhist philosophy. According to them the universe is composed of four basic elements: sa (prithivi-mahabhuta), chu (jala mahabhuta), me (agni mahabhuta), and rlun (vayu mahabhuta). But in Ayurveda the fifth element akasa is also present. The Tibetans also believed that the individual is an exact replica of the macrocosm.

As in Ayurveda, in the Tibetan medicine system also believes that a person suffers from diseases when there is a change (beyond a certain limit) in the equilibrium of Nes pas (dosas) and Lus zuns (dhatus). Drugs and food prescribed by the physician depend on taste and are of six types: sweet, sour, saline, bitter, pungent, and astringent.

The Tibetan system's use of ingredients also bears close resemblance to the Himalayan System. The Tibetan medicine mainly depends on herbal products although many animal products such as musk, bear-bile, cow-bile, and different types of milk, minerals, and metals are also used. Medicine is administered in the form of decoction, powder, pills, syrups, oils, wine, butter, or ash. The medicine may be constituted of a single herb or a hundred of them. For example, a medicine called Agar 35 (Agar sonya) has 35 different kinds of herbs. The physician is expected to be knowledgeable in the herbs, their characters, their potent effects, and their synergy.

The Ayurvedic system was well organized and reduced to writing and therefore was easy to incorporate in the Tibetan System, through the exchange of scholars and translation of texts. But there seem to be some common elements between the Himalayan and Tibetan systems. During their journeys the Tibetan scholars and monks must have come across the Himalayan folk physicians too.

The Traditional Himalayan Medicine System (THMS) was a folk tradition and was transmitted through the word of mouth across the generations. They treat both humans and animals using traditional methods. They generally employ herbal products like resin, bark, and root, as well as soils, minerals, animal products, and tantric (Shamanic) practices. The Himalayan people use magico-religious therapies, like the Tibetans whose medicinal system is also basically based on Shamanic practices.

Thus, Sowa Rigpa is essentially a hybrid Buddhist medicine, an amalgam of the Ayurvedic medical tradition, the Himalayan System, and many forms of Chinese medicine. These different ingredients of medical knowledge and traditions merged with the pre-Buddhist Shamanic traditions. They developed many new concepts of health, disease, and treatment in addition to the ones used in Ayurveda. Their materia medica is a vast collection of many life saving drugs. Like Ayurveda, the Tibetan medicine system is more a way of healthy living than merely a system of treatment of diseases. In other words, Sowa Rigpa is more than merely the study of anatomy, physiopathology, and pharmacopoeia. It is also a guide to 'right living' and involves the spiritual aspects of healing as well.

Modern Manifestations

It is known as the earliest form of mind-body medicine and can lend much of its wisdom to holistic and psychosomatic medicine and nursing, as well as the emerging field of psycho-neuro-immunology. The psychosomatic approaches in India have been of a very ancient origin. The evolution of these approaches started with Ayurveda 1500 B.C. ago and was expanded and spread to other parts of Asia like China. Korea, Indochina, Thailand and eventually Japan by Buddhist medicine in 510 B.C.[2] The Buddhist medicine as originated from the teaching of Lord Buddha and completed by Jivaka spread to the whole of Asia by Buddhist monks and with the spread of Buddhist religion. Philosophy, science, religion, spiritualism and culture merged through the time and greatness of people to make Ayurvedic-Buddhist medicine a holistic one, yet based on bio-psycho-social and ecological concept. With non-pharmacological approaches of Ayurvedic-Buddhist medicine, one can achieve significant therapeutic benefit in the management of psychosomatic diseases. Aurvedic-Buddhist approaches impart information and knowledge concerning the measurable structure and powers of psyche. Ayurvedic approaches clarify the processes by which experiences are apprehended, assimilated, interpreted, and comprehended while Buddhist approaches eradicate the cause of sickly spells, dream of ignorance, and thus to make possible the attainment of serene awakened perfection. The combined approaches of two ancient religions help us to assimilate the foundation of our being without which everything remains stressful and empty. The combined and cohesive approaches produce the state of utter consciousness super-rationally and open the door of self, which is composed of spiritual, physical and emotional joy. Psychosomatic diseases are pathological expressions of biological, psychic and social parameters of health and illness whereas Hindu Buddhist approaches show the way to bind closely the normal interrelationship of the above. The increasing uses of Yoga, Morita, Zen, Monko, Mo-he-zhi-guan, Nai Kan and Kenpo therapies in psychosomatic disorders are consistent and successful examples. Vyasa, Patanjali, Bodhidhara, Chih-i. Morita with their teachings have harmonized the physical, spiritual and emotional parameters of human life.

"It is already becoming clearer that
a chapter which has a western beginning will have

to have an Indian ending if it is not to end in
the self-destruction of the human race...
At this supremely dangerous moment in history
the only way of salvation for mankind is the Indian Way. "

— **Dr. Arnold Toynbee**
British Historian 1889-1975

Notes

1. Central Council for Research in Ayurveda and Siddha, Deptt. of AYUSH, Ministry of Health and Family Welfare, Govt. of India.
2. Amarendra N. Singh FRCP. (C) W.H.O. & A.C.P.M. Professor in Psychosomatic Medicine & Psychopharmacology Programme Director, Hamilton Psychiatric Hospital, McMaster University.

CHAPTER – 1

TRADITIONAL MEDICINE IN INDIA

Historical Background

Contrary to the popular perception that Indian civilization has been largely concerned with the affairs of the spirit and "after-life", India's historical record suggests that some of the greatest Indian minds were much more concerned with developing philosophical paradigms that were grounded in reality. The premise that Indian philosophy is founded solely on mysticism and renunciation emanates from a colonial and orientalist worldview that seeks to obfuscate a rich tradition of scientific thought and analysis in India.

Much of the evidence for how India's ancient logicians and scientists developed their theories lies buried in polemical texts that are not normally thought of as scientific texts. While some of the treatises on mathematics, logic, grammar, and medicine have survived as such - many philosophical texts enunciating a rational and scientific world view can only be constructed from extended references found in philosophical texts and commentaries by Buddhist and Jain monks or Hindu scholars (usually Brahmins).

Although these documents are usually considered to lie within the domain of religious studies, it should be pointed out that many of these are in the form of extended polemics that are quite unlike the holy books of Christianity or Islam. These texts attempt to debate the value of the real world versus the spiritual-world. They attempt to counter the theories of the atheists and other skeptics. But in their attempts to prove the primacy of a mystical soul or "Atman" - they often go to great lengths in describing competing rationalist and worldly philosophies rooted in a more realistic and more scientific perception of the world. Their extensive commentaries illustrate the popular methods of debate, of developing a hypothesis, of extending and elaborating theory, of furnishing proofs and counter-proofs.

It is also important to note that originally, the Buddhist worldview was an essentially atheistic worldview. The ancient Jains were agnostics, and within the broad stream of Hinduism - there were several heterodox currents that asserted a predominantly atheistic view. In that sense, these were not religions as we think of today since the modern understanding of religion presumes faith or belief in a super-natural entity.

That so many scholars from each of these philosophical schools felt the imperative to prove their extra-worldly theories using rationalist tools of deductive and inductive logic suggests that faith in a super-natural being could not have been taken for granted. This is borne out by the memoirs of Hieun Tsang (the Chinese chronicler who traveled extensively in India during the 7th C. AD) who describes the merchants of Benaras as being mostly "unbelievers"! He also wrote of intense polemics and debates amongst followers of different Buddhist sects.

Similarly, there is other evidence that suggests that amongst the intellectuals of ancient India, atheism and skepticism must have been very powerful currents that required repeated and vigorous attempts at persuasion and change. Nevertheless, over centuries, the intellectual discords between the believers and non-believers became more and more muted. The advocates of mystic idealism prevailed over the skeptics, so that eventually, (at the popular level) each of these philosophies functioned as traditional religions with their pantheon of gods and goddesses enticing and lulling most into an intellectual stupor. But at no point were the advocates of "pure faith" ever powerful enough to completely extinguish the rationalist current that had so imbued Indian philosophy.

The Age of Science and Reason

But even amongst those Indian philosophers who accepted the separation of mind and body and argued for the existence of the soul, there was considerable dedication to the scientific method and to developing the principles of deductive and inductive logic. From 1000 B.C to the 4th C A.D (also described as India's rationalistic period) treatises in astronomy, mathematics, logic, medicine and linguistics were produced. The philosophers of the Sankhya school, the Nyaya-Vaisesika schools and early Jain and Buddhist scholars made substantial contributions to the growth of science and learning. Advances in the applied sciences like metallurgy, textile production and dyeing were also made.

In particular, the rational period produced some of the most fascinating series of debates on what constitutes the "scientific method": How does one separate our sensory perceptions from dreams and hallucinations? When does an observation of reality become accepted as fact, and as scientific truth? How should the principles of inductive and deductive logic be developed and applied? How does one evaluate a hypothesis for it's scientific merit? What is a valid inference? What constitutes a scientific proof?

These and other questions were attacked with an unexpected intellectual vigour. As keen observers of nature and the human body, India's early scientist/philosophers studied human sensory organs, analyzed dreams, memory and consciousness. The best of them understood dialectics in nature - they understood change, both in quantitative and qualitative terms - they even posited a proto-type of the modern atomic theory. It was this rational foundation that led to the flowering of Indian civilization.

This is borne out by the testaments of important Greek scientists and philosophers of that period. Pythagoras - the Greek mathematician and philosopher who lived in the 6th C B.C was familiar with the Upanishads and learnt his basic geometry from the Sulva Sutras. (The famous Pythagoras theorem is actually a restatement of a result already known and recorded by earlier Indian mathematicians). Later, Herodotus (father of Greek history) was to write that the Indians were the greatest nation of the age. Megasthenes - who travelled extensively through India in the 4th C. B.C also left extensive accounts that paint India in highly favorable light (for that period).

Intellectual contacts between ancient Greece and India were not insignificant. Scientific exchanges between Greece and India were mutually beneficial and helped in the development of the sciences in both nations. By the 6th C. A.D, with the help of ancient Greek and Indian texts, and through their own ingenuity, Indian astronomers made significant discoveries about planetary motion. An Indian astronomer - Aryabhata, was to become the first to describe the earth as a sphere that rotated on it's own axis. He further postulated that it was the earth that rotated around the sun and correctly described how solar and lunar eclipses occurred.

Because astronomy required extremely complicated mathematical equations, ancient Indians also made significant advances in mathematics. Differential equations-the basis of modern calculus were in all likelihood an Indian invention (something essential in modeling planetary motions). Indian mathematicians were also the first to invent the concept of abstract infinite numbers - numbers that can only be represented through abstract mathematical formulations such as infinite series - geometric or arithmetic. They also seemed to be familiar with polynomial equations (again essential in advanced astronomy) and were the inventors of the modern numeral system (referred to as the Arabic numeral system in Europe).

The use of the decimal system and the concept of zero was essential in facilitating large astronomical calculation and allowed such 7th C mathematicians as Brahmagupta to estimate the earth's circumference at about 23,000 miles - (not too far off from the current calculation). It also enabled Indian astronomers to provide fairly accurate longitudes of important places in India.

The science of Ayurveda - (the ancient Indian system of healing) blossomed in this period. Medical practitioners took up the dissection of corpses, practised surgery, developed popular nutritional guides, and wrote out codes for medical procedures and patient care and diagnosis. Chemical processes associated with the dying of textiles and extraction of metals were studied and documented. The use of mordants (in dyeing) and catalysts (in metal-extraction/ purification) was discovered.

The scientific ethos also had it's impact on the arts and literature. Painting and sculpture flourished even as there were advances in social infrastructure. Universities were set up with dormitories and meeting halls. In addition, according to the Chinese traveller, Hieun Tsang, roads were built with well-marked signposts. Shade trees were planted. Inns and hospitals dotted national highways so as to facilitate travel and trade.

India's rational age was thus a period of tremendous intellectual ferment and vitality. It was a period of scientific discovery and technological innovation. Accompanied by challenges to caste discrimination and rigidity and religious obscurantism - it was also a period of great social upheaval that eventually led to society becoming more democratic, allowing greater social interaction between members of different castes and expanding opportunities for social mobility amongst the population. Social ethics drew considerable attention in this period. Rules of engagement during war were constructed so as to eliminate non-military casualties and destruction of pasture-land, crop-land or orchards. The notion of chivalry in war was popularized - it meant not attacking fleeing or injured soldiers. It also required warring armies to provide safe passage to women, children, the elderly and other non-combatants.

The rational period thus saw progress on several fronts. Not only did it create an enduring foundation for India's civilization to develop and mature - it has also had it's impact on the growth of other civilizations. In fact, India's rational period served as a vital link in the long and varied chain of human progress. Although colonial history has attempted to usurp this collective heritage of the planet and make it exclusively euro-centric, it is important to note that fundamental and important discoveries in science and innovations in technology have come from many different parts of the globe, albeit at different times and stages of world civilization. India made significant contributions in this regard. If India is to fully recover from the depredations of colonial rule, it is imperative that we don't forget the achievements of this inspiring epoch.

Origin of Medicine

BUT on that account, I say, we ought not to reject the ancient Art, as if it were not, and had not been properly founded, because it did not attain accuracy in all things, but rather, since it is capable of reaching to the greatest exactitude by reasoning, to receive it and admire its discoveries, made from a state of great ignorance, and as having been well and properly made, and not from chance. (**Hippocrates**, *On Ancient Medicine*, Adams edition, Vol. 1, 1849, p. 168.)

The true and lawful goal of the sciences is none other than this: that human life be endowed with new discoveries and powers. (**Francis Bacon**, *Novum Organum, Aphorisms, LXXXI*, Spedding's translation.)

For the mind depends so much on the temperament and disposition of the bodily organs that, if it is possible to find a means of rendering men wiser and cleverer than they have hitherto been, I believe that it is in medicine that it must be sought. It is true that the medicine which is now in vogue contains little of which the utility is remarkable; but, without having any intention of decrying it, I am sure that there is no one, even among those who make its study a profession, who does not confess that all that men know is almost nothing in comparison with what remains to be known; and that we could be free of an infinitude of maladies both of body and mind, and even also possibly of the infirmities of age, if we had sufficient knowledge of their causes, and of all the remedies with which nature has provided us. (**Descartes:** *Discourse on the Method, Philosophical Works.* Translated by E. S. Haldane and G. R. T. Ross. Vol. I, Cam. Univ. Press, 1911, p. 120.)

Medicine arose out of the primal sympathy of man with man; out of the desire to help those in sorrow, need and sickness.

In the primal sympathy
Which having been must ever be;
In the soothing thoughts that spring
Out of human suffering.

The instinct of self-preservation, the longing to relieve a loved one, and above all, the maternal passion—for such it is—gradually softened the hard race of man—tum genus humanum primum mollescere coepit. In his marvellous sketch of the evolution of man, nothing illustrates more forcibly the prescience of **Lucretius** than the picture of the growth of sympathy: "When with cries and gestures they taught with broken words that 'tis right for all men to have pity on the weak." we heard the well-known medical historian, the late Dr. Payne, remark that "the basis of medicine is sympathy and the desire to help others, and whatever is done with this end must be called medicine."

The first lessons came to primitive man by injuries, accidents, bites of beasts and serpents, perhaps for long ages not appreciated by his childlike mind, but, little by little, such experiences crystallized into useful knowledge. The experiments of nature made clear to him the relation of cause and effect, but it is not likely, as **Pliny** suggests, that he picked up his earliest knowledge from the observation of certain practices in animals, as the natural phlebotomy of the plethoric hippopotamus, or the use of emetics from the dog, or the use of enemata from the ibis. On the other hand, **Celsus** is probably right in his account of the origin of rational medicine. "Some of the sick on account of their eagerness took food on the first day, some on account of loathing abstained; and the disease in those who refrained was more relieved. Some ate during a fever, some a little before it, others after it had subsided, and those who had waited to the end did best. For the same reason some at the beginning of an illness used a full diet, others a spare, and the former were made worse. Occurring daily, such things impressed careful men, who noted what had best helped the sick, then began to prescribe them. In this way medicine had its rise from the experience of the recovery of some, of the death of others, distinguishing the hurtful from the salutary things" (Book I). The association of ideas was suggestive—the plant eyebright was used for centuries in diseases of the eye because a black speck in the flower suggested the pupil of the eye. The old herbals are full of similar illustrations upon which, indeed, the so-called doctrine of signatures depends. Observation came, and with it an ever widening experience. No society so primitive without some evidence of the existence of a healing art, which grew with its growth, and became part of the fabric of its organization.

Development of Traditional Medicine in India

All human societies have *medical* beliefs that provide explanations for *birth, death,* and *disease.* Throughout history, illness has been attributed to *witchcraft, demons,* adverse *astral influence,* or the will of the *gods.* These ideas still retain some power, with *faith healing* and *shrines* still used in some places, although the rise of scientific medicine over the past millennium has altered or replaced many of the old beliefs.

Although there is no record to establish when plants were first used for medicinal purposes (*herbalism*), the use of plants as healing agents was depicted in the cave paintings discovered in the *Lascaux* caves in France, which have been *radiocarbon dated* to between 13,000 and 25,000 BC. Over time and with trial and error, over the generations a small knowledge base developed, as tribal culture developed into specialized areas. *Shamans* performed the 'specialized jobs' of healing.

In *Mehrgarh, Pakistan,* archeologists made the discovery that the people of *Indus Valley Civilization* from the early Harappan periods (c. 3300 BC) had knowledge of medicine and *dentistry.* The physical anthropologist who carried out the examinations, Professor Andrea Cucina from the University of Missouri-Columbia, made the discovery when he was cleaning the teeth from one of the men. Later research in the same area found evidence of teeth having been drilled, dating back 9,000 years.[1] *Ayurveda* (the science of living), is the literate, scholarly system of medicine that originated over 2000 years ago in India. Its two most famous texts belong to the schools of *Charaka* and *Suœruta.* While these writings display some limited continuities with very ancient medical ideas known from the religious literature called the *Vedas,* historians have been able to demonstrate direct historical connections between early āyurveda and the early literature of the Buddhists and Jains. It seems that the earliest foundations of âyurveda were built on a synthesis of selected ancient herbal practices dating back to the early second millennium BC, together with a massive addition of theoretical conceptualizations, new *nosologies* and new therapies dating from about 400 BC onwards, and coming out of the communities of thinkers who included the Buddha and others.

Therefore, Medical Science was one area where surprising advances had been made in ancient times in India. Specifically these advances got manifested in the areas of Ayurveda, Yoga, Sowa Rigpa (Buddhist medicine), Siddha, Unani, etc., There is documentary evidence to prove the existence of these practices. Even today, the two nodal agencies in traditional medicine, Central Council For Research in Ayurveda & Siddha, New Delhi and Department of Ayurveda, Yoga & Naturopathy, Unani, Siddha and Homeopathy (AYUSH), Ministry of Health & Family

Welfare, Govt. Of India are involved in propagating and popularizing Ayurveda and Sowa-Rigpa.[2]

AYURVEDA

Ayurveda by definition implies "The Science of Life". (Ayurveda is a Sanskrit word derived from two roots: ayur, which means life, and veda, knowledge.) Its origin is traced back to the Vedic times about 5000BC. Ayurveda is a part of the Atharva Veda which solely deals with medicine. Atharva Veda includes eight divisions of Ayurveda:

1. Kayachikitsa (Internal Medicine)
2. Salakya Tantra (Surgery of Head & neck, Ophthalmology and Otolaryngology).
3. Shalya Tantra (Surgery)
4. Agada Tantra (Toxicology)
5. Bhuta Vidya (Psychiatry)
6. Kaumarabhrity (Pediatric)
7. Rasayana (Anti-aging or Gerontology or Science of Rejuvenation) and
8. Vajkarana (The Science of Fertility)

The Vedic Sages took passages from Atharva Veda and created separate books dealing exclusively with Ayurveda. Atreya Samhita is the oldest medical book in the world. Atreya was the son of Rishi Atri. Atri was the son of god Brahma and one of the seven immortal Rishis in Vedic literature. Rishi Atri was Acharya (Teacher) of Ayurveda. The Vedic Brahmanas were priests who performed religious rites and ceremonies. They were also considered as Vaidyas (Physicians of Ayurveda). These sage physicians were the surgeons in the ancient days. These deeply devoted holy physicians considered health to be an important part of spiritual life. It is believed that the Vaidyas received their training of Ayurveda during meditation which were later transcribed into book form.

Beginning of Medicine and Surgery in India is thought as the gifts from god Indra to Sages Bharadwaja , the patron saint of medicine and Dhanvantari, the patron saint of Surgery. These two main schools made Ayurveda a more scientifically verifiable medical system (around 1500BC). These two scholar passed their knowledge to two worthy men Atreya and Susruta. Both Atreya and Susruta practised around 600BC, nearly 150 years before Hippocrates

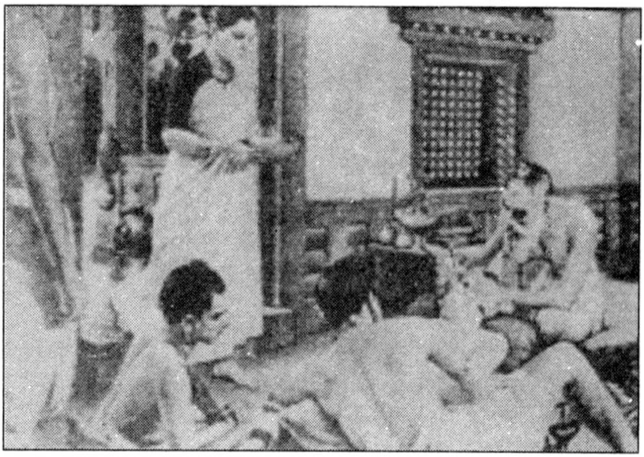

An artist's impression of an operation being performed in ancient India. In spite of the absence of anathesia, complex operations were performed

Shastrakarma- the Art of Surgery

The practice of surgery has been recorded in India around 800 B.C. This need not come as a surprise because surgery (Shastrakarma) is one of the eight branches of Ayurveda the ancient Indian system of medicine. The oldest treatise dealing with surgery is the Shushruta-Samahita (Shushruta's compendium). Shusruta who lived in Kasi was one of the many Indian medical practitioners who included Atraya and Charaka.

Shushruta was one of the first to study the human anatomy. In the ShusrutaSamahita he has described in detail the study of anatomy with the aid of a dead body. Shusruta's forte was rhinoplasty (Plastic surgery) and ophthalmialogy (ejection of cataracts). Shushruta has described surgery under eight heads Chedya (excision), Lekhya (scarification), Vedhya (puncturing), Esya (exploration), Ahrya (extraction), Vsraya (evacuation) and Sivya (Suturing).

Opthalmic Surgery: Shushruta specialised in ophthalmic surgery (extraction of Cataracts). A typically operation per formed by Shushruta for removing cataracts is desired below. "It was a bright morning. The surgeon sat on a bench which was as high as his knees. The patient sat opposite on the ground so that the doctor was at a comfortable height for doing the operation on the patient's eye. After having

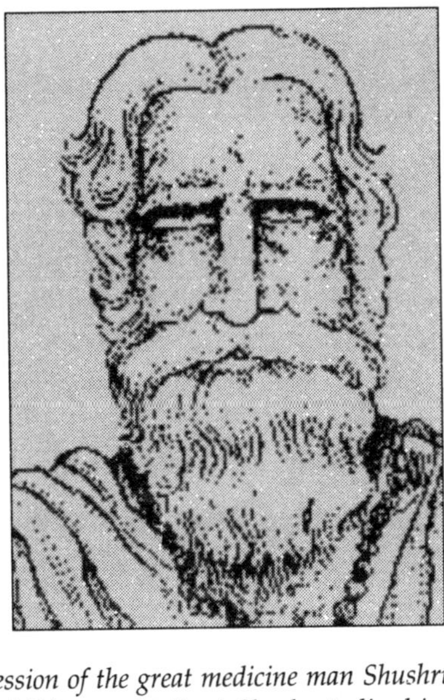

An artist's impression of the great medicine man Shushruta (the term and concept 'Doctor' did not exist then) Shushruta lived in the 8th centory B.C. and has authored the Shushruta Samahita Shushruta's Compendium on Medicine

taken bath and food, that patient had been tied so that he could not move during the operation."

"The doctor warmed the patient's eye with the breath ~ of his mouth. He rubbed the closed eye of the patient with his thumb and then asked the patient to look at his knees. The patient's head was held firmly. The doctor held the lancet between his fore-finger, middle-finger and thumb and introduced it into the patient's eye towards the pupil, half a finger's breadth from the black of the eye and a quarter of a finger's breadth from the outer corner of the eye. He moved the lancet gracefully back and forth and upward. There was a small sound and a drop of water came out.

"The doctor spoke a few words to comfort the patient and moistened the eye with milk. He scratched the pupil with the tip or the lancet, without hurting, and then drove the 'slime' towards the nose. The patient got rid of the 'slime' by drawing it into his nose. It was a matter of joy for the patient that the could see objects through his operated eye and the doctor drew the lancet out slowly. He then laid cotton soaked in fat on the wound and the patient lay still with the operated eye bandaged. It was the patient's left eye and the doctor used his right hand for the operation."

Does this not sound like the detailed procedure and steps of a cataract operation by an ophthalmic surgeon? But this operation was performed around the 8th Century B.C. by Shusruta.

Anatomy : Shushruta was not only one of the earliest pioneers in surgery in the world but also one of the earliest ones to study the human anatomy. In his Samahita, he described in detail the study of anatomy with the use of a dead body.

He has described the following in his Samahita, "For these purposes, a perfectly preserved body must be used. It should be the body of a person who is not very old and did not die of poison or severe disease. After the intestine have been cleaned, the body must be wrapped in bast (the inner bark of trees), grass or hemp and placed in cage (for pro tection against animals). The cage should be placed in a carefully concealed spot in a river with fairly gentle current, and the body left to soften.

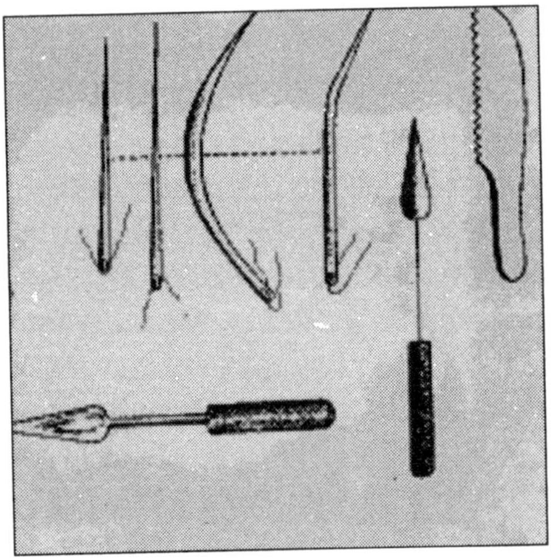

An artist's impression of the surgical tools used in ancient India

"After seven days the body is to be removed from the water and with a brush of grassroots, hair and bamboo it should be brushed off a layer at a time when this is done the eye can observe every large or small outer or inner part of the body, begining with the skin as each part is laid bare by the brushing."

Plastic Surgery : Perhaps the greatest contribution of Shushruta was the operation of rhinoplasty (restoration of a mutilated nose by plastic surgery). The detailed description of the rhinoplasty operation in the Shushruta Samahita is amazingly meticulous and comprehensive. There is evidence to show that his success in this kind of surgery was very high, which attracted people from all over the country and

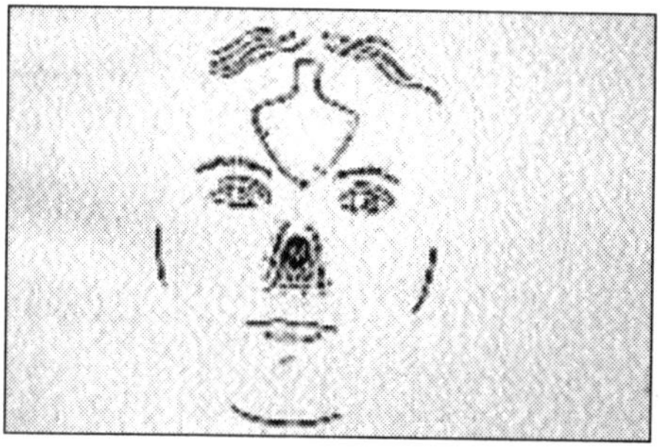

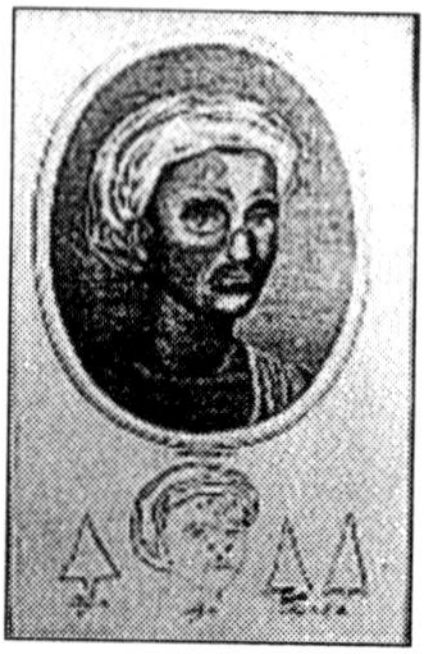

Illustrations regarding the Indian method for plastic surgery for total nasal reconstruction, from an article in Gentleman's Magazine, London

perhaps even from outside. Cutting off of the nose and ears was one of the common modes of punishment in the early Indian kingdoms.

Shushruta moved by his intense humane approach to life and equipped with superb surgical skills, did the operation of rhinoplasty with remarkable skill, grace and success. The details of the steps of this operation, as recorded in the Shushruta Samahita, are amazingly similar to the steps that are followed even to-day in such advanced plastic surgery.

Indian medical tradition also goes back to Vedic times when the Ashwinikumars, who were practitioners of medicine were given a divine status,. We also have a God of Medicine called Dhanvantari. In historic times the earliest recorded treatise on medicine in India viz., the Shushruta Samahita is dated around the 8th century B.C. Plastic surgery dentistry operation of cataracts, were pioneering advances, in the field of medicine.

Basic Principles of Ayurveda

This is the indigenous system of medicine in India. Ayurveda literally means knowledge. The origins of this system of medicine are lost in the hoary past, and the body of knowledge that comes under the heading Ayurveda constitutes ideas about diseases, diagnosis and cure, which have been accumulated over the ages past.

The feature that distinguishes this system of medicines from other systems like Allopathy and Homeopathy is that it is solely based on herbs and herbal compounds. This it shares in common with the ideas on this area in tribal societies. But what makes Ayurveda, a scientific art of healing is its disassociation from the magical aspect which tribal forms of healing normally have. Hence the practitioner of Ayurveda could never degenerate to the level of a shaman or witch-doctor. Hocus pocus and voodoo which are still widely prevalent in rural India could not become a part of Ayurveda as it always retained a physical link between the disease and its cure.

According to Charaka, a noted practioner of Ayurveda in ancient India: "A physician who fails to enter the body of a patient with the lamp of knowledge and understanding can never treat diseases. He should first study all the factors, including environment, which influence a patient's disease, and then prescribe treatment. It is more important to prevent the occurrence of disease than to seek a cure".

These remarks may appear rudimentary today, but they were made by Charaka, some 20 centuries ago in his famous Ayurvedic treatise Charaka Samahita. The treatise contains many more such remarks which are held in reverence even today. Some of them are in the fields of physiology, etiology and embryology. Charaka was the first physician to present the concept of digestion. metabolism and immunity.

According to him a body functions because it contains three dosha or humours, namely, bile, phlegm and wind. These dosha are produced when dhatus, namely blood, flesh and marrow, act upon the food eaten. For the same quantity of food eaten, one body, however, produces dosha in an amount different from another body. That is why one body is different from another. For instance, it is more weighty, stronger, more energetic, Further, illness is caused when the balance among the three dosha in a human body is disturbed. To restore the balance Charaka prescribed medicinal drugs.

Charaka also knew the fundamentals of genetics. For instance, he knew the factors determining the sex of a child. A genetic defect in a child, like lameness or blindness, he said, was not due to any defect in the mother or the father, but in the ovum or sperm of the parents which is today an accepted fact.

Under the guidance of the ancient physician Atreya, another physician named Agnivesa had written an encyclopedic treatise in the eighth- century B.C. However, it was only when Charaka revised this treatise that it gained popularity and came to be known as Charaka-samahita. For two millenniums it remained a standard work on the subject and was translated into many foreign languages, including Arabic and Latin.

The medical system of Ayurveda draws heavily from the doctrines developed in the Charaka-Samahita. The main quality which Ayurveda has borrowed from Charaka is its aim of removing the cause for illness and not just curing the disease itself. In Ayurveda there are no such things as instant relievers, pain killers or antibiotics. The herbs used in Ayurvedic remedies do not operate against the body's metabolism, their effect is registered gradually and hence there are minimum side-effects. The constituents of Ayurvedic medicines are largely based on organic matter. The absence of fast registering inorganic compounds which are at times corrosive, contributes to the absence of side-effects from Ayurvedic medicines.

This art of healing had been held in high esteem in ancient India. It was elevated to a divine status and Dhanvantari the practitioner of this art was deified as the God of Medicine. Even ordinary practitioners of this art - the Ashwinikumars - were given a special status in mythology and folklore. Although very few ancient texts are available today, this method of healing was systematised in early times. The fact that the term Veda was attached to this body of thought testifies to this.

Knowledge of this art was spread among sages, hermits and medicos who roamed from place to place. Those who practiced solely this art were called Vaidyas and they generally belonged to the Brahmin caste. Knowledge of this art was passed from generation to generation. But it remains surprising how this vocation did not obtain the status of a separate caste.

The absence of a caste, wherein this body of ideas could get crystallised and changeless which incidentally could ensure their preservation, along with the absence of a system for regular education and training for practitioners of the art has resulted in its gradual though partial withering over a period of time. The above two lacunae also resulted in the emergence of quackery and made it difficult to distinguish bonafide practitioners from quacks in absence of professional standards. These lacunae have been identified in modern times and recently, organised efforts have been launched to revive and nourish this flagging discipline.

YOGA

Yoga is a system of exercises for physical and mental nourishment. The tradition of Yoga is a hoary one and has been kept alive by ascetics and hermits. The therapeutic qualities of yoga had special relevance for hermits who roamed from place to place, meditating. We normally see an ascetic (Sadhu) meditating in a Yogic pose. Indian classical dance styles also display many Yogic postures. Apart from being a system of exercise, an important aspect of Yoga is that of self-discipline.

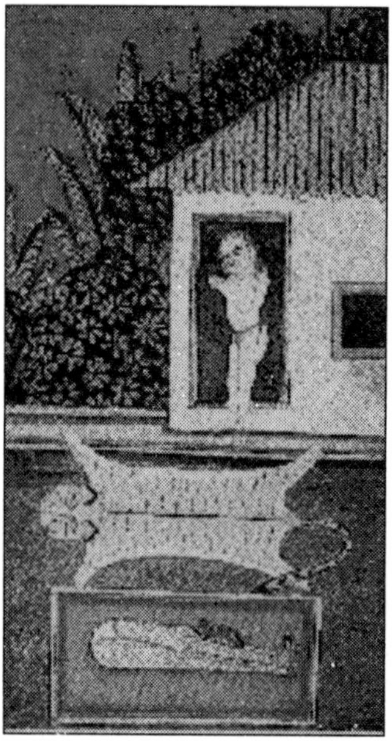

An artist's impression of a Yogi outside a hermitage. The Yogi below is depicted doing the Paschim-ottana-asana

The term Yoga is itself derived from the Sanskrit word "yoktra" meaning a yoke. The etymological closeness of the Sanskrit and English words is striking. They have exactly the same meaning. The self-discipline aspect of Yoga is evident in the qualities of holding the breath (in Pranayama), absolute stilless (in Shavasana), celibacy (Bramhacharya). There are innumerable asanas (poses) in Yoga.

Most of them derive their names from the semblance of the body in those poses to different animals and objects. For instance, there is a Matsyasana (fish pose), Mayurasana (peacock pose), Simhasana (lion pose), Halasana (plough pose), etc. But Yoga is a multifarious system, there are various forms of discipline touching different aspects of human life, which are brought under the heading Yoga. We have Hathayoga (bodily exercise), Gyanyoga or Dnyanyoga (exercise for the mind and intellect), Karmayoga (discipline in our actions in daily life).

It was as early as the 2nd century B.C. i.e. 2100 years ago that the fundamentals of Yoga were systematically presented. The person who is credited with having done this is Patanjali and his treatise is known as Yogasutra i.e. Yoga Aphorisms. According to Patanjali, within the human body there are channels called Nadi and centres called Chakra. If these are tapped, The energy hidden in the body can be released. This energy is called Kundalini. The release of Kundalini enables the body to acquire many powers which are normally beyond its capability.

Patanjali gives eight stages of Yoga viz., Yama (universal moral commandments), Niyama (self-purification through discipline), Asana (posture), Pranayama (breath-control), Pratyahara (withdrawal of mind from external objects), Dharana (concentration), Dhyana (meditation) and Samadhi (state of super-consciousness) .

But though the Yogasutras were formulated two thousand years ago, Yoga has been practiced for countless generations, it is only in the last few years that scientists have begun to recognise the powers of yoga. It has now been established through experiments that by practising Yoga, several ailments can be cured. Tests conducted on Yogis show that they do acquire extraordinary physical powers. For instance, they can live without oxygen for a long time, they can also adjust their metabolism if they have to remain without food for long periods.

Traditionally, Yoga in the strict sense has been practiced by Sadhus and Sanyasis (sages and hermits) who had renounced material pleasures and roamed the country, meditating and spreading the gospel of truth as they perceived it.

In ancient times the teaching of Yoga was also an integral part of the traditional manner of education as imparted in Ashramas and Gurukulas which were presided over by hermits. Though education in these Ashramas was open only to a few, the practice of Yoga in its lesser strict versions has been popular among the common people all through the ages. In the present age though not much is being done officially to promote the practice of Yoga in India and abroad, the spiritual movements originating in India which find many adherents in the West are a medium for the spread of Yoga.

Although the Ashramas are vanishing, Swami Ramdevji Maharaj must be credited for keeping the tradition of Yoga alive in India as well as abroad. He has estblashed **Divya Yog Mandir (Trust)** and **Patanjali Yoga Peeth** at Haridwar (Uttarakhand) for the popularisation of Yoga among the masses. Students of Indian classical dances have to undergo some of Yogic training. But the field where the application of Yoga is being increasingly recognised is physiotherapy, and Pranayam (a sort of breathing exercise).

Divya Yog Mandir (Trust) - Patanjali Yogpeeth : Vision and Objectives:

1. To make a disease free world through a scientific approach to *Yog* and *Ayurved*.
2. To establish a new **World Health Organization** and fulfill the resolution of making a new world order - free from disease and medicine, through research work on the knowledge base of our great saints and

sages viz. **Maharishi Patanjali, Charak** and **Sushurut.**

3. To establish with a scientific approach, *Pran* (breath) as medicine for the treatment of all curable and incurable diseases by extensive research in *Pranayam/Yog*.
4. To propagate *Pranayam* as a " free" medicine for the treatment of diseases across the globe, through in-depth research within the parameters of modern medical science. This will enable both the rich and poor avail its benefits in order to attain sound health.
5. Making the world a peaceful and tranquil place by using Yogic techniques to eradicate fatal effects of medicines and weapons.
6. To study and research the subjects associated with *Yajna*, organic agriculture, cow-urine, nature and environment in addition to the study and research in *Yog* and *Ayurved* at the research centre of the Institution.
7. To form a new integrated system of treatment based on extensive research consisting mainly of the techniques of *Yog* and *Ayurved* but it is Allopathy for Surgery and Emergency cases & others like Homeopathy, Unani and Acupressure to soothe patients suffering from unbearable pains and rid them of disease.
8. To evaluate methods of treatment of the physical body, etheric body, astral body, mental body and causal body beyond the present incomplete system of treatment which cures the physical body alone.
9. To begin degree and diploma courses in disciplines of *Yog* and *Ayurved*.

10. Besides imparting *Yog* and health education, to set up an equalitarian society based on values of spiritualism, nationalism and justice beyond the boundaries of cast, creed, class and religion for the country's development.
11. To create an environment in departments of education, health, armed forces, administration, industry and business that inspires them to adopt *Yog* as a regular & necessary practice.
12. To establish India as the strongest economic and cultural power in the world and provide an environment for every citizen of the world to live with pride.
13. For realization of a dream of a healthy, strong, prosperous and advanced India, free from biases of caste, creed, class, religion, region, corruption and violence through *Yog*.
14. To provide absolutely free lodging, boarding and medical treatment for the economically weaker sections of society.

ALCHEMY AND YOGA IN TAMIL TRADITION (SOUTH INDIA)

> *"Our normal waking consciousness, rational consciousness as we call it, is but one special type of consciousness whilst all about it, parted from it by the filmiest of screens, there lie potential forms of consciousness entirely different."*
>
> —***William James***

This work is a translation of the first eighty verses of the writings of the seventeenth century alchemist-poet Bhogar. Written in Tamil, an ancient language still spoken in the south of India, these eighty verses deal specifically with the Yogic science of re-attuning the flow and distribution of subtle energy in the body.

The flow and distribution of this energy is thought to directly affect consciousness in the most crucial of ways. It is the balance and flow of breath in the two nostrils, which guides the energy through the body. Breath and the movement of subtle energy is said to directly affect how we think and feel.

Any objective observation of the breath as we go about our day reveals that the mind and it's functioning is mirrored in the quality of our breathing process. When we are relaxed and in a calm state of mind, our breathing is slow and even. Breath flows gently into our body and, on a purely physiological level, muscular tension is released with each exhalation. If we are nervous or experiencing stress, our breath is shallow and rapid, often disjointed, flowing in and out in a rather haphazard fashion.

If our mental and emotional state so profoundly affects how we breathe, one can in turn wonder if how we breathe also affects our state of mind and how we feel. Perhaps, it affects not only how we feel but also how we perceive the world, both our outer and our inner life.

The Yogic science, it's practices and philosophy, is centered largely upon altering consciousness and psychological fine-tuning through the conscious control of our breathing process. This was also Bhogar's intention when he composed the eighty-two verses presented in this work. He has distilled the essence of *Kundalini Yoga* into a kind of guided meditation that presents the tradition's set of symbols, sequentially structured for visualization, interwoven with technical advice on regulating the breath.

The key to applying the Siddhar teachings presented in this work begins with a process of objective and unwavering observation of the breath and it's direct relationship to the whole human organism. This practice of objective observation is essential in cultivating the meditative awareness needed to discern the subtle movement of the breath. In order for meditation to truly take place, the subject must identify with the breathing process rather than the mind's erratic wanderings. This allows the practitioner to observe the mind and it's movements without being drawn back into the compulsive identification with thought.

At the initial outset of this practice one inevitably forgets the objective observation of thought, breath, and body again and again, but tradition encourages the practitioner to simply take note of the momentary loss of mindfulness and with persistence and patience return to being conscious of breath. Breath then becomes the anchor of mindful awareness.

Once mindful awareness is established, the meditator widens that sphere of awareness to include thought, emotion, bodily sensation and sound. Here again, the goal is to simply observe phenomena, our mind and bodies response to those stimuli without identifying with that response.

Although Bhogar's work deals specifically with using the breath and various meditation practices to initiate a transformation in consciousness, he seems to have made the assumption that his readers have achieved a certain level of proficiency in the more fundamental of yogic disciplines. This is perhaps a bit of an understatement, in that he does have a tendency to present his system concealed within the language of an adept and, at times, he makes no accommodations for even the practitioners from other schools of Yoga.

Works such as this were encoded in the secret languages of the varying schools to preserve the tradition without revealing the inner mysteries to the uninitiated. After researching other works from Bhogar's school of *Siddha Siddhanta* as well as works from various Tantric Yoga schools, we have presented in the commentary some of the more common and recurring usages of Bhogar's obscure language and what is inferred by the same in the *Kundalini* Yoga and meditation practices of the *Siddha Siddhanta* & *Saiva Siddhanta* schools.

Bhogar, like other Yogis of the various Yoga schools that have grown from tantric roots, employed a language of symbol, myth, and allegory to speak of the transmutation of subtle energy, which leads to the transformation of consciousness.

The complex network of pathways (*nadis)* through which the subtle energy moves, is clearly defined. These pathways, 72,000 in number, are distributed throughout the etheric body double, running parallel to the Central Nervous System. Their location and function are usually presented in a fairly straightforward way. Being closely aligned to the physical body makes them not as abstract as the six nerve plexus' known as *chakras*.

The term *chakra* (literally "wheel") refers to six centers of consciousness that run upwards along the spine at specific points where the *nadis* cluster together. These *nadi*-clusters form jump-points where the frequency of this energy (called "*Shakti*") vibrates on new and higher levels.

As the spine's vibratory frequency is quickened, neuron transmissions reach peak output and brain activity is heightened. The senses are also heightened, pushing thought through new neural pathways, opening up unexplored avenues of perception.

It is in describing these *chakras*, situated at the axis of the etheric body, that Yogis and Mystics have had difficulty in describing their subtle and enigmatic nature. Long ago they discovered symbolism as the most effective tool for conveying their insights and experiences as to how the *Kundalini Shakti* is awakened and caused to propel the human awareness up the spine and through the six *chakra* houses. This journey of consciousness culminates in the *Sahasrara,* the thousand petalled lotus that crowns the top of the head. *Sahasrara* is the seventh and final step of the journey, the fabled "un-*chakra*", where every possible level of consciousness is simultaneously perceived and one is said to perceive the universe from all vantage points at once, fully identified with every aspect of creation.

Contemplation of the symbol, applying the symbolic language to every aspect of life, opens up roads that penetrate into the subtle inner realms. Breath then becomes the vehicle of the undefiled and crystalline awareness that transverses the secret inner terrain, mounting upwards to the blossoming lotus of super-consciousness: *Sahasrara.*

In all languages there have been poets and mystics who have practiced alchemy of words. Poets who have transformed the baseness of a functional system of communication into an expression infinitely more vast; one that strives to enrich humanity in some essential way, breathing new life into human existence.

The Tamil poets have had the added advantage of using a language medium that is perhaps not as heavily encumbered as the rest; where the quality of sound and the impact of meaning seem to share a common ground as far as function is concerned.

Aesthetics and application need not be relegated to opposing ends of the spectrum of necessity. Words are meant to convey both feeling and meaning. Need we set the human heart and mind in opposition of one another when language is adopted as the vehicle of our expression? Poets in all ages, throughout the world, have defied man's tendency to cut asunder the union of heart and mind, and have instead celebrated this marriage as an invaluable asset in reconciling the incongruities of life.

The whole of the Tamil language is the poet's ally. It was born vibrant and malleable, ever ready to be shaped into rhyme or reason. It simply waits for the expelled breath. A breath that is filled with a great passion for life: be it the sighing of heart or the winds of thought.

Even the most dry and linear idea, when voiced with the Tamil tongue, is enlivened by this expelled breath. The sound produced has shape: fine curves & subtle contours, texture & color.

The beauty of Tamil does not rely on any trivial meaning, which the mind might attach to it. The richness of the sound imbues the words with a life of their own, independent of any meaning that our concepts strive to convey. There is an inherent sweetness to the Tamil tongue; and to the Tamil people themselves, "Life" (birth, growth, love, work, death; the struggle of it all) has a sweetness all it's own.

"Like moonlight and the sky,
like the warrior and his sharp sword,
like the beautiful blossom and it's fragrance,
like the crocodile-shaped lute and it's music,
like the eye and it's lustre,
so is my sweet Tamil and I."
"If a stranger asked me, what was the name of my tribe,
an inexpressible joy would arise in my heart.
'I am a Dravidian,' I'd say, and my tongue would be all honey,
and my pride and glory would reach the skies."

—***Bharatidasan***

The origins of these people and their language have been lost in some distant past; only legends remain... a handful of obscure memories. One of which speaks of how the Tamil language came to be...

There were seven great Seers, and one would suppose that they are still around, beyond the realm of form, watching the cogs of time spin round and round. One of them was named Agastya. He knew the secret of language: that all things are vibrating; that the name and its corresponding form are closer than we think.

Agastya paid a visit, long long ago, to the Sanskrit College at Benares, but he being a wandering hermit, clad in rags, humble-hearted, and having the pompous airs and assumptions of the scholar conspicuously absent, he was, needless to say, rejected outright. Distraught and forsaken, he returned to his little hut feeling very sad and terribly alone in the world. There he sought solace by praying to Chandraswami to teach him a language that was even sweeter than the sacred Sanskrit.

All of a sudden his house became fragrant. The God spoke softly, "Look in the corner". Agastya rushed to the corner of his house, and in a nook in the wall he found a small package. He unwrapped it and therein found a stack of Cadjan volumes.

His eyes darted over the inscribed words and he dropped to his knees shouting, "Tamil! Tamil!" ("Sweetness! Sweetness!"). The God taught Agastya the language of sweetness, which he brought to the south and taught to the Dravidian people.

Thousands of years later the Siddhar alchemist Bhogar sat at a small shrine on the top of Palani Hill in the colonial days of 17th century Tamil Nadu. They say he had come to Tamil Country from China and crafted the icon of the Murugan of Palani Hill out of nine arsenics. Water poured in worship over that Murugan is credited with mysterious healing properties. He is said to have attained perfection through yoga, discovering the entire universe hidden in the depths of consciousness. With a mind immersed in silent meditation, he related, in flowing verse, how the ensuing serenity he enjoyed became the gate to life's mysteries.

"Having become calm...
I perceived the accompanying experience.
Having experienced...
I have composed 7000."

Seven thousand verses poured forth gracefully from a foreigner's hand. A foreigner who rejected much of grammar's laws; letting sound run wild in places, letting Tamil's sweetness speak for itself of Life's secrets.

These seven-thousand verses flow in graceful rhyme, a complex echoing of sounds whose meanings convey a flux of images: some humorous or straight forward, brimming with a simple wisdom; others enigmatic, encoded in the secret language of the mystic, haunting if not bizarre.

"My fine fellow,
If you see Nandi,
then you will know alchemy.
"To say even one word
is just noisy useless talk.
"It's like having a chat
with a corpse in the burning ground.
"Only by seeing the light
of the jewelled root
will the golden chain
of the Circle's End
come open."

As this preceding verse infers, Bhogar makes little attempt to explain the Siddhar mysteries. His work reads like a narration of his own free-flowing chain of consciousness, as if he embarked upon some journey through the tangled forest of his own subconscious, mapping out the landmarks along the way, as he propelled himself deeper and deeper into the soil of human existence trying to ferret out the very root of consciousness. With each line he digs up another shovelful of the mind's soil, peeling back layer after layer of thought, of ways of perceiving "reality", until he could reveal the essential living root of being.

Bhogar's work is completely spontaneous. Not a slave to order, wonder explodes as verse in the deceptive guise of a child's conspiratorial mid-night whisperings upon waking from a dream. He tells his secrets with gravity, a touch of humor, and a wealth of unrelenting paternal warmth. Bending the laws of grammar, he even rejects being encumbered by the weight that our rigid meanings attribute to words. Discarding reason, he paints in sound and image an ancient uphill path to freedom.

He cast aside logic, dismissing it as empty noise, he sought essence. He makes no pretence that the mind's ceaseless ramblings bear any real fruit. As he so pointedly puts it:

> *"With words and logic*
> *you get nothing."*

Bhogar has made no attempt whatsoever to make his experience of these altered states of consciousness at all intelligible to the common man. Over vast centuries of experimentation with Yogic disciplines and meditation, people like Bhogar have reported their experiences in their own unique way. Oddly enough, there is a staggering consistency to these reports, that, particularly over the last hundred and fifty years, has attracted the attention of western scholars and scientists. Unfortunately though, they have always encountered some inherent difficulty in finding a way to apply the findings of these mystics to the existing models of the objective scientific world.

Tirumoolar

Bhogar's approach to meditation and *Kundalini yoga*, as well as his application of mythic images and Hindu ritual are by no means revolutionary. He followed so closely in the footsteps of *Saiva Siddhanta's* 8th century founder *Tirumoolar* that one is often amazed at the continuity of teaching and principle preserved and sustained over a period of one thousand years.

Between the 7th-11th century A.D, a strange synthesis of Indian esoteric schools was taking place. Saivite Tantrism, alchemy, magic, *Vajrayana* Buddhism, and *Hatha* Yoga began to merge. The Tantric mysteries, drawing together the entire mystic's tools under one roof, made such distinctions obsolete. Function over form became the rule. Mystics were no longer concerned with postulating the nature of the universe, nor with philosophical concepts and the like; they sought only that which produces a tangible effect, only that which transforms consciousness in an unshakable way. Intellectual theories proposing some "empirical truth", and the debates that ensued, lost their predominance and credibility, as an emphasis on the purely experiential became the rule.

It is impossible to paint an accurate historical picture of this era of cataclysmic transition in India's philosophical arena. The writings of this period pay no mind and render no aid to chronological accuracy, and scholars, both east and west, endlessly propose a vast and conflicting array of dates for these works.

Not wanting to flog a dead horse, we make no attempt at proposing a way out of this historical maze, but one thing can be said for certain: after centuries that stretch back into pre-history, living secluded on the furthest outskirts of society, yoga came down out of its Himalayan sanctuary and entered the mainstream of Indian thought.

Yoga Comes Down

Sometime in the 8th century (and even this vague date is subject to much dispute) there was a high yogi, said to have reached the very precipice of perfection, who came wandering southward from his home on the holy mountain Kailash in Tibet. Legend has it that his name was Sundarar and that he came to Tamil country in search of his friend and fellow-yogi Agastyar who had taken up residence in the Pothiya Hills. After joining his friend for a time, Sundarar wandered deeper into the south.

One evening just after dusk, on the outskirts of a little village called Tiruvavaduthurai, he came upon a small herd of cows lowing and bellowing mournfully.

As he came nearer he saw that the cows, obviously very upset, were standing round the dead body of a cowherd. A few hours earlier, Moolan the cowherd, was stung on the heel by a serpent. His soul had gone to pasture, and his body lay crumpled in the grassy field.

It was getting quite dark and Sundarar, taking pity on the poor cows, shifted his awareness into the body of Moolan. Leaving his original body hidden in the hollow of a log Sundarar brought the much-relieved cows home wearing the guise of the cowherd Moolan.

The new? Moolan' was no longer your average cowherd, but a great yogi. You can imagine the consternation of his wife when Moolan refused to return home. In frustration, she called together the village elders who examined Moolan. They found that the little cowherd had become a saint. They had no recourse but to advise Moolan's wife to let the sage wander as he like.

When the yogi went back to the grassy field in search of his body... it had disappeared. The saint disregarded this minor inconvenience as Siva's grace. He went to Chidambaram, Dancing Siva's holy city, and seated himself at the base of a *pipal* tree. People began to flock there to see the holy man.

Most often he was lost in the trance-like ecstasy of *samadhi*, but every now and again he would look out at the world and utter a few words about the wonders to be found inside. His words always came out in verse.

"The brinjal seeds were sown
and the bitter gourds grew;
when I dug out the dust,
I found the pumpkin blossoming."
—Tirumantiram: 2869

One legend says that only once a year the saint would leave his meditation and speak that one precious verse that the faithful would note down. *Tirumantiram*, the book that has compiled these utterances, is three thousand verses long. So the people say that the sage sat under that pipal tree for three thousand years.

Perhaps this seems a little far-fetched, but it may very well be true from Moolan's (Tirumoolar's) point of view. You see, what the people don't take into account is the Tirumantiram's description of the Tantric Buddhist concept of *Kaalachakra*. *Kaalachakra* is a system of yoga which stresses that (a) the universe, with all it's objects and localities, is situated in the body and (b) time with all it's varieties (viz., day, night, month and year) exists in the body in its process of the *prana vayu* (the vital wind). It believes that by *pranayama* (the controlling of the *prana vayu*) time could be controlled."

As in this case, problems of interpretation are always evident when one tries to apply one's own sociological conventions and cultural predisposition to the obscure musings of the mystic. Naturally a pursuit of a more scholarly interpretation of mystical poetry is no different.

Understanding Tamil Poetry

In *Songs of Experience* Norman Cutler discusses the problems that western critics have in applying their western set of literary values to the Tamil Bhakti poetry (from which Bhogar's style ultimately develops): "Because Bhakti poetry disrespects and even undermines distinctions, it is subversive to certain hallowed principles favored by many literary critics in the West."

In the West poetry generally takes an array of words and phrases, and through extensive ornamentation weaves them together by relying on their decoration to create a sense of order and unity in the work. The ideas and images find integration by dilution, by dulling the sharp-edge of the words with rhetoric. The stark impact of the idea or image is sacrificed when the author employs his lavish display to convey a sense of cohesiveness to his audience.

The western critic lets some Classical sense of order be the judge of beauty. He can rarely penetrate the gaudy mask of ornamentation and discern what substance is there, the many stark and coarser parts of the skeleton that support a shroud of order.

"The Bhakti poet and, even more so, the sectarian interpreters of the saints poems offer a challenge to this way of looking at literature. Unlike many Western critics who find multiplicity underlying the superficial appearance of unity, the commentators find unity underlying a seemingly multiple surface."

Just look at our Bhogar: shooting out in rapid fire, a jumble of images that makes the mind's train jump its tracks and go speeding off into the wilderness of the human psyche. His poetry seems but a barrage of images, terse and sharp, that gather momentum in the stillness and silence that frames them on the page. It is the economy of language that empowers the idea and makes the words resonant. Better still are those chasm-like spaces between words that make an image tower over the clutter of our mind's empty noise. The space between words provides us with an opening through which we can escape the tyranny of the mind.

The Gateway of Earth & Stone

At the top of Palani Hill, near the holy Murugan which Bhogar had crafted from nine arsenics, there is an opening in the Earth; it is a hole in the ground; the mouth of a cave which lies below. Bhogar often lowered himself into the Earth, sat in the cave, accessing Life's hidden secrets. He performed great austerities there, the magnitude of which very few in this modern age can fathom.

There at the opening Bhogar erected a humble shrine to the Great Mother: a few yantras, a couple of five-metal icons baring the form of the Mother and her son Murugan. He worshipped a small emerald lingam there, about ten inches in height. His one and only disciple, Pulipani (perhaps the only one who truly understood the sage), kept him company at the entrance to the underground cavern on the top of Palani Hill.

When Bhogar felt that his outer work was done, he entered the gateway of earth and stone and sat down in the darkness of the cave. Faithful Pulipani heaved a stone slab over the entrance, sealing Bhogar forever in the blackness of his earthen womb.

For thirteen generations Pulipani's descendants have watched over that stone slab that marks the gateway to the underground chamber. Long ago, Bhogar's little shrine was set atop that hallowed spot, and even today, is still worshipped by the vigilant sons of the faithful Pulipani.

They say that Bhogar is seated quietly in meditation even now; alone in the darkness; watching the slow passage of time.

His breath is still. His mind is quiet, his heart unwavering; but through the dense dark matter of his earthly form stabs the vibrant & relentless flame of the Kundalini Shakti. There he waits...

In most cases, we have resisted the temptation to rearrange the order of Bhogar's words. This refusal on our part may make the translated portion of this work seem more choppy and disjointed in places, but we feel that the sequence in which Bhogar presents these words and images is important, and that any attempt on our part to make Bhogar's 7000 "more readable" would subvert the effect that his work was intended to instill in the reader.

This is more that just a map of consciousness or a technical manual on Kundalini Yoga. What may at first appear as Bhogar's inability to be clear and concise, we assure you, is neither empty embellishment, nor the rantings of a madman. The images, which he uses, are not digressions in the narrative, but a carefully structured stream of ideas and symbols.

This is not just a poem, but also a guided meditation, where Bhogar presents more than just a map of the inner terrain: He specifies what the tools are, when & where they are to be employed. All is given freely... encoded within the context of these haunting visions with which the mind must busy itself by conjuring up, lest the journey's momentum be lost in clinging to paltry matters of technique.

All the three traditional systems, namely, Ayurveda, Siddha and Unani are based on common principles of understanding the human body. Diagnosis and treatment are also done on similar grounds - checking the pulse as a part of diagnosis, laying emphasis on diet regulation in treatment, use of herbs and medicinal plants for preparing drugs, etc., all focussing on treating the 'patient' and not the 'disease'.

SIDDHA

This system, which has been in practice since 750 A.D. is also based on the Tridhatu physiology and the Tridosha pathology similar to Ayurveda. Treatment involves use of mineral compounds in preparing medicine. Herbs and medicinal plants are used to a limited extent.

Siddha medicine is the oldest and the foremost of all other medical systems of the world.

The Siddha System of medicine is the oldest in the world. There are two ancient system of medicine in India. The Siddha, which flourished in South India and Ayurvedha prevalent in North India.

The word Siddha comes from the word *Siddhi,* which means an object to attain perfection or heavenly bliss.

Siddha generally refers to *Athma Siddha* that is the 8th supernatural power. Those who attained or achieved the above said powers are known as *Siddhars.*

There were 18 important *siddhars* in olden days and they developed this system of medicine. Hence, it is called Siddha Medicine.

Basic Principles

Siddha science considers nature and man as essentially one. Nature is man and man is nature. Man is said to be the microcosm and Universe is the macrocosm because what exists in the world exists in man. Man is nothing but a miniature world containing the five elements of the various principles, which constitute the minerals, vegetables and the animal kingdom. According to Siddha medical science, the Universe originally consisted of atoms which contributed to the five basic elements, viz., earth, water, fire, air and sky which correspond to the five senses of the human body and they were the fundamentals of all the corporeal things in the world.

A close relationship is found to exist between the external world and the internal system of man. *Siddhars* (practitioners of Siddha) maintain that the structure of the human body is a miniature world in itself. Man consumes water and food, breathes the air and thus maintains the heat in the body. He is alive on account of the life force given by ether. The earth is the first element, which gives fine shape to the body including bones, tissues, muscles, skin, hair etc. Water is the second element representing blood, secretions of the glands, vital fluid etc. Fire is the third element that gives motion, vigor and vitality to the body. It also helps digestion, circulation and simulation besides respiration and the nervous system. Above all, ether is the characteristic of man's mental and spiritual faculties.

Siddha system of medicine is based on *Saiva Siddhantha. Siddha* is a Tamil word that is derived from its root *'chit'* which means perfection in life or "heavenly bliss".

The fundamental subjects of Siddha methodology are:

1. *Vadham* (Alchemy)
2. *Aithiyam* (Medicine)
3. *Yogam* (Yoga)
4. *Gnanam or Thathuvam* (Philosophy)

Siddhars, spiritual scientists of Tamil Nadu explored and explained the reality of Nature and its relationship to man by their yogic awareness and experimental findings. They postulated the concept of spiritualism for self-improvement and the practices propounded by them came to be known as the "Siddha System".

The eight mighty Siddhic Process or Octomiracle (*"Att-ma-siddhi"*) which could keep the body strong and perfect for External Life, where there is no death or rebirth.

Att-ma-siddhi

Anima

The faculty of reducing gross body to the size of an atom and to enable him to fly in space.

Mahima

Power of expanding oneself without limit.

Karima

The power of reducing the primordial elements within himself to a point desired.

Lahima

The power of becoming as light as feather.

Prapthi

Faculty of knowing everything; Past, Present and Future and to secure everything as desired.

Prahamiyam

The power of penetration like rays by which one can attain immortality.

Esathwam

Supreme power over animates and inanimate in the universe.

Vasitham

The power of securing any object.

UNANI SYSTEM

The **Unani system** owes its origin to Hippocrates who laid the foundation for it in Greece between 460 and 377 B.C.

The Arabs later developed it into an elaborate medical system. It travelled through Central Asia imbibing various traditional concepts of medicine and reached India around 10th Century A.D. Unani medicine is ancient Greek medicine that has evolved within the Muslim world for the past 13 centuries (Unani is an Arabic spelling of Ionian, meaning Greek). Greek medicine, greatly simplified for presentation here, was based on the concept of balancing body humors. They either fell out of balance, which might yield diseases (depending on circumstances), or were restored to balance to heal diseases. The system involved four elements, thus differing from the Ayurvedic system of three *doshas* and the Chinese system of five elements. The original Greek and the resulting Unani systems involve these four elements: earth, air, water, and fire; along with four natures: cold, hot, wet, and dry; and four humors: blood (which is hot/wet), phlegm (cold/wet), yellow bile (hot/dry), and black bile (cold/dry). Unani medicine, like Western medicine (which also arose from the Greek background) owes its origination to Hippocrates (460-377 B.C.) and his numerous followers. Other Greek medical masters, such as Dioscorides and Galen, who we recognize as the forerunners of Western herbal medicine, are also considered founders of Unani medicine.

The adoption of Greek medicine into the Islamic culture was depicted by Husain F. Nagamia MD, Chairman International Institute of Islamic Medicine, and former President of the Islamic Medical Association, as arising in the ancient city of Jundishapur (near Baghdad). The timing of events is described in relation to rule of caliphs, the civil and religious leaders of Muslim states, who are considered to be successors of Mohammed:

Jundishapur (or 'Gondeshapur') was a city in Khuzistan founded by a Sasnid Emperor Shapur I (241-272 A.D.) before the advent of Islam. It was to settle Greek prisoners....The town was taken by Muslims during the caliphate of Hadrat Umar, by Abu Musa Al-Ashari in 738 A.D. At this time it already had a well-established hospital and medical school.

It was during the Abbasid Caliphate (754-775 A.D.) that Caliph al-Mansur, the founder of the city of Baghdad, invited the then head of the Jundishapur School to treat him. This physician was Jirjis Bukhtishu, a Christian whose name meant 'Jesus has saved.' He treated the Caliph successfully and got appointed to the court. He did not stay permanently in Baghdad, returning to Jundishapur before his death, but the migration to Baghdad had begun. Thus, his son Jibrail Bukhtishu established his practice in the city and became a prominent physician [he was invited to head the first Islamic hospital, built under direction of the Caliph]. Another family that migrated from Jundishapur to Baghdad was that of Masawayh, who went at the invitation of Caliph Harun-ul-Rashid (786-809 A.D.) and became a famous ophthalmologist. Most famous amongst his three sons who were all physicians was Yuhanna ibn Masawayh (known as Mesue Senior in the West). He wrote prolifically and 42 works are attributed to him [he also translated the Greek works into Arabic]. By this time (the 8th century A.D.) the fame of Baghdad began to rise, as did the political power of the caliphate. Many hospitals and medical centers were established and tremendous intellectual activity was recorded. This culminated into the period of Islamic Renaissance and the golden era of Islamic Medicine.... One of the largest hospitals ever built was the Mansuri Hospital in Cairo, completed in 1248 AD under the rule of the Mameluke ruler of Egypt, Mansur Qalaun...The Mansuri Hospital had its own pharmacy, library and lecture halls. There was also a mosque for Muslim patients and a chapel for Christian patients.

The most influential historical figure in this golden era of Unani medicine was Avicenna (980-1037 A.D.), born in Kharmaitan. He began studying medicine at the age of 13 and started treating patients three years later. He gained a very good reputation, such that the ruler of the Samanid Empire (in what is now Iran), Nuh ibn Mansur (reign: 976-997A.D.), sought him out to treat an illness that was unsuccessfully treated by his court physicians. Avicenna was successful and stayed on as court physician; however, the Empire soon fell, and Avicenna became a wandering physician and teacher. Eventually, he moved to Hamadan (in west-central Iran), where he worked as a court physician. He began writing several works on philosophy and medicine, and, through further political upheaval, ended up in Isfahan, where he was able to complete his books. He died soon after, while serving as a court physician on a military campaign back to Hamadan, suffering an illness he was unable to cure. His writings included diverse subjects such as mathematics, astronomy, geology, and logic. His most important medical work was The Canon of Medicine (*Qunun*), which remained a valued text throughout Europe and the mid-East for several centuries after his death.

The Unani medical system flourished in Persia and India. Today, it is strong in India and Pakistan. The Unani system is sometimes called Hikmat or Unani-Tibb. Its medical practitioners are called Hakims.

Hakim Abdul Majid (1883-1922) founded an organization called Hamdard in Delhi in 1906; at the time, it was a small clinic and herbal medicine shop. Abdul had come from a family that included many herbal doctors, and he joined the herbal pharmacy of the renowned Unani physician Ajmal Khan. As he developed his knowledge of medicine, he too became a doctor (Hakim) and decided to establish his own pharmacy and clinic, which he called

Hamdard Dawakhana. Hamdard, meaning sympathy, refers here to "one who shares the pain of others and is willing to mitigate it" (Dawakhana means clinic). As a result of Hamdard's success, it was moved to a new larger building in 1922; unfortunately, Abdul suffered a serious illness and died that year. The responsibility for Hamdard fell to his wife and his eldest son (in a family of five children), Abdul Hamid, who was only 13 at the time and already studying medicine. Hakim Abdul Majid

Hamdard would undertake its biggest growth and development once Majid's youngest son, Mohammad Said, agreed to study medicine (he had originally wanted to be a journalist). In 1940 he undertook studies of both Ayurvedic medicine and Unani medicine. After graduation, he participated in the Hamdard pharmacy and clinic with his older brother. Soon, however, the state of Pakistan was formed and many Muslims from India migrated there, including Mohammad Said, who was a devout Muslim. In 1948, he moved to Karachi, and set up a branch of Hamdard there, with both clinical facilities and herb manufacturing. In keeping with its aim to serve the people, it was turned into a charitable trust in 1953. Meanwhile, the original facilities in India, devoted exclusively to Unani medicine, continued to expand; under its director, Hakim Abdul Hamid, it became world famous and is likely the largest facility on earth for research and training in herbal medicine.

One of Hamdard's first products formulated in 1907 and commercially produced since 1908, was a beverage made of herbs, fruits, and vegetables called Rooh Afza. The drink derived its name from its function of giving enlightenment (Afza) to the soul (Rooh). It became a major product in India and Pakistan and remains well known today, having worldwide distribution. Among Hamdard's other products are Ayurvedic and Unani internal remedies and topical applications for dozens of common ailments

Unani Medicine Resources in India

India has 18 colleges of Unani medicine, two of them with postgraduate departments (one being Hamdard Tibbi College in Delhi; The annual new admissions in the undergraduate courses is about 700 students, and 30 students in the postgraduate courses. A National Institute of Unani Medicine is in Bangalore. There are about 100 Unani hospitals in India, with nearly 1,400 beds for inpatients. In addition, there were nearly 900 dispensaries of Unani medicines and about 30,000 registered practitioners.

Unani Herbs in Indian clinics

Botanical Name	Common Name	Unani Class*
Terminalia species	Beleric myrobalans	Cold 1, Dry 2
Emblica spp.	Myrobalans	Cold 2, Dry 3
Ptychotis ajowan	Ajowan	
Cassia angustifolia	Senna	
Foeniculum vulgare	Fennel	
Cinnamomum zeylanicum	Cinnamon	Hot 2, Dry 2
Sesamum indicum	Sesame seed	
Piper nigrum	Black pepper	Hot 2, Dry 2
Coriandum sativum	Coriander	
Glycyrrhiza glabra	Licorice root	Hot 2, Dry 1
Mentha spp.	Peppermint	
Viola odorata	Violet	
Rosa damascena	Red rose	
Zingiber officinale	Ginger root	Hot 2, Dry 2
Malva sylvestris	Mallow leaves	
Adhatoda vasica	Malabar nut, adhatoda	Hot 2, Dry 2
Nymphaea lotus	Water lily	

Rheum emodi	Rhubarb	
Cuminum spp.	Cumin seed	Hot 2, Dry 3
Elettaria cardamomum	Cardamom seed	
Althea officinalis	Marshmallow	

Nadkarni presents the Unani classification of the herb where available from Indian Materia Medica. The herbs are classified by the four natures of hot, cold, dry, or moist, and then by degrees, which can range from 1 to 4. Common foods and very mild herbs are usually classified as being in the first degree; the frequently used herbs of relatively mild nature (such as those listed above) are usually classed in the second degree, strong-acting herbs are classed in the third degree, and toxic herbs reach the fourth degree. These depictions, especially of hot and cold, differ from those used in the Chinese system, and refer to the effects on the four humors. One of the more extreme natured herbs is *Ipomoea turpethum* (not commonly used), a powerful purgative, rated as 3rd degree hot and 3rd degree dry. The wet quality is usually attributed to things that are actually wet, such as fresh fruits and vegetables and beverages; cucumbers, for example, are both cold and wet. The herbs for which classification is available in the table above are all of dry nature. Most of the herbs are of hot nature; there are relatively few that are cold. An example of a cold natured herb is white sandalwood, which is classified as 3rd degree cold and 2nd degree dry; it is used for high fevers. The myrobalans fruits (first two items in the table above) are by far the most commonly used cooling herbs. The hot and dry natured herbs help to dispel excess of the phlegm humor, which is cold and moist. In the Ayurvedic system, it is common to use spicy herbs to stimulate the digestive system, and these same herbs, being hot and dry, are used extensively in the Unani medicine of India and Pakistan with a similar benefit attributed to them. The disorder of the humors is diagnosed through questioning, examination of pulse and tongue, and urine and stool analysis. Appropriate food preparation and selection is an important first step to correcting an imbalance in the humors. If the condition is more advanced, a series of herbal formulations are employed to "ripen" and then "purge" the offending humor.

Hakim Ajmal Khan

Ajmal Khan was born in India in 1864, and is generally acknowledged to be the most significant 20th Century contributor to Unani medicine in India. His life in India was something like that of Mohammed Said's in Pakistan; both were humanitarians of the first order who became important leaders and were versed not only in medicine, but in other academic areas, with an intense interest in providing educational opportunities. Ajmal Khan came from the famous Sharif Khani family of Delhi, known best for his great grandfather who made an immense contribution in keeping alive the two age-old native medical systems of India-Unani and Ayurveda-at a time when these systems were in decline as a result of widespread introduction of Western medicine by India's British rulers. Ajmal Kahn established the Hindustani Dawakhana in Delhi in 1905 to manufacture Unani and Ayurvedic medicines (thus, it was founded at about the same time and in the same city as Hamdard was founded by Abdul Majid). The dispensary took out patents for 84 herbal formulas. From the 1930s through 1960s, the Dawakhana employed up to 300 workers; today, it is in serious disrepair, and there are calls to preserve it as a magnificent historical structure.

Three years after founding the Hindusutani Dawakhana, Ajmal Kahn started a Unani Medical School for Women, and after many years more of hard work he helped establish

Jamia Millia Islamia (National Islamic Univeristy, in Delhi) and also established the Ayurvedic and Unani Tibba College (pictured above left), inaugurated by Mahatma Gandhi in 1921. These organizations were partly funded by the proceeds from the Dawakhana. Ajmal Khan also worked politically in close association with Mahatma Gandhi as well as Motilal Nehru and many others and emerged to be a symbol of Hindu-Muslim unity. As a result, in 1921 he also rose to become the President of Indian National Congress.

The herb *Rauwolfia serpentina*, which Ajmal Kahn had used extensively, was analyzed under his supervision, with the contribution of Dr. Salimuzzaman Siddiquil, the primary research scientist. This work eventually led to the production of modern drugs of great importance, such as reserpine (a sedative and antihypertensive agent that was highly effective, though no longer available in North America). Another compound isolated that has anti-arrhythmia activity is named Ajmaline, in commemoration of Ajmal Khan, who died at the end of 1927 after having lived a life of great accomplishments.

An Ajmal Khan Memorial Society has been established. Zafar Ahmad has written a book about his life and works in English. An award given to dedicated physicians of highest quality (in Ayurvedic, Unani, or Allopathic medicines) and for high quality manufacturers of Ayurvedic and Unani medicines in India is named after Ajmal Khan and awarded by the Memorial Society. One of the recipients of the award, Universal Medicaments, provides medicinal materials to ITM.

Unani medicine takes a holistic view and treats the patient in relation to the environment. Diet, regular exercise and proper rest for the body are also stressed. It is based on the Hippocratic theory that a perfect balance of elements (*arkan*), humours (*akhlat*) and temperaments (*mizaj*) helps in keeping the body healthy. A distinctive feature of Unani medicine is the emphasis on diagnosing disorders primarily through the pulse *(nabz)*. Pathological tests on urine and stools are also done.

Treatment in Unani is done mainly through diet control for simple diseases in initial stages, followed by the administration of a single drug, failing which compound preparations may be administered. Every single drug is divided into categories from I to IV according to its potency and efficacy.

ACUPUNCTURE/ACUPRESSURE

This 4000-year-old system is derived from the theories of the Father of Chinese Medicine, Shen Nung. It views disease as excess or deficiency of energy along various meridians in the body and by using needling techniques or by applying pressure the imbalance is rectified.

According to Acupuncture/Acupressure, disease arises when energy is either blocked or deficient. If energy is blocked, it means that it is in excess in one place and deficient in another. The treatment involves moving the energy by inserting a needle in an acupuncture point or applying pressure to remove the block in the flow of energy.

REIKI

Allowing energy to flow through us and directing the excess energy either to ourselves or to others, is the essence of Reiki. It is similar to *Pranic* healing, in the sense that this also used *Prana* or energy to effect cure. But only the technique varies. '*Re*' means 'universal' and '*khi*' means 'vital like force'. Here, the healer draws the *Prana* or energy through his or her crown *chakra* and allows the energy to flow out through the hands or the bro *chakra*. The healer or therapist is the energy channel. Disease is caused by energy imbalance - depletion or congestion of energy. Treatment consists of correcting the imbalance.

The lay people often get confused when doctors of diverse 'pathies' fight and blame each other. (Western medicine dismisses traditional systems of healing as being unscientific and not open to general scrutiny; traditional systems view allopathy as being too reductionist and more interested in the parts rather than in the individual as a whole.) To a sick person, what matters is a relief from suffering. He does not care about what 'pathy' procures it. As a consequence, our people with a robust common sense have developed strategies for health care, which, though far from perfect, are quite functional. People's medicine in India is a strange mixture of home remedies, faith healing, witchcraft and diverse medical systems. How do we transform such a potboiler health system into a scientific, culturally acceptable, and organisationally effective new system? We have to deeply explore the anthropology, sociology, and economics of diverse medical systems and evolve workable adaptations compatible with the human and humane aspects of patient care.

No single system of medicine is able to provide universal cure for the entire spectrum of problems. Also, each system has its own strengths and weaknesses. There needs to be evolved an integrated methodology by which we can blend the best of each of these systems and provide holistic treatment. The biggest question here is whether these diverse healing traditions can sink their differences, concentrate on their strengths and provide a synergy that would be greater than the sum of the parts.

Scientific Basis of Indian Systems of Medicine

The question of "scientific" examination and assessment of traditional medicine has been with us for well over a century.

There have been extensive debates and scholarly discussions but for the purpose of this article, we will just focus on the following:

> *Are there any general criteria based on which we can call a knowledge system as being scientific and if so can traditional medicine be called scientific based on these criteria?*

*Most of us who are brought up on a diet of modern western scientific theory and ways of thinking notice that there are a number of factors in traditional medicine different from what we can expect a scientifc system to be. How do we come to terms with this? Is Ayurveda a science? Let us take the example of Ayurveda as an illustration of traditional medical systems. What are the criteria based on which we can consider Ayurveda as scientific? There can be three types of criteria namely:

Methodological Criteria - It should be based on a sufficiently large body of observational data, and have a comprehensive and rigorous theoretical framework and the basis of legitimisation of all theory should be observation.

Epistemological Criteria - This presupposes that the above method is a legitimate method to acquire knowledge about the subject and the knowledge acquired is always limited and subject to modification in the light of new data.

Sociological Criteria - Society must have a professional community with practitioners of knowledge in the above sense.

Let us have a brief overview to examine Ayurveda based on the above criteria.

The Ayurvedic texts mention of a large number of plants and plant products. The three major texts of Ayurveda list about 700 plants and 1,900 formulations. They discuss animal products from 165 species and a large number of mineral preparations are also mentioned. Quite often we find specific properties given for different parts of plants such as roots, fruits, oils etc. Animal products also encompass a range of animal parts including milk, flesh, urine etc. In fact the Ayurvedic classic *Ashtanga Hrdaya* states that - "There is nothing in this universe which is not medicinal ..."

Ayurveda has developed its own theoretical framework to understand the structure and properties of all material things based on the theory of *Pancha Mahabhutas* (the five primordial elements) which analyses all the constituents of the universe based on the sensory organs that are employed to detect them. They have a theoretical framework based on the three doshas namely *Vatha, Pitta,* and *Kapha* to understand health and disease. The Ayurvedic *Materia Medica* lists the properties of literally thousands of plants as well as hundreds of animals and mineral products based on Ayurvedic concepts.

Ayurvedic literature contains adequate recognition and explicit statements on the limitations of the knowledge systems and its domain of applicability. Ayurvedic texts give indication that this knowledge system is the product of an active community of physicians that has well-established norms to govern itself. There are rules regarding discourses between physicians, admission of students into the fold, ethics of practitioners and manners of settling disagreements and disputes. In fact it is interesting to see that much of the treatise of Charaka Samhita is in the form of a symposium wherein groups of Ayurvedic scholars take up a series of topics for discussion.

Thus there is every indication that Ayurveda is indeed a scientific knowledge system by all the above criteria.

However, to the modern trained mind there are a lot of questions and doubts since the manner of discourse and presentation of knowledge in Ayurveda is vastly different from modern sciences. Some of these pertain to issues such as - can we examine Ayurvedic tenets by modern scientifc systems and validate them, what kind of experiments do people make in Ayurveda, how do they measure and quantify things and above all are traditional medical theories changing and evolving to meet the changing situation in the manner of modern medical theories. We shall try to answer some of these questions.

Is it possible or necessary to test and verify the truth of Ayurvedic prescriptions based on modern medical research? A classic example is the study of the root *Sarpagandhi* (Rauwolfia serpentina) by modern chemical methods. This research succeeded in isolating an alkaloid, which was named as Reserpine. Observations have shown that Reserpine has several side effects, which are not observed with the Ayurvedic preparation using the root. Simultaneously, the use of huge amounts of this root for extracting Reserpine on a commercial scale has rendered this plant scarce and has put it outside the reach of the ordinary village Vaidya and Ayurvedic practitioners. Hence the use of - modern research techniques must be taken up with due caution.

The "Stagnation of Theory" in Traditional Sciences

A feature of Ayurveda (or for that matter, many traditional scientific systems) that often puzzles anyone trained in modern science is the apparent constancy of the theories. It appears that in key areas nothing has changed for centuries or millennia. It is sometimes said that theories have been fossilised because no growth took place after some "dark ages." It has often escaped the observer that there may be a different approach to a scientific endeavour or a different way of organising science, which may lead to a certain "constancy" of the fundamental theories.

The subject of Etiology provides us with a striking illustration of this characteristic feature of Indian thought. That causation of diseases can be by agencies outside of oneself is common ground between Etiology of both Ayurveda and Allopathy; but the analysis of such agencies by Ayurveda and Allopathy shows the characteristic features differentiating the two viewpoints. An analogy may perhaps serve a useful purpose in this context.

Buddhist Medicine[5] and its relation with Ayurveda

Buddhism and Ayurvedic medicine originated in India and both aim at eliminating suffering. Buddhism primarily concerns with the well-being of the mind and Ayurveda deals with the well-being of the body. While treating one aspect of a person, one cannot neglect the other because both are inseparably linked together. Both systems regard the body and the mind as interdependent and inter — linked. This relationship has been illustrated with a picture of a boat and a boatman. Body is the boat, mind is the boatman. The boat cannot go anywhere without direction from the boatman, but the boatman relies on the boat in order to make his journey. Similarly, with body and mind, both are interdependent and rely on each other. Let us look at the relationship between the medical profession and teaching of Buddhism. Both have healed the ailing mind and body throughout their history and will continue to do so in the future.

The Buddha said that his main concern was the problem of human suffering and how it could be eliminated. The term the Buddha used to convey the concept of suffering in Pali is "Dukkha". His whole effort was directed towards finding a way out of dukkha. It is very difficult to find a single English word which conveys the meaning of dukkha, but it has variously been translated as suffering, pain, sickness, unsatisfactoriness, imperfection and so on. It includes all ills of the mind and the body.

The Buddha said, "Monks, there are two kinds of disease. What are they? Bodily disease and mental disease. People are seen who say they have been physically healthy for a year, for two years, for three years....or more, but beings who say they are mentally healthy for even a moment are rare in the world."

The Buddha was teaching his disciples to discipline their minds as an aid to overcome the effects of physical illness. He was very much aware of the intimate relationship between mind and body. Once an old decrepit man named Nakulapita, came to see the Buddha and asked for some solace in his old age. The Buddha, agreeing with him, said that his physical state was poor and that he was getting very old and decrepit. He advised him to train his mind in the following way: "May my mind not be ill, though my body is ill."

The mind has a powerful influence on the well being of the individual. Because it is so closely linked with the body, its mental states affect physical health . The Buddha said, "Mind is the forerunner of all mental states. Mind is chief, mind made are they." (Dh. 1 & 2) Modern psychological studies reveal that -

Fear: lowers resistance, leads to a feeling of weakness and exhaustion.

Anger: results in muscular unco-ordination.

"Mind not only makes sick, it also cures", "One who wishes to succeed in life must treasure good health".

The first task of the doctor is to discover the cause of the patient's sickness. Buddhism too is very much concerned with causation. The Buddhist approach to medicine is entirely in line with the doctrine of Dependent Origination (Paticcasamuppada) i.e. that all happenings are due to a cause or many causes. The attempts of the physician to heal the body is considered in Buddhism as a noble act based on universal love and compassion because it results in the alleviation of suffering. Buddhism, too, is primarily concerned with the alleviation of suffering.

The Ayurvedic approach to life advocates following the very same Noble Eightfold Path as taught by the Buddha. The eight factors of this path are, Right understanding, Right thought, Right speech, Right action, Right livelihood, Right effort, Right mindfulness and Right concentration.

In one of the discourses known as Girimananda Sutta, the Buddha talks about the causes of sickness and disease as originating from an imbalance of bile, phlegm, wind, from conflict of the humours, from changes of weather, from adverse condition (which here means faulty deportment), from devices (practiced by others such as black magic, poisoning and so on), from the result of kamma (kamma-vipaka); cold, heat, hunger, thirst, excrement, and urine. We believe that Ayurvedic medicine is prepared on the grounds of ill-balance of these constituents in a person .

Both Buddhism and Ayurveda maintain a "holistic" approach to life.

For Buddhists this means the doctrine of the "middle way", an avoidance of all extremes and moderation in all things. Ayurvedic principles fully support this Buddhist doctrine, and both systems teach the same method of ethical life. Buddhists call it the five precepts, which are; Abstaining from taking life, Abstaining from taking what is not given, Abstaining from sensual impropriety, Abstaining from unskillful speech, Abstaining from taking intoxicants.

"Of gains, gain in health is the highest and best" (Dhp. 204)

"If one wishes to have along life, one cannot obtain it by prayers or vows.

Instead one should follow a path of life conducive to longevity"

(An. wheel 208 BPS 1975)

Three types of patients: (An. 1. 120)

(a) There are some patients who do not recover even though they get the best medical attention and nursing. (b) There are some who recover whether or not they get medicine and nursing care. (c) There are some who recover only if they get proper medicine and nursing care.

In the recent past the conviction has steadily grown in the medical profession that very many causes of disease, organic as well as functional, are directly caused by mental states. An optimistic patient has a better chance of getting well than a patient who is worried and unhappy.

At the popular level in Buddhist countries one part of the Buddha's teaching has been cultivated with great devotion and used for remedial purpose by the followers. This is the chanting of Paritta. Paritta means discourses for protection and are certainly part of teaching of the Buddha himself. Most chanted discourses are not only of philosophical value, but also have a direct psychological effect. This Piritta charting purifies the mental state of the listeners especially of those who are suffering from physical ailments.

It is certain that paritta recitation produces mental well-being in those who listen to them with confidence in the Dhamma which is truth. Such mental well being can help patients to recover from their illness. The Buddha himself had paritta recited for him and he also requested others to recite it for his disciples when they were ill. Unless the illness is caused as a result of one's own unskillful acts, it is possible to change these mental states to bring about mental and physical healing. But both Buddhism and Ayurveda teach that we live a succession of lives and we bring with us into our present life a karmic inheritance based on our actions in previous lives including some disabilities and diseases.

Some selected sermons of the Buddha are chanted for various reasons such as to recover from illness, to avert danger, to ward off the influence of malignant beings, to obtain protection and deliverance from fear and evil and to promote welfare and well-being. One day Ven. Angulimala came upon a woman in labour and was so moved by compassion for her that he asked the Buddha's advice. The Buddha told him to recite some Piritta verses for the woman to hear. When he did so, the woman immediately and painlessly delivered her child. Since then this verse has always been chanted near the time of labour. The Buddha exhorted his disciples to cultivate loving kindness (metta) towards listeners while reciting these sermons.

Buddhist meditation acts directly on the mind. It has a significant role to play in improving the mental states. Meditation is of two kinds, calming (samatha) and insight (vipassana). The samatha meditation calms the emotions, worries, tensions, anxieties and all that upsets the balance of mind. The Insight Meditation gives one the ability to see things objectively as they really are. Meditation is a universal method of healing, transcending all boundaries of race, creed, colour and nationality.

Following the teaching of the Buddha, rulers actively promoted healing activities by building hospitals and establishing free dispensaries. The well-known Indian Buddhist Emperor, Asoka, of the 3rd century B. C. carved the following edict on a rock (Girnar text 11) "Everywhere in the dominions of King Priyadarsi (Asoka), Beloved of Gods, and likewise in the bordering territories has arranged for two kinds of medical treatment viz. medical treatments for people and medical treatments for animals. And wherever there were no medical herbs beneficial to people and beneficial to animals, they have been caused to be imported and planted. On the roads, wells have been caused to be dug and trees have been caused to be planted for the enjoyment of animals and humans". This is the first record of the establishment of government hospitals not only for human beings but also for animals.

This example was faithfully followed by the kings in Sri Lanka after the introduction of Buddhism. King Gamini provided free food and medicine to the sick as prescribed by his physicians. Venerable Welivita Saranankara Sangha Raja of Sri Lanka is reported to have composed a book on medicine which is known as Bhesajja Manjusa. Thus the well-known Buddhist statement "Health is the highest gain" (arogya parama labha) stands established both in theory and practice. In the Vinaya pitaka (disciplinary code) monks are allowed to treat medically certain people. The Buddha himself ministered to a suffering monk and declared the following memorable words, "He who tends the sick, respects me". Thus we see the close connection between Buddhism and Ayurvedic medicine.

"Whosoever would wait upon me,
Whosoever would honour me,
Whosoever would follow my advice,
He should attend on the sick"
(Mahavagga Bodhi leaves B 76, 1977, BPS)

Tribal Medicine

Tribal traditions and practices pervade all aspects of Indian culture and civilization, yet this awareness is often lacking in popular consciousness, and the extent and import of Tribal contributions to Indian philosophy, language and custom have often gone unrecognized, or been underrated by historians and social scientists.[6]

Although popular myths about Buddhism have obscured the original source and inspiration for it's humanist doctrine, it is to India's ancient tribal (or Adivasi) societies that Gautam Buddha looked for a model for the kind of society he wished to advocate. Repulsed by how greed for private property was instrumental in causing poverty, social exploitation and unending warfare - he saw hope for human society in the tribal republics that had not yet come under the sway of authoritarian rule and caste discrimination. The early Buddhist *Sanghas* were modelled on the tribal pattern of social interaction that stressed gender equality, and respect for all members. Members of the *Sanghas* sought to emulate their egalitarian outlook and democratic functioning. It was the simplicity, the love of nature, the absence of coveting the goods and wealth of others, and the social harmony of tribal society that attracted Gautam Buddha, and had a profound impact on the ethical core of his teachings.

Tribal who developed an intimate knowledge of various plants and their medicinal uses played an invaluable role in the development of Ayurvedic medicines. In a recent study, the All India Coordinated Research Project credits tribal communities with the knowledge of 9000 plant species - 7500 used for human healing and veterinary health care. Dental care products like *datun,* roots and condiments like *turmeric* used in cooking and ointments are also tribal si discoveries, as are many fruit trees and vines. Ayurvedic cures for arthritis and night blindness owe their origin to tribal knowledge.

India will document, validate and popularise folk medicine practices of tribals across the country and even start institutes for their study to save these traditions from extinction.

"Folk medicine is different from ayurveda, homeopathy or unani. These are local medicinal procedures practised by tribals across India. We are trying to document, digitise and scientifically validate them," said Verghese Samuel, joint secretary, Ministry of Health and Family Welfare[7]. "Due to modern systems of medicine, this health heritage is losing its popularity. We are trying to save these good practices through the initiative," Samuel said. Sanjeev K. Chadha, director, department of AYUSH (Ayurveda, Yoga and Naturopathy, Unani, Sidha and Homeopathy) in the ministry, said: "Because of folk medicine practices, tribals in India have a very good immune system. If they are getting benefits out of these practices then there must be something good about these practices.

"These age-old traditions should not be lost in the wilderness. We will do research on these practices and record them. All the good practices would also be considered from patenting." There are over 130 tribal groups in India, many from north eastern states.

Chadha said the health ministry had decided to establish a North Eastern Institute of Folk Medicine at Pasighat, Arunachal Pradesh. The state government has already given over 40 acres of land for the purpose and the institute will come up at a cost of nearly 330 million.

"The institute will dedicate itself to the cause. Research and scientific validations will also be done there. The institute may soon have branches in states like Orissa, Jharkhand and Chhattisgarh among others." Talking about the institute's location, he said north eastern states were full of folk medicinal practices. "From malaria, to diarrhoea to wounds, people in this region use folk medicines and it's better to start from there."

Chadha said folk medicine was "a pool of knowledge" that had to be tapped. "The practices are very utilitarian. We as a nation with diverse culture can't allow a body of knowledge to perish. Like manuscripts, here is a pool of knowledge that needs to be tapped for a greater cause, for betterment of millions of people.

"Who knows it may give India a different pedestal in the health community of the world."

In recent years, uncontrolled exploitation by Multinationals has resulted in the loss of the rich biodiversity of India, which has an immense wealth of about 45,000 species of wild plants of which 7500 species are used for medicinal purposes. The tribal people are the real custodians of medicinal plants. Dr. Vedavathy (2002) has recently reported the results of a study carried out between 1994-1998 in Andhra Pradesh. From the Chittoor district alone they have documented more than a thousand therapies and 500 medicinal plants. The predominant tribal populations in the district comprise the *yanadi, yerukala, nakkala* and the *irula* tribes.

In a recent study, the All India Coordinated Research Project credits tribal communities with the knowledge of 9000 plant species - 7500 used for human healing and veterinary health care. Dental care products like *datun,* roots and condiments like *turmeric* used in cooking and ointments are also tribal discoveries, as are many fruit trees and vines. Ayurvedic cures for arthritis and night blindness owe their origin to tribal knowledge.

Ethnobiology and Tribal Medicine

It could well be one of the most exhaustive scientific pursuits undertaken in post-independence India. The All India Coordinated Research Project on Ethnobiology (AICRPE) has unearthed a large spectrum of uses that tribal populations of the country make of plants and animals.

Home to some of the world's most diverse ecosystems, India has a similar diversity of ethnic groups, characterised by its tribal populations. Bypassed by the march of modern civilisation, some tribal communities still live in rock crevices — in the hunter-gatherer stage of human evolution — while others fall in stages further down the evolution path. Termed 'primitive', these communities have long been neglected by the modern age. But after perpetuating severe deforestation and ecosystem damage, modern civilisation is revising its attitude. The linear notion of history and evolution is being questioned. Primitive, for once, is understood differently. Tribal knowledge and ways of life are serious subjects of analysis now.

With India's tribal communities assimilating into mainstream society, their knowledge and practices needed to be documented. In 1976, M S Swaminathan, the then director general of the Indian Council of Agricultural Research, initiated consultations to this effect. A working group under T N Khoshoo, now a research fellow at the Tata Energy Research Institute, drafted a proposal. Consequently, AICRPE was launched in 1982 under the Man and Biosphere programme of the United Nations Economic, Scientific and Cultural Organisation (UNESCO) by the department of science and technology.

AICRPE was transferred to the department of environment when it was created, and later to the ministry of environment and forests (MEF). P Pushpangadan, then at the Regional Research Laboratory of the Council of Scientific and Industrial Research (CSIR) at Jammu, was posted chief coordinator in 1983. AICRPE was to be multi-disciplinary, multi-institutional and action-oriented. The research project took stock of India's tribal panorama.

The project involved as many as 27 institutions from across the country, including the Botanical Survey of India (BSI), the Zoological Survey of India (ZSI), the Central Drugs Research Institute (CDRI), Lucknow, and the Birbal Sahni Institute, Lucknow. More than 400 investigators took part, representing diverse fields such as anthropology, sociology, modern medicine, *Ayurveda*, botany, zoology, pharmacology and chemistry. After more than 16 years of untiring effort, the exercise concluded in March 1998.

According to the 1991 census, there are 67.8 million tribals in the country. They come from 550 communities and 227 ethnic groups living in more than 5,000-forested villages or in forests. The task was Herculean. The places were mostly inaccessible and the communities spoke 116 different dialects, apart from the known languages. The effort was of seminal importance as the tribal knowledge systems are in the form of oral traditions and are disappearing fast.

The comprehensive database was kept confidential during the project in light of the increasing interest in ethno biology for commercial uses. It is now available with the MEF for planners to be used for pragmatic development models for the tribals and the country in the first place. It also highlights areas where immediate conservation inputs and studies are needed.

Ethnobotany: What Plants Mean

Over 10,000 wild plants used by tribals for varied uses have been recorded. Of these, 8,000 are used for medicinal purposes, with 2,000 new claims warranting scientific scrutiny. As many as 4,000 plant species are used by the tribals for food, with 800 new findings of edible use. "That means alternate food sources for the future," Pushpangadan told *Down To Earth*. "The number of edible species is shrinking through time. People used thousands of plants earlier. This has now reduced to a handful, the majority depending on just four species, namely rice, wheat, maize and potato, which are called staple food," he added. This can affect human health, as the body needs many specific ingredients according to the ecosystem. Many of the above-mentioned edible species can be restored and many others can be used commercially. These options can give incomes to tribals without damaging the ecosystem.

The tribal populations also use plants for fibre and cord, for fodder and for pesticidal and pesticidal uses. Uses for dyes, resins, perfumes and incense are also widespread. With the demand for natural products rising, proper planning can bring rich dividends, said Pushpangadan. The AICRPE team also took stock of the endangered plant species and the reason for their being so. Over-exploitation by tribal people is affecting several plants in the Western Himalaya, the Western Ghats and Andaman and Nicobar Islands.

The study team also found primitive cultivars and wild relative of crop plants being cultivated by tribals in exclusion from the outside world. About 250 such rare cultivars were deposited with the National Bureau of Plant Genetic Resources (NBPGR), New Delhi. Precious gene pools and germplasms of some of these are preserved in various AICRPE centres. Archeo-botanical investigations as part of the AICRPE were undertaken by the Birbal Sahni Institute of Palaeobotany, which threw up important findings about the uses of plants in ancient days.

Ethnozoology: Animal Medicine

Studying the tribals' use of animals is ethno zoology. The first attempt of its kind in the country, it was carried out for AICRPE mainly by ZSI. The project found that more than 100 animals are used for food. Over-hunting is remains a problem as many of these are threatened. Non-tribals also use tribals to hunt the animals. However, with adequate conservation inputs and captive breeding, many of medicinal uses of animals can be continued without causing any significant harm to their populations.

AICRPE found that 76 animals are used for medicinal purposes. Body parts, such as blood, skin and skeleton, and products such as milk, urine and faeces all have medicinal uses. More than 25 animal products have been short-listed for scientific investigation. The hen's egg had maximum number of uses - 36 applications in various tribal communities. Peacock is another bird with several utilities.

Understanding the Mystic

Though there can be differences of opinion, the AICRPE exercise tries to enable the modern world to accept and understand the mystic world of tribals through the medium of modern science. Where a number of "deities and spirits nestle in the old trees and rivers, hills and streams", as the AICRPE report notes. It is a world where one is answerable to the omnipresent and the omnipotent. For most of the tribes the forests are sacred and harm done is punishable.

The tribal healer is also the medium through which they know what is happening. Different tribes use their own theories, like the concept of *tijio* among the Santhals of central India, which is similar to the modern day concept of 'bacteria'. Among the Kanis of Kerala, the concept of *visham* explains cause of disease and it they are expelled by steam with medication.

Despite a rich cultural kaleidoscope the plight of tribals in most areas is poor, except in places where forests are still healthy, notes the report. Malnutrition is rampant. Proselytisation to Hinduism and Christianity are also threatening the customs and practises of the tribals, apart from modernisation. Christianisation is severely damaging as the tribal culture is grounded in faith in several gods, which Christianity negates. Their message is that homogenisation is the only means to livelihood security.

The massive database built up ought to help the tribals earn a living and retain the positive attributes of their life. This possibility of that is proved — though not totally — in the case of the herb arogyapacha and the Kani tribals of Kerala. A series of such steps will change the face of tribal India.

Tribals also played an important role in the development of agricultural practices - such as rotational cropping, fertility maintenance through alternating the cultivation of grains with leaving land fallow or using it for pasture. Adivasis of Orissa were instrumental in developing a variety of strains of rice.

The Herbal Folklore Research Center (HFRC) with a small multi-disciplinary team comprising an ethno-botanist, a social anthropologist, two trained taxonomists, an Ayurvedic doctor and four field assistants, made enthno botanical surveys during 1994-1998 in the Chittoor district, in Andhra Pradesh. The surveys were carried out with a non-random purposive sample of the rural population. 'Snowball and judgmental' selection methods were used to identify community members who are knowledgeable in medicinal plant identification and usage. Vedavathy noticed that there is a strong belief among the tribal people that the efficacy of the therapy is lost if it is revealed to strangers, who have no faith in nature and their medicine.

The tribal people divide the diseases into two categories:

(1) Related to the body;

(2) Related to mind and divine powers.

The bodily ailments are treated using herbal medicines, coupled with animal parts, and psychosomatic diseases using magico-religious practices coupled with herbal medicines.

We will now discuss some of the remedies for main ailments:

Fever: If the ailment is followed by fever the first precaution is to avoid intake of solid food. During the survey the team documented six types of antipyretic agents such as the decoction of root tubers of (*shatavari*), *Asparagus racemosus* Willd or *Cyprus rotundus* used by the Yanadi tribe. The Sugalis used the garlic bulb (*Allium sativum* Linn), and dry ginger. And the Nakkala tribe used the decoction of garlic mixed with *Andrographis paniculata* and *Morinda tinctoria* root.

Headache: For headache the tribals use either dry ginger or sandal wood paste as topical application on the forehead and for pain in the scalp region they bandage either leaves of *Delonix elata* Gamble or *Vitex negundo* Linn. For chronic cases they make a paste of *Achyranthes aspera* Linn, earthworm and *Ocimum basilicum* Linn seeds mixed with a pinch of camphor, which is applied on the head and forehead. If the headache is followed by fever and eye infection the juice made by pounding ginger, garlic and onion is given to drink.

Indigestion: *Trachyspermum ammi* (Linn.) seed powder with a pinch of rock salt is given for indigestion and for chronic cases *Cassia senna* Linn leaf powder mixed with a pinch of salt are given on empty stomach.

Eye Infection: The primary treatment is to foment the affected eye. If the infection is very painful, the juice of lime or onion or fresh turmeric is dropped in the eyes.

Liver disorders: A paste made from cooked *Cuscuta reflexa* Roxb plant is applied topically on the stomach for liver disorders.

Cough and cold: The parts of plant such as fruits of *Pongamia pinnata* Pirre, leaves of *Datura metel* Linn, roots of *Solanum surattense* are used for cold, cough and bronchitis.

Sexual potency: The tribes have many drugs for sexual potency. They use snails, pigeons and sparrows along with food and herbal drugs such as *Mucuna prurita, Asparagus racemosus* roots.

Toothache: The latex of *Calotropis procera*, bark of *Acacia* sp, roots of *Achyranthes aspera* Linn are applied for toothache and infection. For brushing they use neem or *Pongamia* sticks.

For easy delivery: Birth of child is an important event in their life. The people of the hamlet take active part. They never go to hospital for delivery. The people generally possess the knowledge about delivery. During the process the birth attendant massages the abdomen and navel region using castor oil or root paste of *Achyranthes aspera* Linn. Herbal decoction made of ginger, coriander, fennel, black pepper and mustard seeds mixed in equal proportions are given to the laboring mother to hasten the pains. To remove the dead body from the womb the *Nakkla* community mix the decoction of bamboo leaves, asafetida, salt and some ganji (rice gruel). Yanadi and Yerukala communities have many therapies such as leaf decoction of jammi (*Prosopis cineraria* Druce) or garlic mixed with millets and black pepper for the expulsion of dead body from the womb. A wick dipped in the root paste of *Boerhaavia diffusa* Linn or castor oil or soap nut juice is inserted in the vagina to hasten the process. After delivery a decoction or extract prepared from root of *Tephrosia purpurea* is given to clean the uterus and to ensure complete discharge of the placenta. The tribes have many post-natal therapies. For the newborn baby the Yanadis administer the paste made from dried stomach of porcupine. The dried stomach that looks like a stone is rubbed with mother's milk and given to baby to lick. This medicine is continued up to one year with gradual increase in dosage.

Cut and fractures: The Yanadis use warmed banyan leaves to bandage the affected part for cuts and for bone setting and for fractures the leaves of *Dodonaea viscose* Linn. And for inflammation, before applying any medicine they wash the affected area either with cow's urine or with their own urine.

Pain: The tribals give fomentation (heat therapy) to the affected area for relief using hot water rinsing or steam, or fomentation with fried salt along with topical application of castor oil for any pain.

Snakebite: They resort to mantras and magic before giving herbal treatment for snakebite and the victim is given the roots of *Aristolochia indica* Linn or bark of *Alangium salviifolium*. The indigenous people believe that man and nature are interdependent. The medicines given during the treatment and the food regimen they follow are marvelous and give quick relief. The belief that the misuse of nature results in punishment and curse becomes a boon to preserve the snakes and other minor animals.

During epidemics the tribals resort to many magico-religious practices and combined herbal treatment and strict food regimen. There is a need for documentation of all the tribal health practices.

Sowa Rigpa (Tibetan Medicine)

Tibetans use an ancient form of medicine known as *Gso-wa Rig-pa (Sowa Rigpa)* or "The Knowledge of Healing" whose origins are believed to be based on the teachings of the historical Buddha. Tibetan medicine is held in high esteem in Tibet and central Asia. *"Sowa-Rigpa"*, commonly known as Tibetan or Amchi medicine, is the traditional medicine of many parts of the Himalayan region. *Sowa-Rigpa* means 'science of healing' and the practitioners of this medicine are known as *Amchi* (superior to all). Tibetan medicine is an admixture of Buddhist, Ayurveda and Tribal medicines. In India, this system of medicine has been popularly practiced in Ladakh and Paddar-Pangay regions of Jammu and Kashmir, Himachal Pradesh, Arunachal Pradesh, Sikkim, Darjeeling-Kalingpong (WB) and now in Tibetan settlements all over India and abroad. *Sowa-Rigpa* originated from India[8].

The Tibetan medicine seems to be a creative combination of the Indian medical traditions, which it imported with Buddhism from India, and many forms of Chinese medicine. The philosophical basis of Tibetan medicine is rooted in Buddhism. Thus, the Buddhist medical system is more than merely the study of anatomy, physiopathology, and pharmacopoeia. It is also a guide to 'right living' and involves the spiritual aspects of healing as well.

The Buddhists believed that Buddha (567 BC) taught medicine to one and all, in the Royal Palace at Udiyana in India, where the test was compiled in *Sanskrit* from the original *Marying* or *Shanshung Yiggen* language, a variation of present day Tibetan language. The 28th King of Tibet, Lhathothori Nyantsen, introduced the medical science along with Buddhism by inviting two Indian physicians, This established the medical practice based on Buddhist teachings. It is said that Emperor Songtsen Gampo (617-650 AD), the most powerful ruler of Tibet, invited three famous medical scholars: from India, from China, and Galenos from Rome. They jointly compiled seven volumes of the medical treatise, *Mijigpe Tson-ja*.

In the 7th century, King Songsten Gampo adopted Buddhism in Tibet. He was responsible for the international medical conference in Tibet, inviting physicians from India, China, Nepal, Byzantium, and Persia to translate their medical texts into Tibetan. The ideas exchanged and knowledge imparted became the foundation of what is now considered one of the oldest complete medical systems in Tibet. The king sent Prime Minister Thon-mi-Sam-bho-ta to India in 645 AD to learn both secular and religious literature. He translated a number of Indian works in the Tibetan language. In the Tibetan medicine system the most popular medical text is called *Rgyud bzi* (lit. *Catus-tantra*, a compendium of four treatises). According to the introductory paragraph in this work, the title of its Sanskrit origin was "*Amrta Hrdaya Astanga Guhyopadesa Tantra.*" Actually, in the 8th century AD a Tibetan scholar, Vairocana, studied this work from Candranandana of India and translated this into Tibetan.

Relation between Ayurvedic and Tibetan Medicine System

The Tibetan medicine system is essentially based on the Buddhist philosophy. According to them the universe is composed of four basic elements: *sa* (*prithivi-mahabhuta*), *chu* (*jala mahabhuta*), *me* (*agni mahabhuta*), and *rlun* (*vayu mahabhuta*). But in Ayurveda the fifth element *akasa* is also present. The Tibetans also believed that the individual is an exact replica of the macrocosm.

As in Ayurveda, in the Tibetan medicine system also believes that a person suffers from diseases when there is a change (beyond a certain limit) in the equilibrium of *Nes pas* (*dosas*) and *Lus zuns* (*dhatus*). Drugs and food prescribed by the physician depend on taste and are of six types: sweet, sour, saline, bitter, pungent, and astringent.

The Tibetan system's use of ingredients also bears close resemblance to the Himalayan System. The Tibetan medicine mainly depends on herbal products although many animal products such as musk, bear-bile, cow-bile, and different types of milk, minerals, and metals are also used. Medicine is administered in the form of decoction, powder, pills, syrups, oils, wine, butter, or ash. The medicine may be constituted of a single herb or a hundred of them. For example, a medicine called *Agar 35* (*Agar sonya*) has 35 different kinds of herbs. The physician is expected to be knowledgeable in the herbs, their characters, their potent effects, and their synergy.

The Ayurvedic system was well organized and reduced to writing and therefore was easy to incorporate in the Tibetan System, through the exchange of scholars and translation of texts. But there seem to be some common elements between the Himalayan and Tibetan systems. During their journeys the Tibetan scholars and monks must have come across the Himalayan folk physicians too.

The Traditional Himalayan Medicine System (THMS) was a folk tradition and was transmitted through the word of mouth across the generations. They treat both humans and animals using traditional methods. They generally employ herbal products like resin, bark, and root, as well as soils, minerals, animal products, and *tantric* (Shamanic) practices.

The Himalayan people use magico-religious therapies, like the Tibetans whose medicinal system is also basically based on Shamanic practices. Among the magico-religious therapies the Himalayan people practice *Jagar*, *Thau-dham*, *Bhabhuti*, and *Tantra-mantra* to placate the local gods and supernatural powers. The mystic-priest, with the help of hymns, drives the spirit away. Before leaving the patient, the spirit may ask for some rice and pulse or for the sacrifice of a cock, pig, or goat.

Thus the Tibetan medicine is an amalgam of the Ayurvedic medical tradition, the Himalayan System, and many forms of Chinese medicine. These different ingredients of medical knowledge and traditions merged with the pre-Buddhist Shamanic traditions. Like Ayurveda, the Tibetan medicine system is more a way of healthy living than merely a system of treatment of diseases. They developed many new concepts of health, disease, and treatment in addition to the ones used in Ayurveda.

Their materia medica is a vast collection of many life saving drugs.

The fundamental text book "*Chatush-Tantra*" of this medicine was delivered by *Bhagwan Buddha* 2500 years ago, and it was further developed by eminent Indian scholars like Jivaka, Nagarjuna, Vaghbhatt and Chandranandan etc. *Chatush-Tantra* (rGud-bZi) was translated into the Tibetan language around the 8th century AD by Kashmiri Acharya Chandranandan and Tibetan Translator *Verochana*, but before introducing this medicine in Tibet.

It was amended and enriched with other medical traditions like Chinese, Persian and Tibetan folk medicine to make it most effective and more suitable to the socio-climatic conditions of Tibet. From Tibet, the impact of *Sowa-Rigpa* along with Buddhism and other Tibetan art and sciences spread to the neighboring Himalayan regions like Mongolia, Bhutan, Nepal, China and some parts of former Soviet Union etc. and to this day, *Sowa-Rigpa* is very popular in these regions. Besides *Chatush-Tantra*, around two dozen Indian Medical texts are translated into Tibetan from Sanskrit, followed by thousands of commentaries and texts written by Tibetan scholars.

In the Tibetan medical tradition, the concept of well being takes into accounts the full dynamics of mind, body and spirit to achieve an effective and comprehensive healing strategy. It is immersed in Buddhist tradition, which differs from non-Buddhist medicine in that it utilizes three types of therapeutic intervention: medicinal entities, the power of *mantra* (a creative, repetitive sound) and the power of meditative stabilization[9]. In doing so, the Tibetan healing traditions transport us into a strange world of interconnectedness between macrocosmic principles and their microcosmic manifestations; harmony and balance between the cosmic macrocosm and the human microcosm is believed to be essential for health and well-being. This is true not only in the sense that balance is required for health, but also in the somewhat deeper sense that such balance is the essence of health; balance among the physical, psychological and spiritual elements of human existence ***is*** health.

In addition to being a relatively secular approach to health and well-being, involving medicines and dietary and practical suggestions, the Tibetan healing tradition is rich in tantric Buddhist ritual and symbolism. Furthermore, ritual and symbol contain multiple levels of meaning which all exist collaterally in a spiritual approach to healing. Iconography, music, chants, *mantra*, symbolic objects such as prayer wheels and prayer flags, *mandalas* (geometric paintings or drawings) and visualizations are utilized in modest to elaborate rituals to focus and objectify the source of healing power. Tibetan symbols and rituals, whose ultimate purpose is to mobilize the *bodhicitta* (aspiration to attain enlightenment in order to free all sentient beings from suffering) in the individual, generate not only cognitive considerations but also encompass subjective meaning for the spiritual, emotional and sensual spheres.

An effort will be made to have a comprehensive discussion on Buddhist Tibetan healing traditions. However, we will consider several aspects of the tradition which are integral for any basic understanding of the subject. First, we will discuss the etiology of illness from a Tibetan Buddhist perspective. Second, we will discuss some of the relatively secular therapeutic approaches to healing. Finally, we will explore the spiritual dimension of healing by focusing our discussion on some of the tantric practices involving the Medicine Buddha. A powerful example of a Buddhist healing ritual, which invokes a "meditative transformation of medicine" as described in the conclusion of Dr. Yeshi Donden's *Health Through Balance,* will conclude this analysis.

Etiology of Illness

In an early Mahayana text, the Buddhist sage Vimalakirti mused that, "All sentient beings are ill"[10]. To the Tibetan, the inevitability of suffering and illness is a reflection of the fact that we are born. The Tibetans believe that we "take birth" because we are ignorant of the true nature of reality and that it is this ignorance that is the cause of all suffering and disorder. Dr. Yeshi Donden remarked that "the root [of illness] is beginningless ignorance" and that "ignorance is with us like our own shadow . . . even if we think that we are in very good health, actually we have had the basic cause of illness since beginningless time"[11].

Tibetans believe that our false perceptions of the world and its projections actually change the world, which is fundamentally neutral. Moreover, people become attached to ego-centered views, which "contain the seeds of profound misunderstanding of what it means to have Being in this world"[12]. Consequently, because "all phenomena are mere reflections and designation of the mind"[13], and the mind is driven by delusional thinking, *saṃsara* (our perception of the phenomenal world) is filled with suffering.

Furthermore, the Tibetan Buddhist believes that *karma* (simply stated, the law of cause and effect) from one's previous incarnations can also be responsible for our illnesses in our present experience. Sakyamuni, the historical Buddha, explained this principle when he said:

In sooth to every man that's born
A hatchet grows within his mouth,
Wherewith the fool, whene'er he speaks
And speaks amiss, doth cut himself . . .[14]

Thus, the distant causes of the diseases are seated in the past mental environment which was influenced by "afflictive emotions"—mental factors that are the root cause of all illness. While these factors are impossible to enumerate, they are all the consequences of ignorance[15]. Ignorance generates other negative states of mind such as desire, hatred, jealousy and pride. Such negative emotions drive our mentations, and our mentations contribute to our suffering.

However, our emotional energies are neither good nor bad in themselves; for example, the energy/intelligence that turns to hatred when siezed in the neurotic grip of ego can also manifest as simple, clear awareness of the true situation—thus it is how we relate to our emotional energies that is crucial to well-ness. Understanding one's emotions is an essential part of the Buddhist journey to full awakening and freedom form unwanted conditions of all sorts. However, since most of us have very little ability to work with our emotional energies without creating negative experiences, medicines and other remedies are required.

While Tibetan notions of the law of *karma* imply infinite interlinked causes for any single event, three emotions, known as the "Three Interior Poisons," are considered to be at the root of all illness. The first poison is desire or passion, which implies grasping at objects or pleasant experiences. Desire is also perceived as "grasping at self" where *self* is our involvement with any object of our desire whether it is a chair, person or idea[16]. And self, which involves a subject grasping an object, is an illusion to which we cling, because we still do not understand that *anitya*(impermanence) is a primordial condition of living in *samsara*. Similarly, hatred, or aversion, regarded as the second poison, consists of pushing away unpleasant experiences or objects. Finally, ignorance, or confusion, which involves misunderstanding the nature of an object or a particular experience, is the third poison of the mind.

Secular Medicine

The physical manifestations of the Three Poisons assume the form of three humors or *nyes-pa* (literally the three "defects" or "faults" or "forms of punishment") (Ragpay, p.32). They have a dual function: when they are in harmony, they maintain well-being, but when they are disturbed or out of harmony, they are the cause of illness (Rapgay, p.33).

Desire corresponds to disharmony of *rlung* (wind; pronounced 'loong'). Both medical and religious texts consider the flow or blockage of *rlung* to be central in pathology. Some symptoms of *rlung* disorder are frothy urine, a rough dry tongue or a "jumpy" pulse.

Hatred corresponds to disharmony of energy, or bile. Some symptoms of a bile disorder include the presence of thick or yellowish-red urine, thick, yellowish fur on the tongue or a "full" pulse.

Ignorance is related to heavy, or phlegm, disorders. The urine is odorless, thin and whitish, and the pulse is "sluggish or heavy"[17].

Tibetan medicine views emotional, physical and cognitive interactions as "essential components in the understanding of the cause, aggravation and duration of virtually all major diseases"[18]. As Patricia Walsh-Frank noted, "Mind (reason) and spirit (in part emotion) co-mingle in this holistic philosophy".Thus, the principal medicine, which frees us from most afflictions and enables us to live in well-ness, must be that which loosens the grip on the "self" and ego-centered thinking. Consequently, to the Tibetan, the mind is the vehicle by which one can enter the world of non-self and become liberated from the self-centered causes of suffering.

Diagnostic techniques necessitate complex calculations in order to reach a diagnosis and formulate a treatment plan. The Tibetan physician must be thoroughly trained in analyzing a large number of complications in the practical application of the complete doctrine. The most popular and widely commented upon Buddhist medical text, which is used in medical training, is the four-part, 156 chapter *rGyud-bzhi* or *TheFour Secret Oral Tantras of the Eight Branches of the Medical Tradition*[19]. Compiled in about the fourth century A.D., the teachings are believed to have been revealed by the Medicine Buddha in the form of four Buddhas[20]. The Tibetan physician-in-training must commit to memory at least three of the four Tantras: the *Root Tantra, Explanatory Tantra* and *Last Tantra.*

The restoration of harmony and order is crucial to the healing process which includes spiritual, social and psychological well-being as well as physical health. The ideal image of a healer, is that of "a man of noble character, but he is also capable of immediately making the right diagnosis of a patient's illness, without any examination or the least assistance"[21]. Needless to say, such physicians are quite rare. Consequently, before a physician acquires credibility, he must train at least twenty years in the tradition.

Tibetan medicine is a holistic tradition, which is "oriented around symptoms, and therefore it is delicately responsive to symptom clusters, no complaint being disregarded"[22]. Since a lasting cure can only take place when the whole psychosocial environment of the patient is accounted for, superficial methods which consider only the outward symptoms of illness are frowned upon. The physician must be willing to consider more than the diseased organ, or even the whole person: "he must view the man in the world"[23]. Consequently, Tibetan medicine is increasingly gaining recognition in the West as particularly effective for patients with "chronic diseases such as hepatitis, certain kinds of mental illness, ulcers, paralysis, gall stones, kidney stones, and arthritis"[24].

In the Tibetan system, regardless of whether or not one is manifesting symptoms of illness, one is still considered to be sick. Disease, if not evident, is in dormant form. Thus the scope of disease is extremely difficult for the physician to fathom[25]. For example, there are 84,000 different "affective emotions" which generate 84,000 types of disorders. These can be condensed and condensed again into 404 specific diseases[26].

In a simplified rendition of Tibetan disease classification, imbalances of three types of humors, wind, bile and phlegm, are thought to occur. The more complex the imbalance, the greater the therapeutic urgency. Diseases are classified into forty-two types of wind disorders, twenty-six types of bile disorders and thirty-three types of phlegm disorders for a total of 101. There are also 101 disorders whose origins lie in the *karma* of the past life. They are illnesses of a serious nature, which are typically considered the consequences of "mistakes committed in a previous life"[27]. Such illnesses are usually considered to be fatal, unless they are treated with meditation and other spiritual practices, such as confession or exorcism. There are 101 disorders caused by "spirits" and 101 considered as superficial; i.e., they are caused by, and cured by changes in, behavioral patterns such as smoking, diet, bathing, and lack of exercise, or activities such as stealing, adultery, lying and dishonesty[28].

Tibetans look at well-ness as a consequence of three integrated types of medical practices: secular therapies, such as medicine, diet, surgery, etc.; spiritual cures; and as a metaphor for spiritual growth, where Buddha is the Absolute healer and the *Dharma*, orteachings of Sakyamuni, is the "King of Medicine"[29]. In the third case, when it is a potential "catalytic factor" which hastens one toward spiritual enlightenment, Tibetans view illness and its consequences more optimistically[30].

Some of the secular methods used in treating illness include pharmaceuticals; moxibustion (burning herbs upon designated areas of the patient's body); wearing gemstones and animal skins, which are believed to have curative powers due to their emanations; burning incense against "air diseases"; acupuncture, which is "practiced with care and reserve"[31]; massage; mineral baths; bloodletting; the occasional use of laxatives and emetics; and behavioral adjustments regulating smoking, diet and sexual activity[32].

Surgery is considered only as a last resort, and it is exceedingly primitive compared to Western standards. Yeshi Donden indicates that surgery is not performed in Tibet, both because "it is better to cure the organ than to remove it" and for religious reasons, since "it is better to undergo the illness and take medicine to cure it than to seek to avoid the illness and be operated on" (p. 183). Consequently, surgery is considered a violent approach to disease, but the "painful removal of foreign bodies, cauterization of abscesses, curetting of severely damaged tissues, etc." is performed after all other options are exhausted[33]. Moreover, in many cases, surgery is performed without the use of anaesthetics, because the Tibetan is thought to be "far less sensitive to pain than the average Westerner"[34].

Spiritual Dimension of Healing

Ron Leifer, a scholar of Tibetan medicine, considered the practice of Tibetan medicine a science because it is based on "observation and logical reasoning rather than faith, scripture or religious authority" (p. 753). However, even though the therapeutic methods described above may appear to be divorced from spiritual implications, they are not. Tibetan medicine typically directs its attention toward spiritual factors regarding the cause and cure of illness which by Western standards would be regarded as the "domain of the priest or psychiatrist"[35].

The Tibetan physician focuses his attention on spiritual factors even in the treatment of the simplest illnesses. Every Tibetan physician vows to "regard medicine as an offering to the Medicine Buddha and all other medicine deities" and considers his "medical instruments as holy objects"[36]. Even the pharmaceuticals, which are mixtures of vegetable, animal and mineral compounds, are prepared with meticulous attention to religious ritual. For example, after the Tibetan physician gathers the dozens of different ingredients that go into the making of the single small pill, he performs a meditative ritual. Before and after the ingredients in the pills have been assembled, the physician imagines himself and the medicine to be *Hayagriva*, a Buddhist deity. The physician and the deity are considered to be consolidated as one inseparable entity. The medicines are further blessed "into a magnificent state through being implanted with *mantra* [a prayerful vocalization]"[37]. Because pills are blessed this way, Tibetans believe that even the dying can benefit from them.

The emphasis on metaphysical principles in Tibetan medicine has its roots in the teachings of the historical Buddha, who lived about 2,500 years ago. The ancient texts of the Pali Canon record that early Buddhist communities believed that the four necessities of life are food, clothing, shelter and medicine. Since illness tended to weaken the focus of the mind, which was the liberating faculty, concepts of healing were important in the earliest Buddhist communities.

In the teachings of the Pali Canon, a person "who is not liberated, who is still subject to the sufferings brought on by insatiable craving, is considered ill."[38]. Sakyamuni Buddha was portrayed as the Supreme Physician who used two basic healing methods: healing by means of instruction and healing by means of miracles. Sakyamuni Buddha, who was considered a link between humanity and myriad celestial beings, repeatedly reminded his disciples that they should diligently seek to be healed. And Sakyamuni Buddha proclaimed that "Lo, I am physician without peer . . . "[39]. Consequently, his disciples could turn to the *King of Medicines*, (the *Dharma*, or Buddha's teachings) or the Supreme Physician himself for relief.

Those whose illnesses were perceived to be fatal received lessons on impermanence as a fact of the natural world, whereas those who were curable were encouraged to meditate on the seven limbs (*bojjhangas*) of enlightenment: mindfulness, his teachings (*dharma*), striving, joy, tranquility, meditative trance and equanimity[40]. From the traditional perspective the ***bojjhangas*** are considered a method for overcoming the"Three Interior Poisons": desire, hatred and delusion. The emphasis on Buddha as the Supreme Physician, a model of selfless compassion who devoted his life to easing the pain and suffering of others, indicates a fundamental attitude regarding the nature of Buddhist medicine: "dispassionate compassion"[41]. This attitude serves as a behavioral prototype for contemporary Tibetan physicians.

The Medicine Buddha

About the third century A.D., the Medicine Buddha, also known as *Bhaisajya-guru*, was recorded in Buddhist texts as an emanation of the historical Buddha, who was considered the preeminent healing deity in the Mahayana Buddhist tradition. *Bhaisajya-guru*, also known as "Master of Healing, the Lapis Lazuli Radiance Tagatha," is one of a number of emanations of Buddhist deities whose purpose is to open the imagination of the supplicant to expanded understanding and empowerment. The teachings of the Medicine Buddha have been handed down throughout the centuries by means of oral tradition and practical applications gleaned from written works such as *The Medicine Guru Beams of Lapis Lazuli Sutra* and *The Four Secret Oral Tantras on the Eight Branches of the Essence of Nectar*—both works were attributed to Sakyamuni Buddha. Sakyamuni is recorded as saying that by uttering the *Bhaisajya-gurumantra*, one is free of the nine untimely causes of death and of all suffering. All subsequent reincarnations will be "peaceful and joyous"[42].

One can also petition the healing powers of the Medicine Buddha by visualization practices to "invoke the spiritual force of that deity, in order to heal all diseases, inner and outer"[43]. Intense identification with various characteristics associated with the emanation of the *Bhaisajya-guru* invokes a spiritual attitude which generates healing action along the devotee's psychosocial continuum. Even the name of the Medicine Buddha is believed to have the power to free one from the pattern of negative thoughts and emotions. Healing can occur just by speaking, hearing or concentrating on his name. Thus, for example, conceited persons will become humble, greedy persons will become charitable and those who cause dissent will become cooperative and loving just by hearing or saying his name.

Every morning, the Tibetan physician reintegrates into his consciousness the spiritual, intellectual and practical teachings of the Medicine Buddha through visualization and prayers. The rituals enable the practitioner to "ward off any spiritual obstacles to the correct diagnosis and cure . . . as negative spiritual entities can either cloud the diagnosis or prevent the medicines from working properly in the patient"[44].

As I explained above, the mind is considered the origin of all illness and spiritual afflictions. Consequently, much of the healing that the Medicine Buddha promises lies within the mind. The mystical revelations into esoteric teachings regarding compassion, healing and enlightenment are too profound to express in ordinary speech or writing. Tibetan Buddhist art has transcendental implications which are "conveyed through the formal language of symbols, colors, gestures, and attributes [and] cause hidden chords to resonate in the depths of our being"[45]. Because art and ritual surrounding the Buddha focus and uplift the mind, the devotee's consciousness is transformed as he becomes sensitive to the healing rays of the Buddha as Absolute Truth. Thus, Tibetan art possesses incalculable value as a support for private meditative practices and as an agent for ritual devotions related to healing.

Artistic depictions of the *Bhaisajya-guru*, which are rich in symbolism, reveal a deity whose skin is the deep, blue color of the gemstone lapis lazuli. The gemstone, which is very precious to central Asians, is considered to have divine origins. The deity is sometimes depicted holding myrobalan fruit called *dug-bcom*, which means "that which renders poison inactive"[46]. *Dug-bcom* is a Tibetan healing symbol and a metaphor for the Three Poisons: desire, hatred and confusion.

Since every detail of the iconography associated with the image yields a teaching which is integral to the healing process, many elaborate forms of ritual worship have crystallized around the *Bhaisajya-guru*. Some examples of ritual involving the Medicine Buddha which are believed to have a curative or strengthening influence for the ill include meditating upon the deep blue color of lapis lazuli; making *puja* offerings of flowers and incense to the image of the deity; mentally or physically constructing an image of the deity; playing musical instruments and chanting; reading sutras; constructing altars, *mandalas* or banners; and lighting lamps. According to Birnbaum, the response will either be "dramatically immediate" or result in "improved *karmic* circumstances in the next incarnation" (p. 84).

The following ritual, which illustrates the Medicine Buddha's imagery as a dynamic conduit for invoking spiritual healing forces, is typically performed by a Tibetan lama/physician. Seated in a lotus position and repeating *mantra*, the lama/physician either actually or symbolically places medicinal pills in a begging bowl. Then he "generates an altruistic intention to become enlightened"[47]. The physician meditates on the lapis lazuli image of Bhaisajya-guru. He visualizes the Medicine Buddha's right hand as forming a "gesture of meditative equipoise" and his left hand as holding a lapis lazuli begging bowl filled with *amrta* (healing nectar)[48].

The lama/physician now meditates or visualizes a similar Medicine Buddha in front of himself. The physician then dissolves into "the emptiness of inherent existence" and re-emerges as Bhaisajya-guru with a complete *mandala*[49]. At this point the healer believes that he has actually become the Bhaisajya-guru. The Bhaisajya-guru in front of him emits rays of light which gather and dissolve medicinal essences into the medicine in the physician's begging bowl. The *mantra* is repeated endlessly. After more complex visualizations are performed, the invocation of *mantra* and "meditative stabilization" ultimately impart highly potentialized medicines.

Notes

1. BBC NEWS | Science/Nature | Stone age man used dentist drill.
2. Visit websites of Central Council for Research in Ayurveda & Siddha, New Delhi Or Department of Ayurveda, Yoga &

Naturopathy, Unani, Siddha and Homoeopathy (AYUSH), Ministry of Health & Family Welfare, Govt. of India

3. *Sunday Island*, Ven. Pandit Medagama Vajiragnana, Sangha Nayake of Great Britain.
4. See Shishir Thadani's *South Asian History, Pages from the history of India and the subcontinent.*
5. Science section, *Times of India*, 28-2-2008.
6. Central Council for Research in Ayurveda and Siddha, Deptt. Of AYUSH, Ministry of Health and Family Welfare, Govt. of India.
7. Donden, p. 215.
8. Birnbaum, p. 13.
9. Donden, p. 26.
10. Walsh-Frank, p. 8.
11. Thonduk, p. 193.
12. *Samyutta-nikaya* in Birnbaum, p. 9.
13. Donden, p. 15.
14. Tsarong, p. 17.
15. Rapgay, p. 17, p. 20, Thondup, p. 12-13.
16. Rapgay, p. 10.
17. Rapgay, p. 32.
18. Donden, p. 23.
19. Burang, p. 12.
20. Donden, p. 8.
21. Harvey Cushing as quoted in Rapgay, p. 8.
22. Donden, p. 8, p. 20.
23. Donden, p. 16.
24. Donden, p. 56.
25. Burang, p. 2.
26. Donden, p. 16.
27. Birnbaum, p. 13.
28. Birnbaum, p. 9.
29. Burang, p. 64.
30. Burang, p. 60.
31. Burang, p. 67.

32. Burang, p. 60.
33. Burang, p. 59.
34. Dummer, p. xix.
35. Donden, p. 214.
36. Birnbaum, p. 15.
37. As translated by E.M. Hare in *Woven Cadences of the Early Buddhists* in Birnbaum, p. 16.
38. Birnbaum, p. 10.
39. Birnbaum, p. 17.
40. Birnbaum, p. 88.
41. Birnbaum, p. 89.
42. Gold, p. 89.
43. Birnbaum, p. 78.
44. Dummer, p. 26.
45. Donden, p. 216.
46. Donden, p. 216.
47. Donden, p. 216.

CHAPTER – 2

BUDDHISM AND MEDICINE

It is believed that Lord Buddha showed the path of liberation from disease and death and due to this reason he is also known as the great physician (Mahabhisak). He propounded the four noble truths that are nothing but medical logic. These four noble truths include disease, its cause, treatment and its ways and are collectively known as *Aryasatyacatustaya*. Diagnosis of disease and charitable distribution of medicines among the sick people were the regular programmes of the Buddhist sanghas. Buddhist monks and nuns also implemented the same in Buddha-viharas. Emperor Asoka who adopted the Buddha religion after the Kalinga war not only established many hospitals and dispensaries for the treatment of the sick but also ordered planting of medicinal plants at different places.

Medicine in Buddhist Literary Tradition[1]

The oldest source of literature that gives a glimpse of Indian medicine in the Buddhist tradition is the *Tripitaka*[2]. *Tripitaka* mentions *tikiccha* in place of Ayurveda and disease is mentioned as *gilana* instead of *atura* as in medical text. This book also gives some references that suggest that *tikiccha* was one of the most important subjects of learning in Taksasila.

P. V. Sharma[3] says that there are five well-known *bhutas*, but the Buddhist texts mention only four of them, excepting *akasa*. Cullavagga has got enough material that gives a good view of daily life of monks and nuns, health and hygiene and the arrangements in the *viharas*. In the *viharas*, there were systematic arrangements for the maintenance of privies and bathrooms. Personal cleaning as well as cleaning of the surroundings was strictly observed. A special care was also taken for water. A number of diseases are mentioned in *Tripitaka* texts while *kustha, ganda, kilasa, sosa* and *apasmara* are said to be the five prevalent *abadhas*.

Mahavagga (MV) gives valuable information regarding diseases and their treatment in the book (vi) on medicaments. This book provides us very useful information particularly on the treatment of diseases. Some of the treatments contained in this book are described here in brief. To treat headache the drug was administered through nose and oil was also applied on the head. In the case of jaundice, *Haritaki* impregnated with cow's urine was prescribed. In the case of snakebite, four types of filth - dung, urine, ashes and clay were prescribed. For eye-disease, eye ointments and collyriums were also mentioned. Similarly a lot of other treatments are described in that book.

Drugs have been classified in the beginning of *MV* (VI). Here fat of animal is first described, and then the vegetable drugs are mentioned in the given groups:

1. Roots- turmeric, ginger etc.
2. *Kasaya* (bark?)- *nimba, kutaja* etc.
3. Leaves- *patola, tulasi* etc.
4. Fruits- *vidanga, pippali* etc.

5. *Niryasa- hingu, sarjarasa* etc.

At the end an inorganic substance salt is also mentioned. A large number of medicinal plants are also referred but in different contexts.

Mahavagga (viii. 1.1-29) contains a detailed account of the renowned scholar Jivaka and his amazing medical and surgical cures. He performed a large number of miraculous cures. He was born of Salavati, a courtesan of Vaisali. He learnt this medicinal science from Atreya at Taksasila. Atreya was himself a renowned scholar of medicine during the Buddhist period. Later, he became a physician in the court of Bimbisara.

Dhammapada – *Dhammapada* mentions freedom from disease as the highest gain. It advises to avoid two extremes - *ayoga* and *atiyoga* and to adopt the middle path. In *Dhammapada*, the word *'atura'* has been used for diseased; although in the Buddhist texts word *'gilana'* is used.

Apadana- Avadana is the other name of *Apadana*. There are many texts on this topic of which *avadanasataka* and *divyavadana* are more popular.

Avadanasataka is an interesting text dated about 100 CE. According to this text, cloth, food, beddings, appliances for diagnosis and treatment of the sick were offered to Lord Buddha. Several types of diseases, their symptoms and methods of their treatment are also described in it. The case of pregnancy in terms of drugs, diet and behaviour is described in a systematic manner. A pregnant woman was advised to avoid all the six tastes and any kind of unpleasant sound. Once, while operating a women's abdomen to deliver the foetus, Jivaka advised the lady to take five parts of a plant as a drug.

Different types of houses for different seasons (winter, summer and rainy season) are mentioned in *Divyavadana*. Application of *gosirsa candana* is suggested in case of fever with burning sensation. *Sammohini* and *sanjivani osadhi* are also referred to in this text. The *Jyotiskavadana* text gives references about *Jivaka*.

In *Sardulakarnavadana*, plants are referred to in a classified way and divided in to seven different groups such as *phalguvrksa, sthalaja vrksa, ksiravrksa, phalabhaisajya vrska, sthalaja puspavrksa* and *jalaja puspa*. Herbs growing in the villages as well as in the hills are also mentioned. Some diseases like *Apasmara, kilasa* and *kustha* are also described. At the end there is also a topic based on dreams. According to this text, constellations (*Naksatras*) also play a role and it is said that the collection as well as the administration of drugs should be started in *Satabhisa*.

Kunalavadana contains an interesting anecdote about a disease of King Asoka and its treatment with onion by his wife. Initially, his wife experimentally observed the effects of onion on intestinal worms.

Milindapanha is one of the non-canonical Pali texts. It originated in northwest India by about beginning of the Christian era. It holds some precious knowledge about Buddhist traditions. This text is in the form of dialogues between Nagasena and king Milinda. This text also holds some significant information about the Buddhist tradition. According to this text, medicine was one of the most important subjects of teaching during the Buddhist times. There is also a reference that king Milinda himself learned *cikitsa* along with other eighteen subjects. Treatment of wounds with paste, application of oil and dressing is preferred for better and early healing of the wounds. In the case of poisoning, a mixture of ghee, butter, oil, honey and jaggery is suggested. A very interesting connection of urine with reproduction is shown in a story where a fakir or ascetic was born by intake of urine of an ascetic or fakir. According to Nagasena the disease is caused by eight factors – *vata, pitta, slesma, sannipata,* seasonal imbalance, irregular diet, improper treatment and past deeds. Nagasena further narrates the aggravation of *vata, pitta* and *slesma* in ten, three and three ways respectively. According to him *vata* is aggravated by cold, heat, hunger, thirst, overeating, sedentary habit, anxiety, exertion, treatment and past deeds, while *pitta* and *kapha* are aggravated by cold, heat and irregular diet.

Saddharmapundarika is a work that belongs to first century CE. It is one of the most sacred Mahayana texts. This text mentions that followers of the Buddhist tradition established many *viharas* that were well equipped with food, drinks, appliances for diagnosis and treatment of the sick and other comforts. One of the chief characteristics of these *viharas* was that these were attached with a flower garden and park. According to this text diseases were classified into four types- *vatika, paittika, slaismika* and *sannipatika.* Along with the classification of diseases a large number of diseases are also mentioned such as *kustha, kilasa* etc. Deformity in the various body parts and different types of continuous and intermittent fevers are mentioned too. Plants are classified into four types – *trna, gulma, osadhi* and *vanaspati.* The parts of the plant are mentioned as *nala, sakha, patra, puspa* and *phala.* Drugs were taken in various forms such as juice, paste, decoction, infusion, after combining with other drugs, by injecting through needle or cauterization or mixing with food.

Mahayana texts contain some valuable information about the Buddhist tradition. *Lalitavistara* is one of the important texts that deal with the advent of Lord Buddha and his teachings. Lord Buddha is mentioned in this text by several names such as the king of physicians, best among physicians, the great surgeon etc. Several types of diseases are also mentioned here.

According to *Suvarnaprabhasasutra*, two factors play a vital role in the longevity of life – avoiding exertion and proper nutrition. Here, four *dhatus* (*bhutas*) are mentioned out of which two are said as moving upwards and the other two going downwards and thus they neutralize each other. The most interesting and important medical document in *Suvarnaprabhsasutra* is chapter 17. In this chapter, a great and well-informed man in all the branches of Ayurveda taught *Astanga Ayurveda* to his son and the discussion between them exposed some very interesting and valuable information about medicine. Four different seasons (rainy season, autumn, winter, and summer) and four different types of disorders (*vatika, paittka, sannipatika* and *kaphaja*) are mentioned that occur in these four seasons respectively. The pacification of these disorders is also given in the text.

The poetic works of Asvagohsa (2nd Cent.CE), Buddhacarita and Saundarananda, also contain some valuable information related to Buddhist medicine system.

Vinaya Sutta is an important source of information regarding Buddhist Medicine.

Buddha taught Eight Medicine Buddha Suttas (Eight Bhaisajya Suttas), which is still widely practiced in Mahayana Buddhist countries for the treatment of patients, for the stability of ecological balances and also for the prevention from natural calamities. Buddha in Golden Sutta discourse (gser-od-dumpa) has narrated the story of his previous life, where he became a physician.

The Four Tantras or Gyud-shi

According to Tibetan source, before the 'Golden Discourse' Buddha transformed the venue (a forest near Varanasi) into the pure medicine land of Tandadug, It led to the creation Bhaisajya Buddha Mandala and transformed himself into Medicine Buddha Beduga (aquamarine colour).

Representatives of the four medical traditions gathered in four directions of the mandala and looked at the Bhaisajya Buddha waiting for the sermon from Buddha.

A. Non-Buddhist Physicians: like Brahma, Vishnu, Mahadeva, Kartika

B. Buddhist Physician: Manjushri, Avalokiteshwara, Vajrapani, Ananda, Kumar Jeevaka.

C. God's Physician: Indra, Aswin, Lhamodutsima.

D. Rishi Ayurvedic Physiciaan: Atreya, Panaravasu, Ajnivesha, Kashyapa, Dhanavantri.

Then, Buddha gave the discourse of Four Tantra (Gyud-shi). The knowledge was transferred in India through an unbroken lineage till the 8th century A.D. It was developed in Afghanistan, Kashmir, Nepal and finally reached Tibet. The whole collection was translated into Tibetan in the 8th century, by the great translator Vairochana and Chandranandana of Kashmir.

According to the Kagyur and Tengyur Collection, there are numerous teaching of Buddha on medicine and alchemy.

Kumara Jeevaka- The most interesting story is on the life of Kumara Jeevaka and his service to Buddha. Kumar Jeevaka, contemporary of Buddha and son of Bimbisara king of Magadha and his courtesan, was an all rounder: a physician, a surgeon and a paediatrician. He studied medicine in Taxila and was capable of performing brain surgery. He learnt this art from Atreya, a renowned physician of that time. Kumara Jeevaka was also crowned three times the 'King of the Physician', because of his extraordinary feats. He successfully treated his father Bimbisara, his stepmother and others. He became ambitious and went to Buddha to learn the technique of curing mental illness. He attended Buddha's preaching session but couldn't decipher any meaning. Buddha on his introduction asked Jeevaka to go to the Snow Mountain and fetch him some herbs. Jeevaka was accompanied by another illustrious disciple of Buddha, Vajrapani. They brought many plants, herbs and minerals. Later, Buddha categorically explained the medicinal values of those substances to Jeevaka.

Buddha was an expert in four branches of medicine. They were :

1. examining the disease
2. diagnosing the disease
3. pacifying the disease
4. preventing the disease.

According to Buddha- The physician who is adept in all the 4 branches deserves to become a court physician. Kumara Jeevaka became the disciple of Buddha and offered Buddha his mango orchard, where Buddha stayed for several years.

Vinaya Sutta records many stories pertaining to Buddha and Kumara Jeevaka. According to the Tibetan Legend Jeevaka achieved immortality and is believed to be still alive somewhere in this world.

The Buddhist "Medicine King," Jîvaka Komarabhâcca

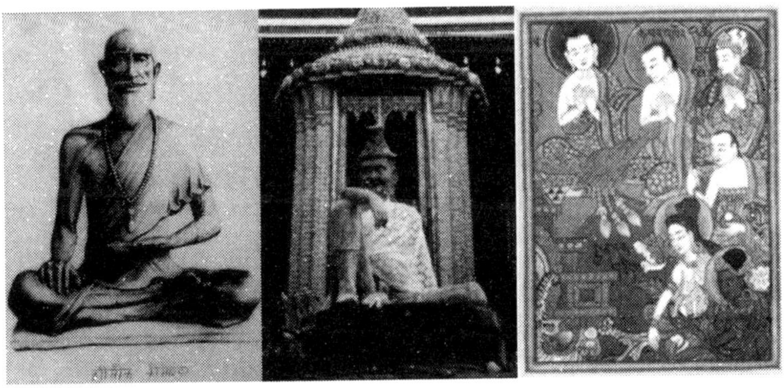

Tradition holds that Jīvaka Komarabhācca was the personal physician of the Buddha. A biography of Jīvaka is found within the Buddhist scriptures in multiple languages. In this story, it is said that Jīvaka was an orphan who was raised by Prince Abhāya. When he came of age, he studied medicine with a well-known master in northwestern India, apprenticing with this teacher for a period many years before returning back home. Different versions of the biography then relate up to a dozen instances where Jīvaka healed different individuals, including instances of major surgeries like the opening of the abdominal and cranial cavities. Among Jîvaka's patients were merchants and their wives, kings, and in some editions even the Buddha himself, who came to him for a purgative of powdered lotus flowers.

In the Theravada Buddhist canon, the biography of Jîvaka is found in the Mahavāgga section of the Vinaya, the monastic basket of discipline composed from the fourth to the first century BC. In addition, the Theravada Buddhist canon mentions Jīvaka in several places as a wealthy lay-physician and the donor of a mango grove called Jīvakarama, which he gave for the use of the Buddha's order of monks as a retreat for the rainy season. Jīvaka also appears in Tibetan translation, where he is an expert in trephination, or the surgical opening of the skull to extract parasites. In the Chinese, where Jīvaka is known as Qipo or Qiyu, he is born with acupuncture needles in his hands, and performs various Chinese medical diagnostic procedures. (These sutras are found at T. 553 and 554, as well as in the Dharmaguptaka Vinaya T. 1428). Several Chinese medical formulas have been named after Jīvaka since the medieval formularies of Sun Simiao. Although in most of the Buddhist world he is a forgotten figure, Jīvaka is actively worshipped in Thailand as the "Father Doctor." Many Thais believe that Jîvaka developed herbal medicine, therapeutic massage, and other healing practices himself, and taught these to future generations.

Although historians long have considered the biography of the Medicine King to be an important example of the introduction of Indian medicine to China, in an upcoming article in *History of Religions* I present a reappraisal of the authorship, dating, and genre of the hagiography, and come to a different conclusion of the text's importance by prioritizing local processes of cultural translation in the reception of Indian religion and medicine. Analyzing the early medieval Chinese sources of Jīvaka's biography, it appears that, in Chinese translation, the Medicine King was recreated as a model Chinese physician and as the founder of a Buddhist medical lineage that could rival the classical medical tradition. The texts also mobilize language from popular literature to transform the Medicine King into a familiar figure from the medieval anomaly tale genre: the miracle-healing wonder-worker. The purposes of the texts were not medical but hagiographic. Employing both classical frames of medical authority and popular literary conventions, the text demonstrates the importance of medical hagiography to Buddhist proselytism and legitimization in China. Claims for the Medicine King's supremacy and efficacy, by extension also applied to those who invoked his name, leading Buddhists to adopt Jîvaka as a source of authority for a wide range of medical activity throughout the medieval period.

From Jeevaka, Gyud-shi (the Four Tantras) after passing through several generations was transmitted to Nagarjuna (1st century A.D.), the founder of Madhyamika Philosophy.

Nagarjuna became rasayansiddha. According to Tibetan Leagend Nagarjuna lived for 600 years and his body sparkled like a gem. He composed several treatises on medical science like Yoga sataka and alchemy. After

Nagarjuna Gyud-shi was passed on to Vagabhatta the author of Astanga Hridaya Sangraha. His descendant was Physician Chandranandana of Kashmir. From Chandranandana, Vairochana translated and compiled Gyud-shi in its present form in the 8th century A.D.

The following authors representing the Buddhist tradition are significant in the field of Ayurveda:

1. Vagbhata-Vagabhata composed the *Astangasangraha* and the *Astangahrdaya.* These books not only contain the *Samhitas* of Caraka and Susruta but also include many Vidyas and mantras as well as a large number of medical formulae prevalent in the Buddhist tradition.

2. Ravigupta-Ravigupta, a Buddhist scholar, composed the *Siddhasara* that also contained a *nighantu* at the end. The date of Ravigupta is fixed as 650 CE, viz. after Vagbhata and before Madhava. The *Siddhasara* contains 31 chapters and the *Siddhasara-nighantu* as appendix. First four chapters of this book are based on *Tantra, dravyagana, annapanavidhi* and *arista,* while chapters 5 to 25 deal with individual diseases. Further chapters are based on *Varna, Salakya, Visa, Rasayana- Vajikarana, Kumaratantra, Pancakarma* and *Kalpa.*

3. Nagarjuna- A large number of works was produced by Nagarjuna in different periods. *Yogasataka* is such a work by Nagarjuna that represents work of this tradition. Apart from *Yogasataka* following works of Nagarjuna are incorporated into the Tibetan Tanjur:

   (a) Avabhesajakalpa

   (b) Arya raja name vatika

   (c) Arya mulakosamahausadhavali

4. Candranandana-The following works of Candranandana are incorporated in the Tibetan Tanjur:

(a) *Vaidya-Astangahrdayavrtti*

(b) *Vaidya-Astangahrdayavrttau bhesajanama-paryayanama*

(c) *Padarthacandrika...... Astangahrdaya-vivrti*

School of Thangka Painting depicting Bhaisajya Buddha or Buddha of Medicine and Bhaisajyaguru Mandala[4]

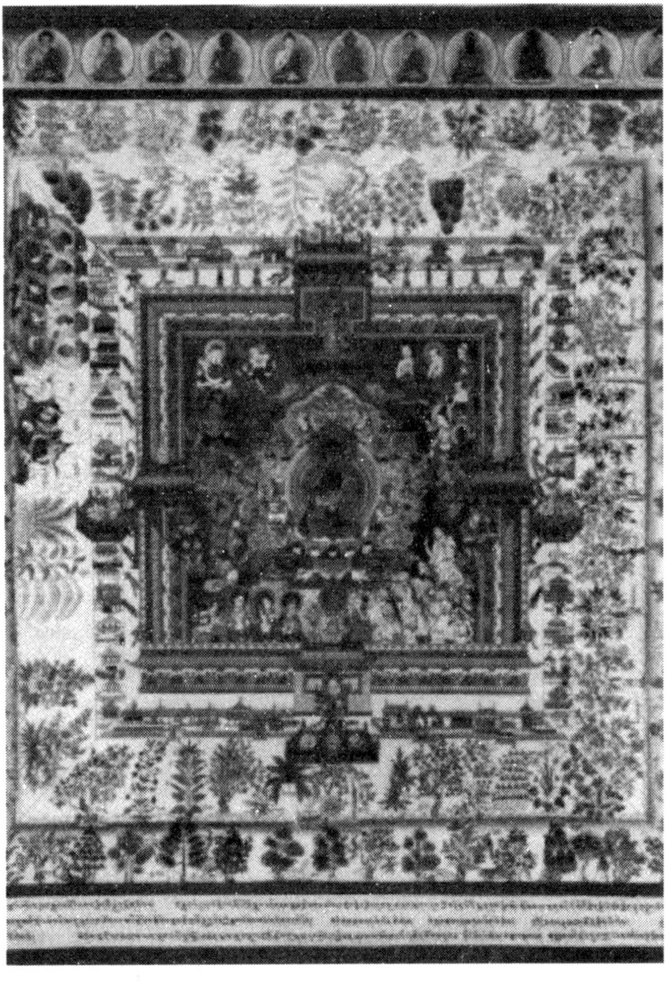

Palace of Buddha Bhaisajyaguru, Master of Remedies

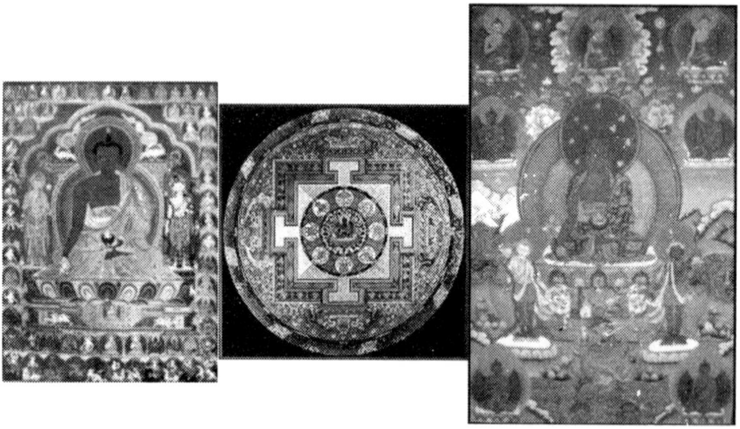

Bhaisajyaguru and Mandala

This is the first painting in the series of medical training paintings that provide illustrations for the basic Tibetan medical text, the "Blue Beryl" tantras. In this painting, Bhaisajyaguru, the Medicine Buddha, indirectly teaches the science of healing to his followers. The dieties in the upper section are representations of the lineage of medical teachings, including the 5th Dalai Lama, the eight Buddhas of Medicine, and several medical scholars.

This central palace of the Mandala of the Medicine Buddha is the site where the science of medicine is taught. Shakyamuni Buddha, as Bhaisajyaguru, the Medicine Buddha, sits on a throne engraved with gems at the center of the palace, at the center of Sudarsana, the city of medicine. In attendence are gods of the devaloka, hermit scholars, Hindu dieties, and Buddhist followers, including bodhisattvas and devout students. While holding his seat on the central throne, Bhaisajyaguru also manifests as the four sibling hermit scholars who instruct all types of students at the same time.

Each class of students receives teachings appropriate to their own level of understanding of the fundamental nature of reality and the lives of beings.

The central figure is Bhaishajyaguru (Menla), the buddha of medicine, the physician of human passions, the unfailing healer of the ills of samsara. He is dark blue like lapis lazuli and hence called Vaidūryaprabharaja. As blue is also well known as Akshobhya's color, Bhaishajyaguru receives some of the attributes of Akshobhya, who presides over the east. Bhaishajyaguru holds the myrobalan (arura) plant in his right hand; his left hand cradles a bowl of amrita - medicine. The bowl is made of lapis lazuli and is dodecagonal in form, symbolising his twelve resolutions to help human beings. His expression is calm and serene, and he does not wear a crown on his head.

According to Hsuan Tsang and I-tsing, his paradise in the east is called "pure world created in lapis lazuli." He is flanked by the two chief Bodhisattvas of his cycle: Suryaprabha, Solar Radiance, to the right and Chandraprabha, Lunar Radiance, to the Left.

Sixteen Bodhisattvas are depicted along both sides of the Thangka's vertical panels. At the time of death, when a dying person invokes the Buddha in earnestness, these Bodhisattvas appear and help the dying person obtain birth on a lotus flower in Vaidurya-nirbhasa Heaven.

The twelve yaksha generals are charged to protect adepts by the divine grace of Bhaishajyaguru. Each yaksha general reigns over one of the twelve months and twelve parts of the day, while Suryaprabha and Chandraprabha rule over day and night. The yaksha generals hold an animal, probably a mongoose, the symbol of Vaishravana, who is the king of the yakshas.

There are seven emanations of Bhaishajyaguru including himself. Besides the main figure, the six emanations can be seen on the top panel, to which Shakyamuni Buddha has been added in the center. The emanation of this buddha into seven arises from the invocation - practiced with the aim to be freed from disease and untimely death - that uses seven images and lasts for seven consecutive days.

The four guardians of the world (catur-maharajika) are illustrated in the corners of the Panel under the throne. The bottom panel depicts the ten keepers of the directions (dikpala). They are, from left to right: Brahma on a goose, Indra on an elephant, Agni on a goat, Yama on a buffalo, Nairrita on a corpse, Varuna on a sea-monster, Vayu on a deer, Kubera on a horse, Ishana on a bull, Prithivi on a boar.

The scroll shows all the 51 deities of the mandala of Bhaishajyaguru:

1 central deity

2-9 his seven emanations and Shakyamuni

10-25 sixteen bodhisattvas

25 - 35 ten dikpalas

36-47 twelve yaksha generals

48-51 four guardians of the world.

Sakya Pandita and inscriptions of his name are depicted on the tapestry hanging from Bhaishajyaguru's throne. This clearly indicates that the scroll was painted in Sakya circles. A number of lamas with red caps can seen on the top panels as well as below the throne. Donors are painted at the top.

Significance of the Mandala

The mandala–a mystical diagram composed of geometrical shapes (usually a circle within a square)–is used to aid meditation and is prevalent in both Hindu and Buddhist art.

A mandala, which is Sanskrit for "circle," is an ancient form of Tibetan art and a symbol which is integral to Tibetan Buddhism. Mandalas can be painted, made of particles, or produced in three-dimensional forms. In general, all mandalas have outer, inner, and secret meanings. On the outer level, they represent the world in its divine form; on the inner level, they represent a map by which the ordinary human mind is transformed into the enlightened mind; and on the secret level, they depict the perfect balance of the subtle energies of the body and the clear light dimension of the mind. The creation of a sand painting is said to effect purification and healing on these three levels.

The mandalas are created whenever a need for the healing of the environment and living beings is felt. The monks consider our present age to be one of great need in this respect and, therefore, are creating sand mandalas where requested throughout their world tours.

Tibetan Sand Mandala of Bhaishajyaguru

(Medicine Buddha)

Created by Tenzin Shakya and Geshe Lobsang Kunga, monk-artists of the Drepung Gomang Monastery in Mundgod, India

Not all monks learn to make sand mandalas. Only those who show a special interest and aptitude are chosen by senior monks to carry on the tradition. Training often lasts two years during which time they construct the mandala again and again until they memorize the design.

The mandala that is being created for the University is a Medicine Buddha mandala. In Tibet the Medicine Buddha, called Bhaishajyaguru, is revered as the source of the healing arts. It is through him that the teachings embodied in the Four Medical Tantras, the basis of Tibetan medicine, came into being. The Buddha transformed himself into a deep blue Buddha, emanating healing rays of light, and taught an assembly of men and gods the science of medicine. The

Buddhist orders valued medicine to alleviate suffering and prolong human life, to improve the human opportunity to attain enlightenment.

The central figure of the mandala represents Bhaishajyaguru. He is surrounded by five other iconographic groups: his seven emanations and Shakyamuni, sixteen bodhisattvas, twenty-four more bodhisattvas, and the four guardians of the world.

The Process of Creating a Sand Mandala

The mandalas made with colored sand are unique and exquisite. In Tibetan, this art is called *dul-tson-kyil-khor* which literally means "mandala of colored powders."

The mandala sand painting process begins with an opening ceremony during which the monks consecrate the site and call for the forces of goodness. This is done by means of chanting, music, and mantra recitation.

The monks then begin by drawing an outline of the mandala on the wooden platform. Millions of grains of colored sand are then painstakingly laid into place over a period of days or weeks. The sand, colored with vegetable dyes or opaque tempera, is poured on the mandala platform with a narrow metal funnel called a "chakpur" that is scraped by another metal rod to cause sufficient vibration for the grains of sand to trickle out of its end. The two chakpurs are aids that symbolize the union of wisdom and compassion. The exact proportions and all the details of the design are laid down in ancient Buddhist texts on the creation of mandalas. The monks carefully follow the canonical iconography. Since each mandala is extremely complex, monks specialize in the construction of only one or two kinds.

When finished, to symbolize the impermanence of all things, the colored sands are swept up and poured into a nearby river or stream where the waters carry the healing energies throughout the world.

Painting of Bhaisajyaguru

This colorful thangka, or scroll painting, represents the Buddha as the master of medicine and teacher of healers. As the patron deity of Tibetan medicine, he is a healer of both the body and spirit. The figure of the Medicine Buddha dominates the center of the painting. He is depicted with bright blue skin, seated in meditation on elegant red-and-gold robe. His eyes are partly closed, as if in deep concentration, and the palms of his hands and the soles of his feet are a brilliant orange color. In his right hand, the Buddha holds a flowering plant believed to have healing properties. Not only is this painting rich in meaning; it is a beautiful aesthetic achievement, and the harmonious use of bold, vibrant colors is characteristic of Tibetan art. Thangkas are intended to serve as a guide for contemplative experience and to focus the mind during meditation. They also enrich religious ceremonies with color, and provide devotees with depictions of the Buddha, other important deities, and *lamas*, or highly respected teachers from the past. Buddhists might imagine themselves as the Buddha figure in the painting, using the thangka as a reference for the details of posture, attitude, color, and clothing. *The Spread of Buddhism* This thangka painting was created over 600 years ago by an artist in Tibet, part of the Himalayan region in Southeast Asia that is made up of high plateaus and some of the world's tallest mountains, including Mount Everest. Previously an independent country, Tibet was annexed by China in 1951 and its official name is now the Tibetan Autonomous Region of the People's Republic of China. As a part of southwest China, Tibet is bordered by Myanmar, India, Bhutan, and Nepal. It has always been a relatively isolated country because of its mountainous geography, but Tibetans have had continuous contact with China and India, as well as other cultures throughout thousands of years of their history. Buddhism spread to Tibet from India in the 7th century, and it soon became the most important religion in the region. It also spread to China and other surrounding countries in part due to the movement of merchants and traders along the Silk Road, a series of trading routes that crossed central Asia. Buddhism changed and adapted to local beliefs as it spread throughout Asia, and so Tibetan Buddhist culture is somewhat different from that of other countries. The type of Buddhism practiced in Tibet is called Vajrayana Buddhism, and one of its unique characteristics is the importance of lamas, or highly respected teachers. The Dalai Lama, a leader whose name means "ocean of wisdom," has traditionally been the religious and political leader of Tibet. There have been fourteen Dalai Lamas in succession, and each one is considered a reincarnation of his predecessor. The current Dalai Lama lives in exile in India, where he is free to practice his religion without the oversight of the Chinese government. Siddhartha Gautama, the man who came to be known as the Buddha (he is also known as Buddha Shakyamuni), was born a young prince in northeastern India (now Nepal) in the 6th century b.c. After seeing human suffering around him, he renounced the privileged class he was born into in favor of living an ascetic life. During his lifetime, he discovered a means to escape the endless cycle of death and rebirth that, according to his teachings, is determined by an individual's karma, their accumulated actions. Through meditation, the Buddha attained a state of enlightenment, the end of reincarnation and suffering; in fact the name Buddha means "the enlightened one." After his enlightenment at the age of 35, Buddha traveled around India for 45 years teaching others what he had learned and suggesting a code for living. He developed guidelines for thoughts and actions to help all beings reach this state of absolute peace. In his first speech, given in 528 b.c. to a group of his followers in Sarnath, in northeast India, Buddha introduced his understanding of the Four Noble Truths:

- All life is suffering.
- Suffering is caused by desire.
- To eliminate suffering, eliminate desire.
- To eliminate desire, follow the Noble Eightfold Path.

In Buddhism, morality is left up to the individual and is expressed through accumulated actions, or karma. The Noble Eightfold Path is at the center of daily Buddhist practices. It is not a ritual performed by priests but a guide for all people to live by, known as the dharma. It means adopting right (true or correct) views, right thoughts, right conduct, right speech, right livelihood, right effort, right mindfulness (putting aside greed and distress), and right meditation. The reward for following the Noble Eightfold Path is the achievement of enlightenment.

Buddhist Art

One important aspect of traditional Tibetan Buddhist culture is the practice of creating images to be used in worship, like this thangka painting. A thangka is a painted or embroidered Tibetan banner that was hung in a monastery or over a family altar and was also carried in ceremonial processions. In Tibetan the word "than" means "flat" and the suffix "ka" means "painting." A thangka is usually painted on cotton and framed in silk brocade, and is meant to be a portable icon. Because thangkas can be rolled, they can travel easily with monks who move from village to village. Their vibrant colors brightened the often dark interiors of temples and monasteries. Thangkas are created in a careful and systematic way, involving six steps.

1. The first step is to apply a priming layer of paint to the cloth to prepare the surface to be painted. Then the artist creates a separate sketch, laying out the figures and structure of the design in great detail. After that, the artist draws a grid of lines onto the cloth and transfers his design. The artist then applies the first layers of paint; the pigments are ground from semiprecious stones and other natural materials. Gradually more layers of paint are added for shading and outlining until the painting is complete. Artists throughout Asia have created a standard way to depict the Buddha, so that people could always recognize him when looking at a painting or sculpture. The Buddha can be recognized by his ushnisha (prominent bump on the top of his head) and urna (dot or mole on his forehead), signifying his extraordinary wisdom. Short hair and elongated earlobes represent his renunciation of the princely life in which long, beautiful hair and heavy earrings (which stretched the earlobes) were desired. Although images of the Buddha have similarities, artists have created many versions, and if you look closely no two depictions are exactly alike.

2. Other typical characteristics of the Buddha include mudras, or hand gestures that signal his various roles of teaching, meditating, protecting, and urging generosity. Every mudra symbolizes something different. In this painting, the Medicine Buddha's right hand is in the meditation mudra, resting in

his lap. His left hand rests upon his knee with the palm facing outward in the mudra granting blessings, and holds the stem of a flowering plant believed to have healing properties. In this work of art two bodhisattvas, or compassionate beings, flank the Buddha. A bodhisattva is a person who has attained enlightenment, but chooses to remain in the cycle of life and death in order to help others escape the cycle of human suffering. A bodhisattva provides help to other beings over a series of lifetimes, transferring his own karmic merit, or buildup of good deeds, to other beings. Their gold and silver complexions represent the bright splendor of the sun and the moon, and they act as the eternal helpers of the Buddha. These figures wear the sparkling gold jewelry of princes, showing that they still reside in the earthly realm. A number of other figures of deities surround the central figure of the Medicine Buddha, arranged in neat rows. Seven more Medicine Buddhas, a goddess, and a sword-carrying god are directly above the Buddha's head, in the top center.

3. Below them a number of bodhisattvas wearing elaborate crowns gather in adoration. The side edges of the thangka are patrolled by two vertical rows of protective deities riding various animal mounts. These figures are directly derived from Hindu gods who have been incorporated into the service of the Buddha. Along the bottom of the thangka are two rows of Jambhala wealth deities who hold jewel-spitting mongooses, and four armored figures in the two lower corners represent the cardinal directions—North, South, East, and West. At the base of the Buddha's lotus throne a

green carpet overflows behind a small figure. This is Padmasambhava, a legendary mystic who formally introduced Buddhism to Tibet from India. The whole composition is set in shallow space almost like a stage, and all of the figures appear very close to the picture plane in their own small red niches. There is no signature on this painting, and we do not know the name of the artist who created it. Buddhist art is made primarily for religious ceremonies and meditation, and for many Tibetan painters individual expression is not as important as following traditional designs and depicting a particular deity correctly. The artist's goal is to complete a painting that includes the details necessary to serve its proper religious function.

Bhaishajyaguru, The Medicine Buddha

Originally, there was only one Buddha (Shakyamuni). However, according to later Buddhist doctrine an infinite number of Buddhas work in multiple universes (past, present, and future) for the benefit of all beings. Artists have depicted many different types of Buddha images as subjects for devotion, and one of the most popular of these is the Medicine Buddha, who represents the Buddha's ability to embody healing for all beings. The Medicine Buddha is said to "heal humanity of all sins and unpleasant circumstances." He has many of the features of a typical Buddha image, including a lotus flower throne and an urna on his forehead, as well as his own distinctive attributes.

The most distinctive feature of the Medicine Buddha is the deep blue color of his skin, painted from the blue of the gemstone lapis lazuli. Asian and European cultures have greatly prized this semiprecious stone for more than 6000 years. An aura of mystery surrounds it, perhaps because it is very rare and comes from a remote area of northeast Afghanistan. Traditionally this beautiful stone was used to symbolize something that is pure or rare. It is said to have a curative or strengthening effect on those who wear it against the three poisons of desire, hatred, and delusion, and its natural smoothness allows it to be polished to become highly reflective. For all these reasons lapis lazuli is the principal color of the Medicine Buddha.

Medicine Buddha is a fully enlightened being. To understand who he is, what his nature is, what his function is, and so on, we first need to understand what an enlightened being is. Generally, 'being' means any being who experiences feelings – pleasant, unpleasant, or neutral. Thus we are beings, and animals are beings; but houses and plants are not beings because they do not experience any feelings. There are two types of being: sentient beings and enlightened beings. A sentient being, or living being, is a being whose mind is afflicted by the darkness of ignorance. An enlightened being is a being who is completely free from the darkness of ignorance.

Just as sentient beings have many different aspects, so do enlightened beings. Enlightened beings emanate countless different forms for the benefit of living beings. Sometimes they appear as Deities, sometimes as humans, sometimes as non-humans. Sometimes they appear as Buddhist Teachers, sometimes non-Buddhist Teachers, sometimes as crazy people or evil people, and sometimes even as inanimate objects. Emanations of enlightened beings pervade the whole world, but because our mind is covered by ignorance we do not recognize them. We cannot say who or what is an emanation of a Buddha.

Medicine Buddha is an enlightened being who has unbiased compassion for all living beings. He protects living beings from physical and mental sickness and other dangers and obstacles, and helps them to eradicate the three poisons – attachment, hatred, and ignorance – which are the source of all sickness and danger. He is a Buddha Doctor.

At one time Buddha Shakyamuni was staying at a place called Vaishali with thirty-six thousand Bodhisattva disciples. At that time, Manjushri was appearing as a Bodhisattva disciple. Through his compassion, Manjushri realized that in the future the Buddhadharma would degenerate, and the beings of this world would find it very difficult to practise pure Dharma and gain pure realizations. He understood that it would be very difficult for those beings to control their minds, and so they would naturally engage in negative actions such as killing, stealing, and holding wrong views. As a result they would experience horrific illnesses and unbearable mental pain. The world would be full of problems, dangers, and adversity. Finding the thought of all this suffering impossible to bear, Manjushri asked Buddha:

> *In the future when your Dharma and general spiritual practice are in decline, when the human beings in this world are spiritually impoverished, when their attachment, anger, and ignorance are so strong and difficult to control that they experience continual physical suffering, mental pain, fears, and dangers, and especially many incurable diseases, who will release them from this suffering and protect them from danger? Who will help them to overcome the three mental poisons?*

In response to Bodhisattva Manjushri's question, Buddha expounded the Sutra of Eight Thousand Verses Principally Revealing the Instructions on Medicine Buddha. Many beings heard this teaching. In addition to the thirty-six thousand human Bodhisattva disciples, millions of other Bodhisattva disciples came from many Pure Lands, together with beings from other realms such as nagas and givers-of-harm, or yakshas. To this vast assembly of disciples Buddha explained all about Medicine Buddha - his special qualities, his Pure Land, and how in the future by relying upon this Buddha and just hearing his name, living beings could be cured of heavy mental and physical sickness, especially the sickness of delusions. He also explained how to make a connection with this Buddha, the benefits of relying upon him, and how to practise the Medicine Buddha instructions.

While Buddha was giving this teaching, Manjushri realized with his clairvoyance of knowing others' minds that some of the humans and gods in the audience were developing doubts, finding it difficult to believe the Buddha's explanation about the existence of Medicine Buddha. Therefore, again he rose from his seat, respectfully circumambulated Buddha three times, made three prostrations, and then with his left knee on the ground according to tradition, requested Buddha:

To remove doubts from the minds of disciples, please show clearly how this Buddha exists, where he exists, and what his good qualities are.

Buddha immediately entered into an absorption of concentration, and from his heart emanated light rays inviting the seven Medicine Buddhas to Vaishali so that everyone could see them. Medicine Buddha came with his two main disciples, Radiance of the Sun and Radiance of the Moon, as well as a vast retinue of thousands of other disciples. The other six Medicine Buddhas also came with their retinues. Everyone could see the seven Medicine Buddhas with their retinues directly, and their doubts were immediately dispelled. Buddha introduced each of the Buddhas, saying for example "This Buddha is Medicine Buddha. He comes from the eastern Pure Land called Lapis Jewel Land. This Buddha Land is the nature of wisdom with the aspect of lapis lazuli. The entire ground of that Pure Land is illuminated by this Buddha's light," and so on.

Buddha then gave instructions on how to recite the mantra for oneself and for others, for sick and dying people, and so forth, and how to perform many different healing rituals. Everyone rejoiced and developed deep, unchangeable faith. It is said that through hearing these instructions seven million non-human givers of harm gained a direct realization of ultimate truth and promised to help future followers who sincerely relied upon the practice of Medicine Buddha. Twelve chief givers-of-harm who were present later attained enlightenment, and are included within the fifty-one Deities of Medicine Buddha's mandala.

The practice of Medicine Buddha is a very powerful method for healing ourself and others, and for overcoming the inner sickness of attachment, hatred, and ignorance. If we rely upon Medicine Buddha with pure faith we shall definitely receive the blessings of these attainments.

This is a statue[5] of the Medicine Buddha, or Healing Buddha, sitting on a lotus base. He holds a bowl of healing

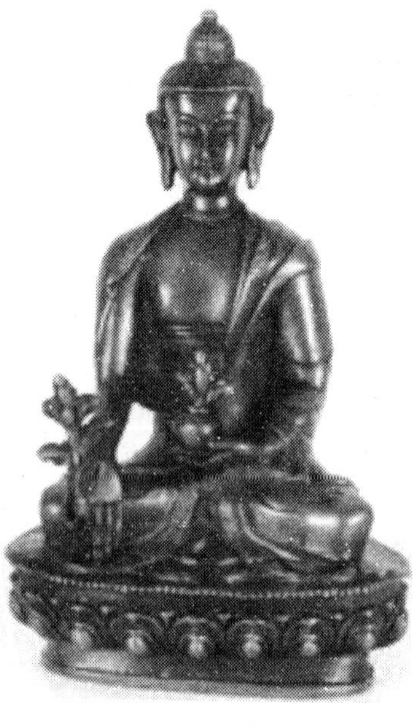

herbs in his left hand, and his right hand is in charity mudra and holds a branch of the myrobalantree, a medicinal plant found in India and other tropical countries.

The Medicine Buddha is said to dispense spiritual medicine to those who properly approach him. Some believe just touching the image brings benefit.

MEDICINE BUDDHA AND TIBETAN MEDICINE

Tibetan medicine is one of the oldest medical systems in the world. It is a science, art, and philosophy that promotes a holistic approach to health care. In Tibetan medical practice, mental well-being is just as important as physical well-being, and the two are believed to be intimately connected. For Tibetan Buddhists, many things in the physical world, including the state of one's body, is determined by a person's mindset. All disease and illness is the result of negative karma from past bad deeds. The role of the doctor is to guide the patient toward greater self-awareness. As one Tibetan philosopher has written, "True healing begins when we discover within ourselves that place where we are linked with the larger forces of the universe."

5. In Tibet, the Medicine Buddha is revered as the source of the healing arts, for it is through him that the teachings embodied in the Four Medical Tantras, the basis of Tibetan medicine, came into being. The practice of the Medicine Buddha is not only a very powerful method for healing and increasing healing powers both for oneself and others, but also for overcoming the inner sickness of attachment, hatred, and ignorance. Tibetans hope for health in order to live a long life and thus have more time to progress on the spiritual journey toward enlightenment.

6. If you are ill, a Tibetan doctor might advise you to change your diet or your behavior. The treatments a Tibetan doctor would prescribe include natural medicines made

from plants, minerals, and animals. From as early as the 7th century, dialogue between the leading physicians of India, China, Nepal, Byzantium, Persia, and Tibet resulted in a large body of accumulated knowledge, making the Tibetan medical tradition one of the richest in the world. Although you cannot usually see it, there is an inscription on the back of this painting in Tibetan that is over 100 lines long. It includes prayers and religious verses that honor the Medicine Buddha. The authors of this poem asked to be liberated from the suffering of the earthy world, reborn in the paradise of the Medicine Buddha, and purified of all sins. They also request to improve their own karma and the karma of all living things, and to be blessed with great compassion.

7. Although we do not know the names of the patrons who commissioned this painting, the inscription tells us how important the image of the Medicine Buddha was to them.

Mantra of the Medicine Buddha

"Therefore the World's Most Venerable entered into a Samadhi called the Removal of Suffering for All Beings. While He was in this contemplation a great radiance of light of light was sent forth from his Ushnisa, and he pronounced the great Dharani as follows:

NAMO BHAGAVATE BHAISAJAYA-GURU-VAIDURYA-PRABHA-RAJAYA TATHAGATAYA ARHATE SAMYAKSAMBUDDHAYA TADYATHA

OM BHAISAJYE BHAISAJYE BHAISAJYA SAMUDGATE SVAHA

When He, in his radiance, had spoken this mystical formula, the earth was shaken and emitted a great light. All beings were delivered from their diseases and miseries, they are now happy because their bodies and minds are at rest. "

The ancient teachings that tell us even seeing an image of the Medicine Buddha can confer inconceivable benefits also reveal that just hearing the name of the Medicine Buddha brings the same benefits.

Mantra of the Medicine Buddha

Sanskrit Pronunciation

d-ya-ta: Om Bhai-sha-jye Bhai-sha-jye Maha Bhai-sha-jye Ra-ja Sa-mud-ga-te Sva-ha

---

Tibetan Pronunciation

Tad-ya-ta: Om Be-kan-dze Be-kan-dze Ma-ha Be-kan-dze Ra-dza Sa-mung-ga-te So-ha!

Tibetan Scrip

ཏདྱཐཱ་ཨོཾ་བྷཻ་ཥ་ཛྱེ་བྷཻ་ཥ་ཛྱེ་མ་ཧཱ་བྷཻ་ཥ་ཛྱེ་
རཱ་ཛཱ་ས་མུདྒ་ཏེ་སྭཱ་ཧཱ།

The sutra of Bhaishajyaguru represents dramatic changes in patterns of life, as illustrated in the life of the T'ang emperor Chung-tsung who lost the throne in 684 to his mother, Empress Wu, and later regained it upon her death in 705. His life was saved by the spiritual force of Bhaishajyaguru, whose name he had constantly repeated. He requested the learned monk I-tsing, who had been on a pilgrimage to India, to translate the Bhaishajyaguru sutra from Sanskrit. The emperor assisted in the translation by acting as the scribe.

In the thousandfold of Myrobalan offering, prayers are offered to generate compassionate energy:

> *By the power of the medicines offered to the conclave, by the far-reaching strength of the oblations. spells, and medicines, may all sentient beings who are tormented by illness be liberated from pain and enjoy happiness. May all sentient beings that are deprived be refreshed by the medicine of commiseration, everywhere be relieved from the two obstacles, and speedily attain the stage of Bhaishajyaguru.*

"All of the Buddha's teachings can be subsumed under the two categories of shamatha and vipashyana— calm abiding and insight."[6]

Some medical traditions focus on material causes of illness and material treatments; other traditions insist on the importance of psychological and spiritual causes and remedies. Various types of conflicts between these two approaches are common. In contrast, Buddhist medicine maintains a deep and powerful integration of spiritual and practical understanding, and the Buddhist healing tradition respects both of these aspects of human nature and their potential for supporting health and healing. In his *Teaching of Medicine Buddha* Venerable Thrangu Rinpoche explains this in terms of the imagery of the hands in the image of the Medicine Buddha (an image like the one at the top of this page):

> *"His right hand is extended, palm outward, over his right knee in the gesture called supreme generosity. In it he holds the arura, or myrobalan, fruit. This plant represents all the best medicines. The position of his right hand and the arura which he holds represent the eradication of suffering, especially the suffering of sickness, using the means of relative truth. Sickness can be alleviated by adjusting the functioning of interdependent causes and conditions by the use of relative means within the realm of relative truth, such as medical treatment and so on. The giving of these methods is represented by the gesture of the Medicine Buddha's right hand.*

His left hand rests in his lap, palm upward, in the gesture of meditative stability or meditation, which represents the eradication of sickness and suffering— and, indeed, the very roots of samsara— through the realization of absolute truth. From the point of view of either relative truth or absolute truth, the fundamental cause of sickness and suffering is a lack of contentment and the addictive quality of samsara. Therefore, to indicate the need for contentment, in his left hand he holds a begging bowl."

Development of Tantricism and Vajrayana Sect

Buddhism was the crowning cultural achievement of Pala period India (eighth through twelfth centuries) and an internationally influential movement that swept throughout Asia, where it has survived in many countries to the present day.

Tantric Buddhism[7] arose when Mahayana Buddhism was enjoying a period of great philosophical productivity and intellectual influence. Flourishing monastic universities offered a life of study and contemplation but also provided a direct route to tremendous wealth, political influence, and social prestige.

A monk who enjoyed a successful academic career might be given land, servants, animals, buildings, precious metals, jewels, furnishings, art, and the privilege of riding on an elephant in official processions.

Admiring patrons offered these gifts as tokens of their esteem and as a way to gain religious merit. One monk was even offered the income from eighty villages by an enthusiastic royal patron. The monk declined.

Building upon the great achievements of Mahayana philosophy, yet impelled by a spirit of critique, Tantric Buddhism arose outside the powerful Buddhist monasteries as a protest movement initially championed by lay people rather than monks and nuns.

Desiring to return to classical Mahayana universalism, the Tantric reformers protested against ecclesiastical privilege and arid scholasticism and sought to forge a religious system that was more widely accessible and socially inclusive.

The Tantrics believed that self-mastery was to be tested amidst family life, the tumult of town and marketplace, the awesome spectacles of a cremation ground, and the dangers of isolated wilderness areas.

The Tantric revolution gained popular and royal support and eventually made its way into the curriculum of monastic universities like Nalanda, Vikramasla, Odantapur, and

Somapur. These institutes of higher learning were patronized and attended by both Hindus and Buddhists. They featured philology, literature, medicine, mathematics, astronomy, and art, as well as the "inner sciences" of meditation, psychology, and philosophy.

While the monasteries served as the institutional strongholds of the faith, wandering lay Tantrics carried Buddhism to the villages, countryside, tribal areas, and border regions, providing an interface at which new populations could bring their practices, symbols, and deities into the Buddhist fold.

Practices that had great antiquity in India's forests, mountains, and rural areas, among tribal peoples, villagers, and the lower classes, were embraced and redirected to Buddhist ends.

The renewed social inclusiveness and incorporation of an eclectic array of religious practices reshaped Buddhism into a tradition once again worthy of the loyalty of people from all sectors of Indian society.

Tantric Buddhism drew adherents from competing faiths, expanded geographically into every region of the Indian subcontinent, and continued outward on a triumphal sweep of the Himalayas, East Asia, and Southeast Asia.

Tantra in both Hinduism and Buddhism, esoteric tradition of ritual and yoga known for elaborate use of mantra, or symbolic speech, and mandala, or symbolic diagrams; the importance of female deities, or Shakti; cremation-ground practices such as meditation on corpses; and, more so in Hindu than in Buddhist tantra, the ritual use of wine, meat, and sexual intercourse.

Mantra in Hinduism and Buddhism, mystic words used in ritual and meditation. A mantra is believed to be the sound form of reality, having the power to bring into being the reality it represents. There are several types of mantras. Sanskrit verses used in the Vedic sacrifice are known as mantras. Bija-mantra or "seed-sounds, used mainly in Tantra, are syllables without semantic value having an occult affinity for particular deities or forces; use of such mantras usually requires initiation by a guru.

Mandala is a concentric diagram having spiritual and ritual significance in Hindu and Buddhist Tantrism. The mandala may have derived from the circular stupa and the ritual of walking around the stupa in a circle. The mandala is seen as a microcosm embodying the various divine powers at work in the universe, and it serves as a collection point for the gods and universal forces.

Tantric practices use both ritual and meditation to unify the devotee with the chosen deity. In Hindu Tantra, practice is graded into three types, corresponding to three classes of devotees: the animal, i.e., those in whom the guna, or quality, of *tamas* (darkness) predominates; the heroic, those in whom the guna of *rajas* (activity) predominates; and the divine, those in whom *sattva* (goodness) predominates (see Hindu philosophy).

The practice of the heroic devotee entails actual use of the five elements, called the *five m's: fish (matsya), meat (mamsa), wine (madya), aphrodisiac cereals (mudra), and sexual intercourse (maithuna).*

The animal devotee, not yet ready for the heroic practice, performs the rituals with material symbols; for the divine devotee the rituals are purely internal and symbolic.

The object of the rituals, attainable only by the divine devotee, is to awaken kundalini energy, which is identified with Shakti, and merge with the Godhead.

In Buddhist Tantra, or Vajrayana, in contrast to the Hindu, the female principle of "wisdom (prajna) is seen as static, whereas the male, or "means (upaya), is active.

In Buddhism, rituals that appear to break basic moral precepts have for the most part been dropped, but the complex meditation practices have been retained.

Meditation

"If one meditates on the Medicine Buddha[8], one will eventually attain enlightenment, but in the meantime one will experience an increase in healing powers both for oneself and others and a decrease in physical and mental illness and suffering. Whether or not we have a very strong motive to attain buddhahood, we all desire these sorts of relative objectives, so deity meditation provides tremendous incentive for the practice of dharma. And yet deity meditation is just another version of shamatha and vipashyana. When one meditates on the form, the attire and other attributes, the entourage and environment, and the internal mandala of a deity, and when one recites the deity's mantra, one is practicing shamatha; and when one realizes that all that one is meditating on is mere empty appearance, one is practicing vipashyana. But because meditation on the deity and on the union of the deity and one's own root lama instantly connects one with the empty clear light nature— which is the essence of the deity, the guru, and the lineage, as well as being one's own essential nature— the power of this form of shamatha to purify the mind of the practitioner of the mental obscurations blocking his or her insight is immeasurably greater than that of ordinary tranquillity meditation on mundane objects like the breath or a flower or a candle flame. And since the forms upon which one is meditating are mere mental fabrications, their emptiness is more immediately apparent than, say, the emptiness of something like the Jefferson Memorial or the Washington Monument.

This is all possible because of the special quality of the vajrayana, which takes enlightenment as the path, rather than seeing it merely as a goal. Through the three processes of abhisheka, which ripens the mental continuum; oral transmission, which supports one's practice; and the teachings, which liberate, one is connected directly to the enlightened state transmitted by the guru and the lineage. Thereafter, when one practices or merely brings to mind those teachings, one is instantly reconnected with that compassionate primordial awareness, and this constant reconnecting then becomes one's path, bringing with it the rapid purification of mental defilements and the rapid accumulation of merit and wisdom. The recognition of this connection is the uncovering of one's own wisdom. If it goes unrecognized, it still exists in the practitioner's mental continuum as a seed, which will gradually ripen according to conditions."

"We might think that fundamentally we are practicing the Medicine Buddha[9] in order to benefit our own bodies, whereas the motivation of bodhicitta is the wish to benefit all beings. But in fact there is no contradiction, because, in order to be effective in benefiting other beings, we need to accomplish an excellent samadhi or meditative absorption; and in order to accomplish that, together with the insight and realization that it brings, we need to have a stable practice. In order to have a stable and profound practice, we need to be physically and mentally healthy or comfortable, because by being comfortable in our body, and comfortable in our mind, we will be free of obstacles to diligence in practice and free of obstacles to the cultivation of meditative absorption. So therefore, we are practicing the Medicine Buddha in order to attain states of mental and physical health or balance, not merely for our own benefit, but for the benefit of others as well."

"The primary technique in the meditation consists of imagining ourself to be the Medicine Buddha, conceiving of yourself as the Medicine Buddha. By replacing the thought of yourself as yourself with the thought of yourself as the Medicine Buddha, you gradually counteract and remove the fixation on your personal self. And as that fixation is removed, the power of the seventh consciousness is reduced. And as it is reduced, the kleshas or mental afflictions are gradually weakened, which causes you to experience greater and greater well-being in both body and mind."

"In most religious traditions, the deities of that tradition, when they are related to or imagined, are imagined in front of one. Then, visualizing the deity or deities as being present in front of one, one prays to them, and by doing so hopefully one receives their blessing, which benefits one in some way. In the vajrayana tradition, however, we regard the blessing and the power and the qualities of the deities as being innate, as being within one's own mind."

"It is through regarding oneself as the deity that defects are gradually eradicated and qualities gradually revealed. The primary technique of visualization is to visualize ourselves as the deity, because the potential to transcend our problems is innate rather than external to us."

"We supplement the visualization of ourselves as the deity with visualizations such as imagining the actual wisdom deities themselves dissolving into ourselves again and again, by means of which we receive their blessing. Sometimes we visualize the deity in front of us, separate from ourselves, thinking that rays of light from the deity's heart engulf and pervade us, granting the blessing of the deity. And sometimes we visualize that rays of light, which embody the blessing of that deity in front of us, strike all beings, removing their obstacles, increasing their longevity, wisdom, and so on."

"The practice of the Medicine Buddha comes primarily from the uncommon tradition of the vajrayana, which means that the transmission of the practice is done using three processes called the empowerment, which ripens; the instruction, which frees; and the reading transmission, which supports. The function of empowerment, the formal ceremony or ritual of empowerment, is to introduce you to the practice and to the process of visualization and so forth, which will make up the practice. The function of the instruction, which frees, is to give you complete access to the practice by means of telling you literally how to do it—what you do with your body, what you say with your speech, and what you think with your mind. The function of the reading transmission, which supports, is to transmit the blessing of the lineage of the practice which serves to consecrate or bless your practice in the form of sound. Because the lineage has been transmitted as the sound of the words of its transmission, when the reading transmission is given to you, you simply listen to the sound and think that by doing so you receive the blessing of the lineage."

"With regard to the empowerment, you should understand that the Medicine Buddha practice is not solely a vajrayana practice. Like the practice of mahamudra, it is a combination of vajrayana [tantra] and sutra. For example, while we could say that mahamudra is primarily taught in the vajrayana, it is also found in certain sutras, such as the Samadhiraja Sutra, and so forth. In the same way, this practice of the Medicine Buddha is a combination of what the Buddha taught about the Medicine Buddha in the sutras of the Medicine Buddha and in various tantras. Because it is connected with vajrayana, it is most appropriate to receive the empowerment to enhance the practice; but because it is also connected with the sutras, it is acceptable to do the practice without the empowerment as well."

The Reading Transmission

Thrangu Rinpoche[10] then gave the reading transmission, or *lung*, for this Medicine Buddha practice, going through the text and explaining for each of the various sections what it's purpose is, what the practitioner should actually be doing at that point in the liturgy, and what the various symbols and symbolic actions mean.

The liturgy begins with a supplication of the Medicine Buddha and his retinue, including the holders of the lineage of this teaching, in order to invite the awareness of and to receive the blessings of the deity and the lineage.

The invocation of the principle Medicine Buddha begins with these lines:

> *You are endowed with an oceanic treasury of qualities and merit;*
> *By the blessing of your inconceivable compassion*
> *You calm the suffering and torment of sentient beings.*
> *I supplicate you, Light of Lapis Lazuli.*

The section of the liturgy on the details of the visualization sketches out the main features of the image of the Medicine Buddha, and Thrangu Rinpoche[11] explains the meaning of each of the important symbols. For example, the description and commentary on the arms and hands points out how they symbolize the Medicine Buddha's mastery of both physical and spiritual aspects of healing:

"The Medicine Buddha has two arms.

His right hand in the mudra of supreme generosity holds an arura. His left hand in meditation mudra holds a begging bowl

His right hand is extended, palm outward, over his right knee in the gesture called supreme generosity. In it he holds the arura, or myrobalan, fruit. This plant represents all the best medicines. The position of his right hand and the arura which he holds represent the eradication of suffering, especially the suffering of sickness, using the means of relative truth. Sickness can be alleviated by adjusting the functioning of interdependent causes and conditions by the use of relative means within the realm of relative truth, such as medical treatment and so on. The giving of these methods is represented by the gesture of the Medicine Buddha's right hand.

His left hand rests in his lap, palm upward, in the gesture of meditative stability or meditation, which represents the eradication of sickness and suffering— and, indeed, the very roots of samsara— through the realization of absolute truth. From the point of view of either relative truth or absolute truth, the fundamental cause of sickness and suffering is a lack of contentment and the addictive quality of samsara. Therefore, to indicate the need for contentment, in his left hand he holds a begging bowl."

Rinpoche points out that the visualization is much more than merely wishful fantasy:

> *"More important than how many deities you visualize is to understand what you are doing. And most important is to understand that by visualizing yourself as the Medicine Buddha you are not pretending to be something that you are not, and that by visualizing the Medicine Buddha and his retinue in front of you, you are not pretending that they are in a place where they are not. By definition, buddhas are omniscient. Whenever someone thinks of them, brings them to mind, or supplicates them, they are aware of it and respond with their compassion and blessing. In the final analysis, the situation is identical to their actually being present anywhere they are thought of. Therefore, it is always appropriate to regard a buddha that is present in one's mind as actually being present in front of one. When you think that the Medicine Buddha, together with his retinue, is present in front of you, it is really true that they are.*

Visualizing yourself as the Medicine Buddha is also appropriate, because your fundamental nature— what you truly are— is buddha nature. Buddha nature is essentially the potential to attain awakening. At some point in the future you will attain the same awakening or buddhahood as the Medicine Buddha himself. By visualizing yourself as the Medicine Buddha, you are assuming the appearance of what fundamentally you are even now and what manifestly you will be upon your awakening. It is to acknowledge this truth that you assume the aspect of the body, speech, and mind of the Medicine Buddha, which is, therefore, entirely appropriate."

"If you can visualize clearly, it is best to do all of this very slowly and gradually. While you continue to say the mantra, you think that rays of light emerge from the self-visualization, go to the front visualization, and then from the front visualization outwards to the pure realms, proceeding gradually and slowly. Especially when the blessings of body, speech, and mind rain down upon and dissolve into you, you can do the visualizations in sequence: first, visualizing the blessings of body raining down, without being in any kind of a hurry and so quite distinctly; and then visualizing the blessings of speech and then the blessings of mind. If you find that the visualization is extremely unclear, if you wish, you can do it all at once. But if you do it gradually and slowly, you will find that you will get a much stronger sense of the blessings actually entering into you. By taking your time with the visualization, you will develop real confidence, a real feeling of the blessings entering into you."

Rinpoche[12] describes a special type of visualization when the main point is the actual alleviation of sickness:

> *"You can visualize yourself as the Medicine Buddha, if you wish, but the main focus is to actually visualize a small form of the Medicine Buddha, no larger than four finger-widths in height, in the actual part of your body that is afflicted. So if it is an illness or pain in the head, visualize a small Medicine Buddha in he head; .... Visualize the Medicine Buddha in that place, and think that from this small but vivid form of*

the Medicine Buddha rays of light are emitted. These rays of light are not simply light, which is dry, but liquid light having a quality of ambrosia. This luminous ambrosia or liquid light actually cleanses and removes the sickness and pain— whatever it is. You can do this not only for yourself, by visualizing the Medicine Buddha in the appropriate part of your own body, but you can do it for others as well by visualizing the Medicine Buddha in the appropriate part of their body or bodies. The radiation of rays of light of ambrosia and so on is the same.

This can be applied not only to physical sickness but to mental problems as well. If you want to get rid of a particular type of anxiety or stress or depression or fear or any other kind of unpleasant mental experience, you can visualize the Medicine Buddha seated above the top of your head and think in the same way as before that luminous ambrosia or liquid light emerges from his body, filling your body and cleansing you of any problem, whatever it is.

You might think that all of this sounds a bit childish, but in fact it actually works, and you will find that out if you try it."

Medicine Buddha and Tibetan Medicine

The full name of the Medicine Buddha is Bhaishajyaguru Vaiduryaprabha, the Healing Master of Lapis Lazuli Radiance. Like Shakyamuni he wears the robes of a monk and is seated in the full cross-legged posture. His left hand is in the meditation mudra, resting in his lap and holding a begging bowl filled with medicinal nectar and fruit. His right hand rests upon his knee with palm facing outward in the mudra granting blessings and holds the stem of a myrobalan plant (*Terminalia chebula*), renowned as the king among medicines because of its effectiveness in treating both mental and physical diseases.

In traditional Tibetan tangkas, the Lapis Healing Master is often shown in the company of seven other Medicine Buddhas, one of whom is Shakyamuni himself. And in depictions of his eastern buddha realm known as Pure Lapis Lazuli, the Healing Master is generally flanked by the two leading bodhisattvas of that pure land, Suryaprabha and Chandraprabha, respectively All-pervading Solar and Lunar Radiance.

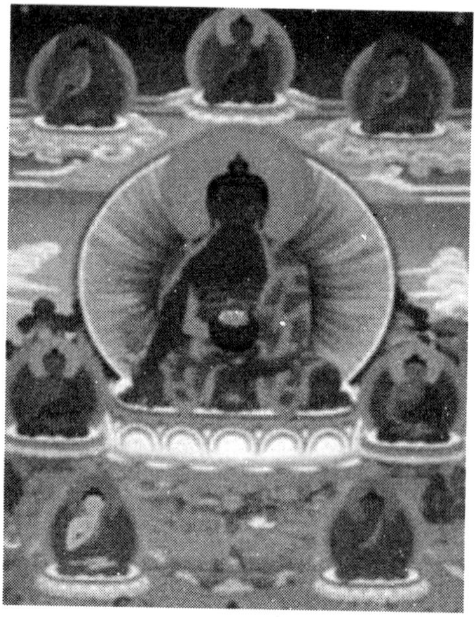

The most distinctive feature of this Medicine Buddha is his color, the deep blue of lapis lazuli. This precious stone has been greatly prized by Asian and European cultures for more than six thousand years and, until relatively recently, its ornamental value was on a par with, or even exceeded, that of the diamond. An aura of mystery surrounds this gemstone, perhaps because of its principal mines are located in the remote Badakshan region of northeast Afghanistan, an all-but-inaccessible area located behind the Hindu Kush. One commentator has written, "the finest specimens of lapis, intensely blue with speckled waves and swirls of shining gold-colored pyrite, resemble the night aglow with myriads of stars." Traditionally this beautiful stone was used to symbolize that which is pure or rare. It is said to have a curative or strengthening effect on those who wear it, and its natural smoothness allows it to be polished to a high degree of reflectivity. For all these reasons - plus the fact that deep blue light has a demonstrable healing effect on those who use it in visualization practices - lapis is the color of the principal Medicine Buddha.

The Lapis Healing Master is one of the most honored figures in the Buddhist pantheon. The sutras in which he appears compare his eastern pure land with the western paradise of Amitabha, and rebirth there is said to be as conducive to enlightenment as is rebirth in Sukhavati. Recitation of his mantra, or even the mere repetition of his holy name, is said to be sufficient to grant release from the lower realms, protection from worldly dangers and freedom from untimely death. In one of the main sutras concerning the Medicine Buddha, Shakyamuni tells his close disciple and attendant Ananda:

> *If these sentient beings [those plunged into the depths of samsara's sufferings hear the name of the Lord Master of Healing, the Lapis Lazuli Radiance Tathagatha, and with utmost sincerity accept it and hold onto it, and no doubts arise, then they will not fall into a woesome path.*

In Tibet the Medicine Buddha is revered as the source of the healing arts for it is through him that the teachings embodied in the Four Medical Tantras, the basis of Tibetan medicine, came into being. As explained in the first of these Four Tantras, the Lapis Lazuli Healing Master was once seated in meditation surrounded by an assembly of four circles of disciples including divine physicians, great sages, non-Buddhist gods and bodhisattvas, all of whom wished to learn the art of healing. Rendered speechless by the radiant glory of his countenance, they were unable to request the desired teachings. To accommodate their unspoken wishes, the Medicine Buddha manifested two emanations, one to request the teachings and the other to deliver them. In this way, then, the Buddhist explanation of the various mental and physical ailments, their causes, diagnoses and treatment and the maintenance of health is said to have originated.

According to the *Four Tantras*, the fundamental cause of every disease is to be found in the three poisonous delusions - ignorant bewilderment, attachment and hatred - occupying the hub of the wheel of samsaric existence. These three root delusions lead to imbalances in three so-called humors (phlegm, wind and bile), the various bodily constituents (blood, flesh, bone, etc.) and waste products, or impurities (excrement, urine and perspiration), all of which are analyzed in twenty-five divisions. The *Root Tantra* says:

> *Thus if all these twenty-five are in balance and the three factors of the (1) tastes and (2) inherent qualities of one¹s food and (3) one¹s behavior are wholesome, one¹s health and life will flourish. If they are not, one¹s health and life will be harmed.*

And further on:

> *Attachment, hatred and bewilderment are the three causes producing imbalances of wind, bile and phlegm. Along with these, the four contributing circumstances of time, spirits, food and behavior cause the humors to increase and decrease. The imbalance then spreads over the skin, increases in the flesh, moves along the vessels, meets the bones and descends upon the solid and hollow organs.*

Treatment of disease and the maintenance of health are therefore primarily a matter of bringing the various elements of the body back into balance and this is accomplished through four progressive types of treatment. The first two involve changes in the type of food we eat and behavior we engage in. Only when these prove ineffective is the physician advised to prescribe medicine and only when this also fails is he or she to resort to external forms of treatment such as cauterization and the like. However, none of these types of treatment will have a lasting effect unless they are accompanied by spiritual transformation. If ignorance and its associated delusions remain festering inside, sooner or later they will give rise to disease and the recurring miseries of cyclic existence. Thus Buddhas such as Shakyamuni and the Lapis Healing Master are referred to as great physicians not because of their medical abilities - as great as these are - but because they have the compassion, wisdom and skillful means to diagnose and treat the root delusions underlying all mental and physical malaise.

The following prayer of request is addressed to the Lapis Healing Master:

I beseech you, Blessed Medicine Guru,
Whose sky-colored, holy body of lapis lazuli
Signifies omniscient wisdom and compassion
As vast as limitless space,
Please grant me your blessings.

I beseech you, Blessed Medicine Guru,
Holding in your right hand the king of medicines
Symbolizing your vow to help all the pitiful sentient beings
Plagued by the four hundred and twenty-four diseases,
Please grant me your blessings.

I beseech you, Blessed Medicine Guru,
Holding in your left hand a bowl of nectar
Symbolizing your vow to give the glorious undying nectar of the dharma
Which eliminates the degenerations of sickness, old age and death,
Please grant me your blessings.

In traditional Tibetan culture, patients and physicians alike, really — shared respect for physical and mental aspects of healing — of any sort of meaningful human life. The doctor recommended adjustments in lifestyle and diet that would help restore the patient's balance, physiologically and psychologically, and worked to prepare and prescribe herbal medicines appropriate to the patient's condition. The patient made the effort to take the medicines according to the doctor's instructions, and make the recommended dietary and behavioral changes. All of these efforts took place in the context of a devotion to spiritual practices and training designed to foster basic sanity and compassion — a devotion shared by the patient and the physician, their families, and the entire community.

May we learn from their example.

Of all the traditional systems of herbal medicine that are still surviving, Tibetan medicine may offer the most promise. Many traditional systems are more environmentally sustainable, more affordable and more free of harmful side effects than our Western system of medication with purified chemicals, but the Tibetan system may be the most effective of all of these.

Tibetan medicine is reputed to be ameliorate psychological problems and diseases of all sorts, including hepatitis, certain kinds of mental illness, ulcers, paralysis, gall and kidney stones (treated without surgery), arthritis, and conditions like certain cancers that Western physicians find very difficult to treat successfully. Tibetan medicine is also reported to resolve many conditions that Western doctors don't even recognize, dismissing patients' complaints with comments like "There's nothing wrong with you. Just take ibuprofen for the pain and don't worry about it."

Are the glowing reports about Tibetan medicine true? Can Tibetan physicians really cure cancer? Are they really developing a cure for AIDS? At this point, it's hard to say: Aschoff's *Annotated Bibliography of Tibetan Medicine* includes hundreds of research reports published in Western languages before 1995, but few of them meet modern standards of evaluation research.

If the research now going on at a number of institutions in various countries gives positive assessments of how effective Tibetan medicine can be with various health problems, more questions will remain to be answered: How can I find a Tibetan doctor? Is this doctor competent? Do I really have to stop drinking coffee? Tibetan doctors, too, will have questions: Why won't these people do what we ask them to do to help them recover? How can we get enough herbs to make medicines for all these patients? How can we keep from driving these wild herbs to extinction?

The health of the billions of people in the world can't be sustained by medicines requiring rare Himalayan plants as ingredients, as the Dalai Lama has pointed out. Already several species of these herbs are in danger of extinction because of the demand for them in medical formulas.

For this healing wisdom to be available to human beings all over the world, Tibetan medicine must be sustained where it is now practiced. That will require preserving the plants and animals that provide the ingredients of the current medicines, and the ecologies that support those organisms, while a new generation of healers and researchers learn which Himalayan herbs can be grown as crops, evaluate the healing properties of plants indigenous to other areas, and learn to formulate remedies for the diseases we know about and new diseases that are emerging.

Perhaps the best beginning would be for interested people to learn about Tibetan medicine and perhaps to explore its use in their own lives, and thus develop confidence in its efficacy and gentleness. Then providing support will follow naturally, support for the training and the work of a new generation of practitioners, and for preserving the medicinal plants and their environments.

Notes

1. P. V. Sharma (Ed). 1992. Medicine in Buddhist and Jaina traditions. In *History of Medicine in India.* New Delhi: INSA. Pp. 117-135.
2. Pankaj Goyal, Lok Vigyan Kendra,Almora 263601 India.
3. P. V. Sharma is a well known historian of Indian medicinal sciences.
4. Prof. Lokesh Chandra.
5. *For A Change* , Alan Channer, Publication, Date: Monday, April 1 1996.
6. Lama Tashi Namgyal (ed.), Thirangpu Rinpoche 'Medicine Buddha Sadhana', & 'Medicine Buddha Sutra' *Shenpen Osel,* Vol. 4, No. 1and 2.
7. *Passionment Enlightment,* Miranda Shaw.
8. Lama Tashi Namgyal (ed.), 'Medicine Buddha Sadhana', *Shenpen Osel,* Vol. 4, No. 1.
9. Thirangpu Rinpoche 'Medicine Buddha Sutra' *Shenpen Osel,* Vol. 4, No. 2.
10. Thirangpu Rinpoche 'Medicine Buddha Sutra' *Shenpen Osel,* Vol. 4, No. 2.
11. Thirangpu Rinpoche 'Medicine Buddha Sutra' *Shenpen Osel,* Vol. 4, No. 2.
12. Thirangpu Rinpoche 'Medicine Buddha Sutra' *Shenpen Osel,* Vol. 4, No. 2.

CHAPTER – 3

BUDDHIST MEDICAL PRACTICE IN MONASTERIES

Buddha, as a young Prince Siddhartha, renounced the worldly goods after realising the existence of sufferings (Dukkha) in human life. A dying man and a corpse of a dead man were some of the few things, which had great impact on Young Buddha's psyche. After renunciation and attainment of the ultimate enlightenment (*Nibbana*), Buddha himself used to nurse the Bhikkus and sick people around him. Some other legends associated with Buddha like convincing Angulimala, the serial killer, to shun his bad practices and making him his disciple; taming of a wild elephant, etc. have prompted many scholars to contend that Buddha was basically a great Psychiatrist, who cured people's mental illness. Moreover, the fact like Buddha himself died due to blood dysentery after consuming pork (shukra kheer) make us feel that Buddha was not very concerned about the physical ailment of the mankind. This contradiction gets manifested in the difference of attitude of the Hinayana and Mahayana doctrines towards medical practice. In older Hinayana writings, medicine had been considered a worldly science that monks were forbidden to learn. Members of the monastic community were expressly prohibited from earning their livelihood by the medical treatment of laymen. Buddha, however, upon finding a sick monk, who had been ignored and neglected by fellow brothers striving for their own personal salvation, had admonished the latter to assist one another in such circumstances. Thus it became the duty of monks to preach brothers who had fallen ill to recite to them the precepts of ancient sages, and if necessary, to summon Buddha himself to the sick bed for assistance. Only a monk, it was claimed, is competent to provide the necessary spiritual assistance – recitations from the doctrine, the encouragement of indifference and patience - the specific remedies an ill monk requires above else. Attendance by anyone other than the monks can only be a temporary measures, for religious support not only possesses moral value but also leads to physical recovery from illness.

According to Vinaya Sutta, Buddha himself did some physical exercises, maintained a very fine physique and he used to walk 60-70 kilomatres regularly for the propagation of his teachings. Vinaya Sutta[1] reveals Buddha's love and compassion towards the patients and his teaching influenced the ancient medical practice. However, Buddha prohibited the use of knife and surgery. He also banned animal sacrifice. Consequently, his followers built many health centres for mankind and animals.

Medicine proved as an effectual tool in the expansion of Buddhism. There are certain examples where people adopted Buddhism only for being treated by renowned physicians like Jivaka. In Buddhist *Viharas* medicine was one of the most important programmes in their daily activities. Indian medicine travelled far and wide and spread to other countries along with Buddhism. A feeling of deep sympathy and sorrow as well as great service towards the sick was a unique feature of Buddhism and because of this reason the sick had a feeling of great respect for Lord Buddha.

Viaharas

Medicine was a popular subject of teaching in the curricula of the *Viharas* and *mahaviharas* as Buddhists treat it as an important tool for missionary service to humanity and animals. Medicine was an important and compulsory subject in all the universities. The University of Taksasila was famous for this subject where Atreya was a renowned teacher. Jivaka was a famous student of this university, who got proficiency in medicine as well as surgery. The Nalanda University had also medicine as one of the compulsory subjects of teaching. Medicine was also taught in Vikramasila University. *Tantras* as well as *Rasasastra* also flourished there in theory and practice.

ROYAL PATRONAGE

During the periods of Kings Asoka, Kaniska and Sri Harsa, the Buddhist tradition flourished side by side with the Vedic traditions. These kings established many *viharas* in various parts of the country as well as far off places. As a result of this Buddhism spread to other Asian countries along with which Indian medicine also reached out there. Some valuable accounts given by Chinese travellers like Fahian, Huan Chwang and Itsing give a detailed view of Buddhist tradition in those periods.

The Great Section on Virtue in the Sâmaññaphala Sutta[2] lists the types of wrong livelihood from which a bhikkhu should abstain. Among them is the practice of medicine, or in the words of the sutta:

> *"administering emetics, purges, purges from above, purges from below, head-purges; ear-oil, eye-drops, treatments through the nose, ointments, and counter-ointments; practicing eye-surgery (or: extractive surgery),*

general surgery, pediatrics; administering root-medicines and binding medicinal herbs — he abstains from wrong livelihood, from lowly arts such as these. This, too, is part of his virtue."

A bhikkhu should not act as a doctor for lay people unless they are:

- his parents, people who care for his parents, his other blood relatives;
- his preceptor and teacher's parents or other blood relatives;
- applicants for ordination;
- his own steward;
- travelers who arrive ill at his monastery;
- people who fall ill while in the monastery.

In none of these cases, however, should he expect material reward for his services.

Bhikkhus are, however, expected to know enough medicine to care for their own and for one another's illnesses. This point is beautifully illustrated by one of the most inspiring passages in the Canon:

Now at that time a certain bhikkhu was sick with dysentery. He lay fouled in his own urine and excrement. Then the Blessed One, on an inspection tour of the lodgings with Ven. Ânanda as his attendant, went to that bhikkhu's dwelling and, on arrival, saw the bhikkhu lying fouled in his own urine and excrement. On seeing him, he went to the bhikkhu and said, "What is your illness, bhikkhu?"

"I have dysentery, O Blessed One."

"But do you have an attendant?"

"No, O Blessed One."

"Then why don't the bhikkhus tend to you?"

"I don't do anything for the bhikkhus, venerable sir, which is why they don't tend to me."

Then the Blessed One addressed Ven. Ānanda: "Go fetch some water, Ānanda. We will wash this bhikkhu."

"As you say, venerable sir," Ven. Ānanda responded, and he fetched some water. The Blessed One sprinkled water on the bhikkhu, and Ven. Ânanda washed him off. Then — with the Blessed One taking the bhikkhu by the head, and Ven. Ānanda taking him by the feet — they lifted him up and placed him on a bed.

Then the Blessed One, with regard to this cause, to this incident, had the bhikkhus assembled and asked them: "Is there a sick bhikkhu in that dwelling over there?"

"Yes, O Blessed One, there is."

"And what is his illness?"

"He has dysentery, O Blessed One."

"But does he have an attendant?"

"No, O Blessed One."

"Then why don't the bhikkhus tend to him?"

"He doesn't do anything for the bhikkhus, venerable sir, which is why they don't tend to him."

"Bhikkhus, you have no mother, you have no father, who might tend to you. If you don't tend to one another, who then will tend to you? Whoever would tend to me, should tend to the sick."

The Buddha then sets out precise duties both for the sick and for those who nurse them:

"If one's preceptor is present, the preceptor should tend to one as long as life lasts (or) should stay until one's recovery. If one's teacher is present, the teacher should tend to one as long as life lasts (or) should stay until one's recovery. If one's pupil is present, the pupil should tend to one as long as life lasts (or) should stay until one's recovery. If one's student is present, the student should tend to one as long as life lasts (or) should stay until one's recovery. If a fellow pupil of one's preceptor is present, the fellow pupil of one's preceptor should tend to one as long as life lasts (or) should stay until one's recovery. If a fellow student of one's teacher is present, the fellow student of one's teacher should tend to one as long as life lasts (or) should stay until one's recovery. If no preceptor, teacher, pupil, student, fellow pupil of one's preceptor, or fellow student of one's teacher is present, the Community should tend to one. If he/it (i.e., the bhikkhu or the Community responsible for the care, as the case may be) does not: an offense of wrong doing.

"A sick person endowed with five qualities is hard to tend to: He does what is not amenable to his cure; he does not know the proper amount in things amenable to his cure; he does not take his medicine; he does not tell his symptoms, as they actually are present, to the nurse desiring his welfare, saying that they are getting worse when they are getting worse, improving when they are improving, or remaining the same when they are remaining the same; and he is not the type who can endure bodily feelings that are painful, fierce, sharp, wracking, repellent, disagreeable, life-threatening. A sick person endowed with these five qualities is hard to tend to.

"A sick person endowed with five qualities is easy to tend to: He does what is amenable to his cure; he knows the proper amount in things amenable to his cure; he takes his medicine; he tells his symptoms, as they actually are present, to the nurse desiring his welfare, saying that they are getting worse when they are getting worse, improving when they are improving, or remaining the same when they are remaining the same; and he is the type who can endure bodily feelings that are painful, fierce, sharp, wracking, repellent, disagreeable, life-threatening. A sick person endowed with these five qualities is easy to tend to.

"A nurse endowed with five qualities is not fit to tend to the sick: He is not competent at mixing medicine; he does not know what is amenable or unamenable to the patient's cure, bringing to the patient things that are unamenable and taking away things that are amenable; he is motivated by material gain, not by thoughts of good will; he gets disgusted at cleaning up excrement, urine, saliva (§), or vomit; and he is not competent at instructing, urging, rousing, and encouraging the sick person at the proper occasions with a talk on Dhamma. A nurse endowed with these five qualities is not fit to tend to the sick.

"A nurse endowed with five qualities is fit to tend to the sick: He is competent at mixing medicine; he knows what is amenable or unamenable to the patient's cure, taking away things that are unamenable and bringing things that are amenable; he is motivated by thoughts of good will, not by material gain; he does not get disgusted at cleaning up excrement, urine, saliva, or vomit; and he is competent at instructing, urging, rousing, and encouraging the sick person at the proper occasions with a talk on Dhamma. A nurse endowed with these five qualities is fit to tend to the sick."[3]

Issues related to two of the last five qualities are discussed in detail in the Khandhakas: competence in mixing medicine and the question of material gain, i.e., the rewards given to nurses who have faithfully tended to the sick. Here we will discuss issues related to medicine, which fall under four main topics: the basic "support" medicine; general classes of edibles that count as tonics and medicines; medical treatments recommended for specific diseases; and medical procedures.

Support medicine. A bhikkhu's basic medicinal support is *pûti-mutta-bhesajja,* which translates literally as "rancid urine medicine"[4] Strangely, none of the texts define the term. The commentaries to the Khuddakapâtha, Udâna, and Sutta Nipâta give an example of this sort of medicine — rancid urine with yellow myrobalan — but without a formal definition to indicate the full range of the term. The Sub-commentary to the Vinaya defines rancid urine as any sort of urine at all, citing as a parallel the Pali expression *pûti-kâya,* decomposing body, which refers to any human body, living or dead, "even one with golden skin." However, it does not say whether rancid urine medicine is the rancid urine itself or, as suggested by the example from the commentaries, rancid urine in which medicinal fruits are pickled.

Because the texts are vague about this term, various oral traditions have developed around it. In Sri Lanka, rancid urine medicine is interpreted as rancid cow's urine, in which different types of myrobalan are sometimes pickled. In Thailand, some Communities interpret it as one's own first urine in the morning, following the ancient Indian tradition of using this urine as a tonic. (Modern scientists have discovered that this urine contains a high level of melatonin.) Given the silence of the texts, the best policy here is to follow the traditions of one's own Community.

The five tonics are discussed in detail, but the issue of flour mixed with sugar bears repeating. The Canon states that if sugar is mixed with flour or ashes as a binding agent and is still called sugar, then it counts as one of the five tonics. Some have argued that this allowance extends to candies that have small amounts of flour or other food starch mixed in, but if the candies are not called sugar they do not meet the terms of the allowance and so should be classed as food.

Life-long medicines. Six types of edibles are classed as life-long medicines: root medicine, astringent decoction medicine, leaf medicine, fruit medicine, resin medicine, and salt medicine. The Canon lists specific examples for each type. Although some of the examples are hard to identify precisely, each of the classes when taken as a whole is clear enough to form a guideline for applying the Great Standards to similar medicines today. Thus we have made no effort to identify the more obscure examples. As the Canon itself makes clear, *any* medicine that would come under these six classes — as long as it does not serve as a staple or non-staple food — is allowed here.

Root medicine. The Canon defines life-long root medicine as follows: turmeric, ginger, sweet flag, white orris root, ativisa, black hellebore, khus-khus, nut-grass, or whatever other roots are medicines and do not serve as staple or non-staple food. With this, and all the remaining classes of life-long medicine, one may keep the medicine for life and consume it when there is a medicinal reason for doing so. If there is no such reason, there is a dukka for consuming it. As mentioned in the preceding chapter, there is a specific prohibition against eating garlic when not ill. In connection with the allowance for root medicine, there is also an allowance for a grindstone and a grinding wheel to reduce the medicine to a powder.

Astringent-decoction medicine. Here the Canon lists astringent decoctions from the nimb-tree (*Azadirachta indica*), from the kumaja (*Wrightia dysenterica*), from the pakkava, from the nattamâla (*Pongamia glabra*), or any other astringent decoctions that are medicines and do not serve as staple or non-staple food.

Leaf medicine. The Canon's list includes nimb leaves, kumaja leaves, cucumber leaves (*Trichosanthes dioeca*), basil leaves, cotton-tree leaves, or any other leaves that are medicines and do not serve as staple or non-staple food.

Fruit medicine. Here the Canon lists vilaEga (*Embelia ribes*), long pepper (*Erycibe paniculata*), black pepper, yellow myrobalan (*Terminalia chebula* or *citrina*), beleric myrobalan (*Terminalia balerica*), embric myrobalan (*Phyllantus embelica*) (these last three form the triphala mixture still used in modern Ayurveda), gomha-fruit, or any other fruits that are medicines and do not serve as staple or non-staple food.

Resin medicine. The Canon lists assafoetida, assafoetida-resin, assafoetida-gum, gum, gum-patti, gum-panni, or any other resins that are medicines and do not serve as staple or non-staple food.

Salt medicine. The Canon allows the following salts: sea salt, black salt, rock salt, culinary salt, red salt (which the Commentary defines as salt mixed with other medicinal ingredients), or any other salts that are medicines and do not serve as staple or non-staple food. The Parivâra[5] mentions both natural and man-made salts as allowable. Modern medicines that are organic or inorganic salts would fit under this category.

Specific treatments. In addition to the general classes of medicines, we have list[6] of allowable treatments for specific diseases. The stress here is on the word *allowable:* A bhikkhu is not required to use these treatments but he might want to familiarize himself with them so that he can apply the Great Standards to modern medicine in an informed way. Historically, this list, together with similar lists in the Vinayas of the other early schools, has played an important part in the spread of medical knowledge from India to the lands to which Buddhism spread in the rest of Asia. At present, it gives a fascinating picture of the state of medical art in the Buddha's time.

For itch, small boils, running sores, an affliction of thick scabs, or bad body odor: One may use powders. To refine the powder, one may use powder sifters, including cloth sifters. The commentary states that for bad body odor all fragrant powders are allowable. The Canon allows the use of (powdered) dung, clay, and dye-dregs for one who is not ill. According to the Commentary, ordinary (unscented) chunam comes under "dye-dregs."

For possession by non-human beings: Raw flesh and raw blood are allowed (!). The texts do not say whether this a medicine per se, or — if the non-human being is blood-thirsty — the bhikkhu should simply not be held responsible for eating such things.

For eye diseases: Ointments such as black collyrium, rasa-ointment (made with vitriol?), sota-ointment (made with antimony?), yellow orpiment (§), and lamp-black are allowed. Sandalwood, tagara (*Tabernaemontana coronaria*), benzoin gum, tâlîsa (*Flacourtia cataphracta*), and nut-grass — all of which are fragrant — may be mixed in with the ointments. The ointments may be kept in boxes made of any of the standard ten materials (except for human bone, says the Commentary) but not in boxes made of fancy materials. The boxes may have lids, which may be tied to the boxes with thread or string. If an ointment box gets split, it may be bound together with thread or string. Ointment sticks may be used to apply the ointments, but again they must be made of one of the ten standard allowable materials. A bhikkhu may keep the ointment sticks in a case, and the ointment box in a bag. The bag may have a string for tying the mouth of the bag as a carrying strap.

For pains in the head: Apply oil to the head; give treatments (such as snuff medicine) up the nose; or have the patient inhale smoke. Nose-tubes (or nose-spoons), double nose-tubes (double nose-spoons), and smoke inhaling tubes are allowed but must be made from any of the standard allowable materials. One may keep lids, bags, and double bags for the smoke-inhaling tubes, and the bags may be tied at the mouth with a string for use as a carrying strap.

For wind afflictions: According to ancient Indian medicine, sharp pains in the body result from the provocation of the wind property. Dizziness is also counted as a wind affliction. The basic treatment is for the patient to drink a decoction of oil. The oil may be kept in a flask made of metal, wood, or fruit (e.g., coconut shell). Alcohol may be mixed in with the decoction, but not so much that the color, smell, or taste of the liquor could be detected. To drink oil mixed with excessive alcohol is violation. If too much alcohol has been mixed in with the oil, it may be determined for use as rubbing oil.

For wind afflictions in the limbs: Sweating treatments, sweating treatments with herbs, and a "great sweating" treatment are allowed. The Commentary gives directions for this last treatment: Use a hole dug lengthwise the size of a human being and fill it with burning embers, charcoal, or coals; cover it with sand or dirt, and then with various leaves that are good for wind diseases. Have the ill bhikkhu cover his body with oil and lie down on top of the leaves, turning over as necessary. Other treatments for wind afflictions in the limbs include hemp water (according to the Commentary, this means water boiled with hemp leaves;

pour it over the body, cover the body with the leaves, and then get into a sweating-treatment tent) and a water tub, which the Commentary says is a tub big enough for a bhikkhu to get into. Hot tubs would come under here.

For wind affliction in the joints: Blood-letting and moxibustion are allowed.

For split feet: Rubbing-oil and foot salves are allowed. The Commentary states that the foot salve may include whatever liquor will help split feet to heal.

For boils: Lancing (surgery) is allowed unless the boil is on the genitals or near the anus (see below). Allowable post-operative treatments include astringent water, pounded sesame paste, a compress, and a bandage. The scar may be sprinkled with mustard-seed powder to prevent itching. It may also be fumigated, and the scar-tissue cut off with a piece of salt-crystal. The scar may also be treated with oil. An old piece of cloth is allowed for soaking up the oil, and every kind of treatment for sores or wounds is allowed.

For snakebite: A medicine may be made of the "four great filthy things": excrement, urine, ashes, and clay (!). If there is someone present to make these things allowable, one should have him/her make them allowable. If not, one may take them for oneself and consume them. The Commentary notes that this allowance covers not only snakebite, but also any other poisonous animal bite. The Sub-commentary adds that *for oneself* here also includes cases where Bhikkhu X fetches these items himself for Bhikkhu Y, who has been bitten. Y, in such cases, is allowed to consume them. None of the texts mention this point, but an oral tradition in Thailand asserts that the excrement to be used in this medicine should first be burnt in a fire.

For drinking poison: Water mixed with excrement (!!) may be drunk. If one receives the excrement while excreting it, it does not need to be formally received again. The

Commentary interprets this last statement by saying that if, while excreting, one catches the excrement before it falls to the ground, one need not have it formally offered. If it falls to the ground, one does. This, however, seems overly scrupulous. The parallel in the case of offering food is that if the food falls to the ground while being offered, it still counts as offered. The same principle should hold here.

For drinking a sorcery concoction: According to the Commentary, a sorcery concoction is voodoo medicine made by a woman to put a man under her power. The antidote given in the Canon is to drink mud turned up by a plow. The Commentary recommends that it be mixed with water.

For constipation: The Canon recommends drinking alkaline liquid, and the Commentary gives directions for how to make it: Take cooked rice, dry it in the sun, burn it, and drink the liquid coming from the ashes.

For jaundice: Urine and yellow myrobalan are allowed, which the Commentary defines as yellow myrobalan pickled in cow urine. This raises the question: If this were the meaning of *rancid urine medicine* in the four supports, why would there be this special allowance?

For skin disease: A scented rubbing is allowed.

For a body full of bad humors: One may drink a purgative. After the purgative has worked, one may take clarified conjey (which, according to the Commentary, is the clear liquid from rice porridge, strained to remove all rice grains), clear green gram broth, slightly thick green gram broth (which the Commentary interprets as green gram broth that is not oily or greasy), or meat broth (which again, the Commentary says, is just the broth without any meat). Some Communities extend these last allowances for any occasion, but the Canon gives them in the context of an antidote to the effects of a strong purgative, so there are those who will extend the allowance only to cases where a bhikkhu is weakened by diarrhea or other similarly severe conditions.

As a general tonic: LoGasovīraka (or loGasocīraka — "salty sour gruel"), is a fermented medicine.

Medical procedures. A bhikkhu who has surgery (lancing) or hemorrhoid removal performed in the crotch or within the area two fingerbreadths around it incurs a thullaccaya. The word for *crotch* (*sambādha*) literally means "confining place," and the area two fingerbreadths around it covers the anus and genitals.

> *Now at that time a certain bhikkhu had a fistula. Ākāsagotta the surgeon lanced it. Then the Blessed One, on a tour of the lodgings, headed to that bhikkhu's dwelling. Ākāsagotta the surgeon saw the Blessed One coming from afar and, on seeing him, said, "Come, Master Gotama. Look at this bhikkhu's anus (§). It's like an iguana's mouth." Then the Blessed One, (thinking,) "This worthless man is making fun of me," turned back right there ((§) — reading* tato'va *with the Thai and Sri Lankan editions). (He then convened a meeting of the bhikkhus, at which he said,) "How can this worthless man have surgery done in the crotch? In the crotch the skin is tender, a wound is hard to heal, the knife hard to guide."*[7]

It is interesting to note that brain surgery[8] was known in the Buddha's time and yet he did not regard it as dangerous as the procedures forbidden here. The Vinaya-mukha maintains that surgical technique has developed to the point where this prohibition is counterproductive, but post-operative complications from hemorrhoid surgery, for example, still arise fairly frequently. The Commentary states that if the scrotum is enlarged, one may apply medicines to it and warm it over the fire. None of the texts discuss alternatives to prostate surgery. Some Communities, following the Vinaya-mukha, would allow it whenever needed.

The Pali term translated here as hemorrhoid removal — *vatthi-kamma* — is a cognate of the Sanskrit term, *vasti-*

karman, usually translated as the administration of an enema. However, the Commentary restricts its meaning to hemorrhoid removal, and it is possible that the Commentary is right, for Pali terms do not always have the same meaning as their Sanskrit cognates, and the idea of administering medicines through the anus may have first developed in the context of hemorrhoid treatment. The Commentary adds that even trying to remove a hemorrhoid by squeezing it with a piece of hide or cloth would come under this prohibition. However, it recommends as a safer alternative that one apply an astringent decoction to the hemorrhoid and tie off the end with string. If the hemorrhoid then falls off on its own, well and good. Furthermore, the Commentary allows any equipment, such as tubes, used to apply medicine through the anus — an explicit allowance for enemas.

As mentioned above, blood letting is allowed as a treatment for wind afflictions of the joints. For some reason, Burmese editions of the Canon contain a separate general allowance for blood-letting. This passage is not in the Thai or Sri Lankan editions.

The Great Standards. Appropriately, the Khandhaka dealing with medicine ends with the Great Standards, as medical knowledge is so changeable over time, and variable from location to location, that there is a need for general principles to apply the rules of the Buddha's time to the modern period. In this chapter, the rules about practicing medicine and the classifications of tonics and life-long medicines are timeless. In the sections on specific treatments and medical procedures, however, the only hard and fast rules are the prohibitions. Outside of the prohibitions, all modern medical procedures are allowed.

RULES

The Five Tonics

"I allow that the five tonics, having been accepted at the right time, be consumed at the right time."[9]

"I allow that the five tonics, having been accepted, be consumed at the right time or the wrong time."[10]

"There are these tonics to be taken by sick bhikkhus: ghee, butter, oil, honey, sugar-molasses. Having been received, they may be used from storage seven days at most. Beyond that, one is to be dealt with in accordance with the rule.[11]

"Even though, to bind it together, they mix flour or ashes (§) into sugar lumps and it still counts as sugar, I allow that sugar be consumed as much as you like."[12]

"I allow sugar lumps for a bhikkhu who is ill, and sugar-lump water for one who is not ill."[13]

"I allow that tallow-medicine — i.e., tallow from bears, tallow from fish, tallow from alligators, tallow from pigs, tallow from donkeys — be consumed as oil if received in the right time, rendered in the right time, and filtered (§) in the right time."[14]

Life-long Medicines (compiled by Thanissaro Bhikkhu from Mahavattu)

"I allow that, having accepted root-medicine — i.e., turmeric, ginger, sweet flag, white orris root, ativisa, black hellebore, khus-khus, nut-grass, or whatever other roots are medicines and do not serve, among non-staple food, the purpose of non-staple food; or, among staple food, the purpose of staple food — one may keep it for life and, when there is reason, consume it. If there is no reason, there is an offense of wrong doing for one who consumes it." — VI. 3.1

"Garlic should not be eaten. Whoever should eat it: an offense of wrong doing." ... "I allow that garlic be eaten in the case of illness."

"I allow a grindstone and a grinding wheel." —VI.3.2

"I allow that, having accepted astringent-decoction medicine — i.e., astringent decoctions from the nimb-tree, from the kumaja, from the pakkava, from the nattamâla, or whatever other astringent decoctions are medicines and do not serve, among non-staple food, the purpose of non-staple food; or, among staple food, the purpose of staple food — one may keep it for life and, when there is reason, consume it. If there is no reason, there is an offense of wrong doing for one who consumes it." —VI. 4

"I allow that, having accepted leaf-medicine — i.e., nimb leaves, kumaja leaves, cucumber leaves, basil leaves, cotton tree leaves, or whatever other leaves are medicines and do not serve, among non-staple food, the purpose of non-staple food; or, among staple food, the purpose of staple food — one may keep it for life and, when there is reason, consume it. If there is no reason, there is an offense of wrong doing for one who consumes it." —VI. 5

"I allow that, having accepted fruit-medicine — i.e., vilaEga, long pepper, black pepper, yellow myrobalan, beleric myrobalan, embric myrobalan, gomha, or whatever other fruits are medicines and do not serve, among non-staple food, the purpose of non-staple food; or, among staple food, the purpose of staple food — one may keep it for life and, when there is reason, consume it. If there is no reason, there is an offense of wrong doing for one who consumes it." —VI. 6

"I allow that, having accepted resin-medicine — i.e., assafoetida, assafoetida-resin, assafoetida-gum, gum, gum-patti, gum-panni, or whatever other resins are medicines and do not serve, among non-staple food, the purpose of non-staple food; or, among staple food, the purpose of staple food — one may keep it for life and, when there is reason, consume it. If there is no reason, there is an offense of wrong doing for one who consumes it." —VI. 7

"I allow that, having accepted salt-medicine — i.e., sea salt, black salt, rock salt, culinary salt, red salt, or whatever other salts are medicines and do not serve, among non-staple food, the purpose of non-staple food; or, among staple food, the purpose of staple food — one may keep it for life and, when there is reason, consume it. If there is no reason, there is an offense of wrong doing for one who consumes it." — VI. 8.

Specific Treatments

"I allow powders as medicines for one who has an itch, a small boil, a running sore, or an affliction of thick scabs; or for one whose body smells bad; I allow (powdered) dung, clay, and dye-dregs for one who is not ill. I allow a pestle and mortar." —VI. 9.2.

"I allow a powder sifter... I allow a cloth sifter." —VI.10.1

"I allow, for one who is afflicted (possessed) by non-human beings, raw flesh and raw blood." — VI. 10.2

"I allow (eye) ointments: black collyrium, rasa-ointment (made with vitriol?), sota-ointment (made with antimony?), yellow orpiment (§), lamp-black." ... "I allow (mixed in the ointments) sandalwood, tagara, benzoin gum, tâlîsa, nut-grass." — VI. 11.2.

"I allow an ointment box." ... "One should not use fancy ointment boxes. Whoever does: an offense of wrong doing. I allow (ointment boxes) made of bone, ivory, horn, reed, bamboo, wood, lac (resin), fruit (§) (e.g., coconut shell), copper (metal), or conch-shell." — VI. 12.1.

"I allow a lid." ... "I allow, having tied it with thread/string, to tie it to the ointment-box." ... "(An ointment box became split) I allow it to be bound together with thread/ string." — VI. 12.2.

"I allow an ointment stick." ... "One should not use fancy ointment sticks. Whoever does: an offense of wrong doing. I allow (ointment sticks) made of bone, ivory, horn, reed, bamboo, wood, lac (resin), fruit (§) (e.g., coconut shell), copper (metal), or conch-shell." — VI. 12.3.

"I allow a case for (ointment) sticks." ... "I allow a bag for the ointment box." ... "I allow a string for tying the mouth of the bag as a carrying strap." — VI. 12.4.

"I allow oil for the head." ... "I allow treatment through the nose." ... "I allow a nose-tube (or nose-spoon)." ... "One should not use fancy nose tubes. Whoever does: an offense of wrong doing. I allow (nose tubes) made of bone, ivory, horn, reed, bamboo, wood, lac (resin), fruit (§) (e.g., coconut shell), copper (metal), or conch-shell." — VI. 13.1.

"I allow a double nose-tube." ... "I allow that smoke be inhaled." ... "I allow a tube for inhaling smoke." ... "One should not use fancy smoke-inhaling tubes. Whoever does: an offense of wrong doing. I allow (smoke-inhaling tubes) made of bone, ivory, horn, reed, bamboo, wood, lac (resin), fruit (§) (e.g., coconut shell), copper (metal), or conch-shell." ... "I allow a lid (for the smoke-inhaling tubes)." ... "I allow a bag for the smoke-inhaling tubes." ... "I allow a double bag." ... "I allow a string for tying the mouth of the bag as a carrying strap." — VI. 13.1.

(For wind afflictions): "I allow a decoction of oil." ... "I allow that alcohol be mixed in the decoction of oil." ... "Oil mixed with too much alcohol should not be drunk. Whoever drinks it is to be dealt with in accordance with the rule. I allow that when neither the color, the smell, nor the taste of alcohol can be detected in the decoction of oil, this sort of oil mixed with alcohol may be drunk." —VI. 14.1.

(When too much alcohol has been mixed with oil): "I allow that it be determined as rubbing-oil." ... "I allow (for oil) three kinds of flasks: a metal flask, a wood flask, a fruit flask." — VI. 14.2.

(For wind affliction in the limbs): "I allow a sweating treatment." ... "I allow a sweating treatment with herbs ... a 'great-sweating' treatment ... hemp water ... a water tub." — VI. 14.3.

(For wind afflictions in the joints): "I allow blood-letting ... moxibustion (§)." ... (For split feet): "I allow rubbing oil for the feet... I allow that a foot salve be prepared." ... (For boils): "I allow lancing (surgery)... I allow astringent water... I allow pounded sesame paste." — VI. 14.4.

(For boils, continued): "I allow a compress ... a bandage ... that it be sprinkled with mustard-seed powder (to prevent itching)." ... "I allow fumigating." ... "I allow that (scar-tissue) be cut off with a piece of salt-crystal." ... "I allow oil for the sore/wound." ... "I allow an old piece of cloth for soaking up the oil and every kind of treatment for sores/wounds." — VI. 14.5.

(For snakebite): "I allow that the four great filthy things be given: excrement, urine, ashes, clay." ... "I allow, when there is someone to make them allowable, that one have him make them allowable; when there is no one to make them allowable, that having taken them oneself one consume them." ... (For drinking poison): "I allow that water mixed with excrement be drunk." ... "I allow (excrement) that one received while making it as having been received in and of itself (§). It does not need to be received again." — VI. 14.6.

(For drinking a sorcery concoction): " I allow that mud turned up by the plow be drunk." ... (For constipation): "I allow that alkaline juice be drunk." ... (For jaundice): "I allow that urine and yellow myrobalan be drunk." ... (For skin disease): "I allow that a scented rubbing be done." ... (For a body full of bad humors): "I allow that a purgative be drunk." ... (After taking a purgative) "I allow clarified conjey... I allow clear green gram broth... I allow slightly thick green gram broth... I allow meat broth." — VI. 14.7.

"I allow that a bhikkhu who is ill may consume loGasovîraka (loGasocîraka) as much as he likes, and that one who is not ill may consume it mixed with water as a beverage." — VI. 16.3.

Medical Procedures

"Surgery should not be done in the crotch. Whoever should do it (have it done): a grave offense." — VI. 22.3.

"Surgery and hemorrhoid removal (§) should not be done within the area two inches around the crotch. Whoever should do it (have it done): a grave offense." — VI. 22.4.

[Included in the Burmese & PTS editions, but not the Thai or Sri Lankan editions: "I allow the letting of blood."] — *Chulavamsa*, V. 6.

The Great Standards

"Whatever I have not objected to, saying, 'This is not allowable,' if it conforms with what is not allowable, if it goes against (literally, "preempts") what is allowable, this is not allowable for you. Whatever I have not objected to, saying, 'This is not allowable,' if it conforms with what is allowable, if it goes against what is not allowable, this is allowable for you. And whatever I have not permitted, saying, 'This is allowable,' if it conforms with what is not allowable, if it goes against what is allowable, this is not allowable for you. And whatever I have not permitted, saying, 'This is allowable,' if it conforms with what is allowable, if it goes against what is not allowable, this is allowable for you." — VI. 40.1.

BUDDHISM AND MEDICINE[15]

It has not gone unnoticed that the Buddhist aim of eliminating suffering coincides with the objectives of medicine (Duncan *et al.*, 1981; Soni, 1976). The Buddhist emphasis on compassion finds natural expression in the care of the sick, and according to the *Vinaya* the Buddha himself stated, "Whoever, O monks, would nurse me, he should nurse the sick" (Zysk, 1991: 41). Buddhist clergy and laity have been involved with the care of the sick for over two thousand years. The Indian Buddhist emperor Asoka states in his second Rock Edict that provision has been made everywhere in his kingdom for medical treatment for both men and animals, and that medicinal herbs suitable for both have been imported and planted.

Birnbaum (1979) and Demieville (1985) provide good general introductions to Buddhism and medicine. Buddhism appears to have played an important role in the evolution of traditional Indian medicine (Zysk, 1991), and there are many parallels between Buddhist medicine, as recorded in the Pali canon, and *Aayurveda* (Mitra, 1985). There are short monographs by Haldar on the scientific (1977) and public heath aspects (1992) of medicine in the Pali sources. It is likely that as Buddhism spread through Asia it would have interacted with indigenous medical traditions promoting the cross-fertilization of ideas. Redmond (1992) discusses the relationship of Buddhism to medicine from Theravaada and Mahaayaana perspectives and compares Buddhist and Daoist concepts of disease. Discussions of Tibetan medicine may be found in Clifford (1984), Dhonden (1986), and Rechung (1976), while Ohnuki-Tierney (1984) discusses illness and culture in contemporary Japan.

Buddhism's holistic understanding of human nature encourages a psychosomatic approach to the pathology of disease (Soni, 1976), something to which Western medicine is now increasingly attuned. It may also be suggested that the Buddhist philosophy of origination in dependence is both a fruitful diagnostic model and a philosophy, which encourages a preventive approach to healthcare. However, disquiet has been voiced recently about how "natural" certain forms of traditional Buddhist medicine are - notably the Tibetan "black pill" - some recipes for which specify rhinoceros horn and bear-bile among the ingredients (Leland, 1995).

MEDICAL ETHICS

Despite Buddhism's long association with the healing arts, little attention has been paid to the ethical issues, which arise from the practice of medicine. A small number of monographs provide introductions to the issues and dilemmas, which arise in medical practice. These are Ratanakul (1986), Nakasone (1990) and Keown (1995), and these volumes should be consulted in conjunction with the sources listed under the specific subject-headings below. Also relevant is the unpublished Masters thesis by Shoyu Taniguchi (1987a). For general discussions in the periodical literature see Taniguchi (1987b), Mettanando (1991), and Ratanakul (1988; 1990). A useful discussion of Buddhism in terms of the "four principles" approach to medical ethics developed by Beauchamp and Childress (1989) is provided by Robert Florida (1994).

The *Encyclopedia of Bioethics* contains articles on medical ethics in India (Jaqqi, 1987), Asia (Unschuld, 1987), and Japan in the nineteenth century (Kitagawa, 1987). Also on Japan see Umezawa (1988). On medical ethics in imperial China see Unschuld (1979) and on Thailand Violette Lindbeck (1984) and Ratanakul (1988; 1990).

The principal issues to be addressed in contemporary medical ethics may be summarised as moral personhood (the question of who is and who is not entitled to moral respect), abortion, embryo experimentation, genetic engineering, consent to treatment, resource allocation, defining death, organ transplantation, living wills, the persistent vegetative state, and euthanasia. Buddhist practitioners or scholars have yet directed little systematic attention to these subjects, and some subjects have not been discussed at all from a Buddhist perspective. The arrangement of the topics below is neither comprehensive nor final. It is inevitable there will be overlap between the sections, and items, which appear under one category, may contain discussion of issues or principles, which have broader relevance.

At this time, however, it seems useful to identify three groups of issues and related literature. These concern: moral personhood, issues surrounding life at its beginning, and issues surrounding life at its end. There is insufficient literature on resource-allocation, socio-economic issues, or other questions about general medical practice to justify a category on those topics in this review. There are signs, however, that a Buddhist perspective on certain aspects of medical treatment is beginning to appear, for example Epstein (1993) and Kabat-Zinn's (1990, 1994) integration of Buddhist meditation into medical practice, and the growing literature on Buddhism and social justice, such as Jones (1989) and Sizemore and Swearer (1993).

MORAL PERSONHOOD

Personhood is both a central problem for Buddhist ethics and Western medical ethics, and consequently a very promising area for a dialogue between the two. The problem for Buddhist ethics has always been why should people act ethically if there is no act, no actor and no consequences of action (Collins, 1982). If there is no self or other, how can there be karmic consequences, responsibility, loyalty, or even compassion? Theravaadin scholars continue to be divided over whether Buddhism suggests different ethics for those who persist in the illusion of self (*kammic* ethics) and for those who would transcend the illusion of self (*nibbanic* ethics). The paradoxical unity of compassionate ethics and nihilistic insight into selflessness has been the central koan of Mahayana Buddhism. Tantra and Zen suggest that the person who sees that there is no "I" is beyond good and evil.

For bioethics, struggles over abortion, animal rights and brain death have brought personhood to the forefront (Nelkin, 1983). Opponents of abortion and euthanasia, and advocates for the disabled and animals, on the other hand, assert that mere humanness or merely being alive should bestow a "right to life." But most bioethicists believe that human beings and animals take on ethical significance to the extent that they are "persons." Some, such as Tooley (1984), would set a standard, which would exclude almost all animals, newborns, and the severely retarded or demented. When they specify which elements of sentience and neurological integrity create the illusion of personhood, Western bioethicists begin to sound remarkably Buddhistic: "the awareness of the difference between self and other; the ability to be conscious of oneself over time; the ability to engage in purposive actions" (see, for instance, Fletcher, 1979).

At the same time, Western bioethicists have become increasingly troubled by questions about the autonomy, continuity and authenticity of the self. Do anti-depressants create an inauthentic self, or is the self more authentic when its cheerful? Is one respecting a patient's autonomy by respecting the treatment preferences they expressed when healthy, or those they express in the throes of illness? Is it ever possible for a patient to give truly free and informed consent to treatment?

The most radical challenge to Western ethics of self-determination came in 1984 with the publication of British philosopher Derek Parfit's *Reasons and Persons*. In this meticulously argued tome, Parfit rejects the existence of continuous selves and concludes that an individual is as discontinuous from itself at some later time as it is from other individuals. Consequently, working for the future welfare of all beings is the same as working for one's own future welfare, since there will be no "I" to benefit in the future.

Bioethicists are only now incorporating Parfit's argument. For instance, researchers find that is impossible to accurately anticipate one's state of mind when one is sick or dying, much less when one is unconscious, undercutting the assumption of continuous personhood undergirding "living wills."

From a Buddhist/Parfitian perspective, the search for "real" preferences, central to the identity of the person, is a pointless one. With this acknowledgement, it is less troubling to place our trust in our family and friends to make decisions for our future selves (Kuczewski, 1994). More to the point, a Buddhist/Parfitian would encourage citizens to look beyond their personal preferences in dying, which may be to "die with dignity" but may also be to use as many resources as possible to stave off death, and instead participate in creating a health care system that served the needs of everyone in society.

Another area of potential dialogue is in the efforts to go beyond Cartesian (and Hindu etc.) mind-body dualism in defining life and death. Over the last twenty years the West has slowly accepted that a "person" is dead if their brain is destroyed, even if the body continues to function. Yet it still troubles many Westerners and Buddhists to declare the permanently unconscious "dead," believing that this is an example of inappropriate mind-body dualism. Other Westerners and Buddhists believe that only a "neocortical" definition of death recognizes the centrality of consciousness and personhood in ethics (Gervais, 1986). More challenging, some Western ethicists have begun to discuss the status of personhood as future technologies make possible the continuity of personality from one body to another (More, 1994). When medical technology offers reincarnation, Buddhist bioethics will certainly flourish.

ABORTION

Buddhism, like all religious and secular philosophies, focuses on two central questions concerning abortion: (a) when does the embryo or foetus acquire the property which makes termination of pregnancy "killing"?; and (b) is termination of a pregnancy, before or after this point, ever justifiable?

While there was a minority tradition in classical Hindu embryology that held that incarnation does not occur till as late as the seventh month (Lipner, 1989), most Buddhist commentators have adopted classical Hindu teachings that the transmigration of consciousness occurs at conception, and therefore that all abortion incurs the karmic burden of killing. Before modern embryology, however, in both Buddhist countries and the West, ideas about conception were scientifically inaccurate, and often associated the beginning of life with events in the third or fourth month of pregnancy (for a discussion of traditional Tibetan embryology, see Dhonden, 1980 and Lecso,1987).

Another problem in early Buddhists' embryology is their assumption that the transmigration of consciousness is sudden rather than gradual. Based on the findings of modern neuro-embryology Buddhists today might maintain that the fetus does not fully embody all five *skandhas* and the illusion of personhood until after birth; this is the argument developed by most Western ethicists to defend abortion (Tooley, 1984; Flower, 1985; Bennett, 1989). If the fetus is not yet a fully embodied person, then the karmic consequences of abortion would be even less than the killing of animals, which Buddhism teaches do have moral status. This neurological interpretation of the *skandhas* may be more consistent with Western Buddhism, which often sees the doctrine of rebirth as peripheral or interprets rebirth metaphorically rather than literally (Batchelor, 1992; King, 1994).

The second question is whether abortion always generates bad karma, or in Western terms, is it ever "justified." This relates to the debate about whether Buddhist ethics are absolutist, utilitarian or "virtuist," i.e. seeing the good in the development of personal qualities. The absolutist would hold that bad karma is incurred from any act of murder, whatever the justifications. The utilitarian would argue that murder can be a compassionate act with positive karmic consequences, taking into account factors such as the health of the fetus or mother, the population crisis, and the readiness of the parents to raise a child.

A virtue-oriented Buddhist would argue that the attitude and motivations of the pregnant woman and her collaborators would determine the ethics of an abortion. Along this line, Tworkov (1992) argues that the karmic skilfulness of an abortion is related to whether the person became pregnant and made her decision to abort without serious mindfulness. From this perspective, aborting a fetus conceived without an effort at contraception would be more karmically significant than an abortion necessitated in spite of contraception.

The much discussed Japanese tolerance for, and ritualization of, abortion appears to combine both utilitarian and virtue approaches. The Japanese believe that abortion is a "sorrowful necessity," and Buddhist temples sell rituals and statues intended to represent parents' apologies to the aborted, and wish for a more propitious rebirth. The Japanese have reached these accommodations consensually, with little debate, and without discussion of the rights of women or the unborn (LaFleur, 1990, 1992).

The Theravaadin commentator Buddhaghosa appears to have combined all three views. He held that killing produces karma jointly through the mental effort and intensity of the desire to kill, and the virtue of the victim (Florida, 1991). Since killing big animals required more effort, and was therefore worse than killing small animals, the karma of feticide would be less than murder of adults, and less in earlier stages of pregnancy. On the other hand, for Buddhaghosa, the karma of feticide would be greater than that of killing villains in self-defence.

Buddhists have thus far given little thought to the third important question, the connection between morality and law, specifically how, and on what grounds, the state should regulate abortion. Some Buddhists have adopted the stance of many moderates in the West: abortion is murder of a person, but women should have that choice (for instance, Imamura, 1984 and Lecso, 1987). Since most Buddhists have no problem with laws to discourage and punish murder in general, implicit in this position is that murder is either justifiable when it conflicts with bodily autonomy or, since few Buddhists would imprison butchers, that fetuses are closer in status to animals. Clearly there is much room for clarification of the relationship between religious ethics and law in pluralistic societies.

Some scholars (such as Ling, 1969, and LaFleur, 1992) have looked beyond the strictly ethical concerns with abortion to examine the cultural aspects of the question. From this perspective it is sometimes pointed out that Buddhism is not "pro-natalist," i.e. does not hold that reproduction is a religious duty - quite the reverse in fact - and does not advocate "family values," at least in the sense that Confucianism did. Buddhist skepticism about family and reproduction was a central cause of Confucian and Shinto persecution. The Sinhalese embrace of contraception and abortion was so enthusiastic in the 1960s, compared to Sri Lanka's Muslims, Catholics and Hindus, that racialist monks began to argue that Buddhists had an obligation to "race-religion-nation" to reproduce.

DEATH, DYING AND EUTHANASIA

The themes of impermanence, decay and death are omnipresent in Buddhist literature. In many Asian cultures Buddhism is identified as the authority par excellence on matters pertaining to death, and is closely linked to the rites and ceremonies associated with the transition from this life to the next. Buddhist literature emphasises the importance of meeting death mindfully since the last moment of one life can be particularly influential in determining the quality of the next rebirth.

General reflections on death will be found in Philip Kapleau's 1972 anthology *The Wheel of Death* and his 1989 *The Wheel of Life and Death*. Stephen Levine is the author of several books dealing with the subject of death from a Zen perspective while a contemporary Tibetan perspective is provided by Sogyal Rinpoche's popular *Tibetan Book of Living and Dying*, Glenn H. Mullin (1986) and John Powers (1995, Ch.10). James Whitehill (1974) discussed what can be learned from the death of the Buddhist masters, and the development of a corpus of "Great Death" stories of various Buddhist masters is examined by LaFleur (1974). Other writings on death in Buddhism include Smart (1968), Amore (1974), and Bowker (1991).

In a 1993 monograph on the subject of death in Buddhism, Becker asserts that the Buddhist tradition, especially in Japan, is very tolerant of suicide and euthanasia. Evidence of this is the Buddha's tolerance of suicide by monks (Wiltshire, 1983) and Japanese stories praising suicide by monks, samurai and laypeople. Becker suggests that Buddhism values self-determination and praises those who decide when and how they will die when they do so in order to have a dignified conscious death. Becker also concludes that the key point is not whether there is still warmth or reflexes (as suggested by some readings of the *Visuddhimagga*) but whether the patient's *skandhas* have permanently left, i.e. the patient is permanently unconscious. In other words, Buddhism would endorse a brain death definition of death. On the understanding of death in Japanese religion see also Picken (1977).

A number of issues in medical ethics turn upon the problem of defining death, but few writers have addressed the question of a Buddhist definition of death directly. Only van Loon (1978), Keown (1995), and Mettanando (1991) have argued for a specific definition: van Loon equates death with neocortical death whereas Keown and Mettanando support the "whole brain" criterion.

There has been considerable resistance to the adoption of the brain death standard in Japan, both from the public and within the medical profession, due in no small measure to its association with organ transplantation. The brain death criterion allows organs to be harvested with the minimum delay, thereby enhancing the prospects for a successful transplant. Japanese tradition, however, requires the performance of rituals over a lengthy period before an individual is regarded as having passed on, and is also reluctant to countenance plundering the bodily organs of future ancestors. Some commentators suggest that public acceptance of brain death is growing as professional groups and universities develop criteria, and as pressure from potential beneficiaries grows. Also, countries such as the Philippines have raised objections to Japanese patients going abroad for transplants rather than building an organ retrieval system of their own. The best analysis available (in English) of the Japanese situation is Hardacre (1994), but relevant material may also be found in Lock and Honde (1990), Feldman (1988), Becker (1990), and Nudeshima (1991). For discussions of the issue outside of Japan see Ratanakul (1988, 1990), Sugunasiri (1990), and Nakasone (1994).

A more positive attitude towards transplantation is revealed in Tsomo (1993). The author surveyed teachers from many different traditions about their attitudes to donation. All were very positive, and emphasized that the corpse is merely an empty vessel, and that to give of oneself is a great thing, and an act of compassion.

EUTHANASIA

There are no monographs devoted specifically to euthanasia in Buddhism. There are a few periodical articles and the subject is dealt within one or two books. Relevant issues are the distinction between various forms of euthanasia (e.g. "active" and "passive") and the use of narcotics in palliative care, which may cloud the mind and interfere with the process of dying (Keown, 1995; Kapleau, 1989; Lecso, 1986; Ratanakul, 1988, 1990).

Kapleau's volume *The Wheel of Life and Death* (1989) contains a short discussion of euthanasia in conjunction with suicide and it is suggested that Buddhism would reject the practice of either. Ratanakul concurs, reporting "a growing consensus among the Thai public that euthanasia (passive or active) is morally unjustifiable" (1990:27). Keown and Keown (1995) explore Buddhist and Christian attitudes to euthanasia and suggest both oppose it for similar reasons. Nakasone, however, is of the opinion that "Evidence indicates that Buddhists would favor the 'right-to-die' position" (1990:76). Jennifer Green's short article "Death with Dignity: Buddhism" (1989:40-41) discusses only the practicalities of funeral arrangements and does not mention euthanasia. Neuberger (1987) is likewise concerned with practical as opposed to moral issues.

Euthanasia has been a special feature in two Buddhist magazines, *Raft*, and *Tricycle*. London-based *Raft, the Journal of the Buddhist Hospice Trust*, devoted its No. 2 Winter 1989/90 issue to Euthanasia. Sixteen pages in length it contains short pieces by authors such as Elisabeth Kubler-Ross, Ajahn Sumedho, Dame Cicely Saunders and David Stott, exploring the cases for, against, and in terms of a middle way. A similar range of opinions will be found in the Winter 1992 edition of *Tricycle*, which contains short articles by Patricia Anderson, Jeffrey Hopkins, Philip Kapleau, Chogyam Trungpa, and an interview with author Stephen Levine.

Notes

1. See Pasang Arya's article titled *Buddhism and Medicine* on *tibetanmedicine.edu.org*
2. Digha Nikaya 2.
3. *Mahavattu*, VIII. 26.1-8.
4. *Mahavattu*, I.30.4.
5. *Digha Nikaya*, VI, 2.
6. *Mahavattu*, VI.
7. *Mahavattu*, I, 2.
8. *Mahavattu*, v.VIII. 1.16-20.

9. *Mahavattu*, VI.1.3.
10. *Mahavatut*, VI.1.5.
11. *Mahavattu* VI.15.10.
12. *Mahavattu* VI.16.1
13. *Mahavattu* VI. 27.
14. *Mahavattu*, VI. 2.1.
15. *Buddhism and Medical Ethics: A Bibliographic Introduction*, James Hughes, Mclean Centre for Clinical Medical Ethics and Damien Keown, Goldsmiths, University of London, *Journal Of Buddhist Ethics*, Vol. II, 1995.

CHAPTER – 4

REGIONAL VARIATION IN BUDDHIST MEDICINE

Among the many types of Buddhism are three overarching categories, all of which developed in India from c. 500 BCE to 1100 CE. The Buddhists consider the historical Shakyamuni Buddha to be the founder of the three main forms or "vehicles" of Buddhism: the Monastic or Individual (Hinayana/Theravada), the Messianic or Universal (Mahayana), and the Apocalyptic or Tantric (Vajrayana). Buddhism based on the Theravada model is found today in Sri Lanka, Thailand, Burma, Laos and Cambodia, while the Mahayana style went north into China and from there to Japan, Tibet, and Korea. Vajrayana Buddhism is a strand of Mahayana that blends the physical and spiritual world and engages both. Vajrayana Buddhism still exists in many countries, but it reached its full potential, and further developed, in Tibet.Buddhism came to the West with an adjective such as Sri Lankan Buddhism, Thai Buddhism, Cambodian Buddhism, Tibetan Buddhism, and Zen or Chan Buddhism. Sometimes Westerners can be confused with this identification as they compare this concept with the hundreds of sects of Christianity. Many people have been misled by misunderstanding the cultural influences on Buddhist teaching in different countries. Even the Theravada traditions in Sri Lanka, Thailand, Myanmar, and Cambodia monks have their own rituals, which are different from each other as well as Mahayana and Vajrayana. Similar pattern is evinced, with respect to the Theravadin medicine (in Thailand, Sri Lanka etc.,), Zen medicine (in China and Japan) and Vajrayana medicine (in Tibet). They are not identical in their respective natures and contents.

To highlight some of the continuities and differences in Buddhist medical practices throughout Asia, we will discuss Buddhist medicine in China, Thailand and Tibet, representing the three major sects in Buddhism. In case of China, we will try to trace the history of Buddhist medicine, as this region witnessed one of the first interactions with the Indian Buddhist monks. However, in this context, we will also like to talk about modern Buddhist medicine in Mongolian China, as both the regions exhibit similar cultural pattern. And, it is also very difficult to make out the modern form of Buddhist medical practice prevalent in communist China. Later, we will try to explore the Theravadin's Thai medicine. Finally, we will discuss Tibetan (Vajrayana) medicine exclusively in a separate chapter, as it deserves such attention. In recent times, the credit of rising popularity of Buddhist medicine, especially in the western countries, goes to Tibet and Dalai Lama. Now, for most people in developed countries Buddhist and Tibetan medicine are almost synonymous. Moreover, in India, this system of medicine (*Sowa Rigpa*) has been popularly practiced in Ladakh and Paddar-Pangay regions of Jammu and Kashmir, Himachal Pradesh, Arunachal Pradesh, Sikkim, Darjeeling-Kalimgpong (WB) and now in Tibetan settlements all over India. It also constitutes one of the missions of Central Council for Research in Ayurveda and Siddha, Deptt. Of

AYUSH, Ministry of Health and Family Welfare, Govt. of India.

Buddhist Medicine in China

History of Chinese Buddhist medicine from the first arrival of Buddhism in China to the early Tang dynasty[1] has important implications for our understanding of the cross-cultural encounter between India and China in the medieval period. Encapsulated within Buddhist texts translated into Chinese, Indian medical knowledge accompanied the transmission of Buddhism from India to China across the Silk Roads and over the sea routes. While Buddhism introduced to China radically foreign models of state, society, and the cosmos, as an integral part of its mission it also forwarded new ideas about disease, healing, and the body. Once arriving on Chinese soil, received Indian medical and religious knowledge merged with local traditions to produce a pluralistic and syncretic body of healing doctrines and practices that are referred to in some Chinese texts as "Buddhist medicine" (*fo yi*).

We treat "Buddhist medicine" as an analytic category[2] separate from Indian or Chinese classical medicine. It is a unique body of hybrid medical knowledge produced through a specific historical instance of cross-cultural exchange between India, China, and several kingdoms in Central and Southeast Asia. Analysis of this distinct and heretofore relatively unstudied medical tradition is possible through the investigation of a number of texts found in the Chinese Buddhist canonical and extracanonical literature. This corpus contains a large amount of new material previously unknown to medical historians that is nonetheless critical for understanding medical theory and practice in China, India, and elsewhere in Asia in the medieval period. Spanning many centuries, these sources include scattered sections and passages from monastic disciplinary codes, philosophical treatises, ritual manuals, hagiographies, spell-texts, commentaries, collectanea, and other genres. Translated into Chinese from a variety of Indic and Central Asian languages or originally composed in China, such sources in their diversity contain divergent or even conflicting medical details. In the aggregate, however, they suggest that medicine was central to the transmission of Buddhism throughout Asia, and that healing was among the principal benefits the new religion held out to converts in new lands.

We focus on the dynamics of this cross-cultural dialogue and the social, cultural, and intellectual contexts leading to the creation of this hybrid medical tradition. However, rather than discuss the impact of Buddhist medicine on China using abstract terms such as "the Indian influence on China" or "the sinification of Buddhism," we will emphasize the concrete textual practices of Chinese translators as they appropriated foreign medical knowledge and adapted it to local conditions and expectations. Buddhist monks[3] offered medical treatment to the inhabitants of their host country for a great variety of reason. In addition to the ethical obligation to provide assistance to all men, the missionary value of such action was recognised early and is mentioned as a reason for therapeutic activity. Fo-tu-teng (fl. 310-349), for instance, realised that the tenets of his religion were too profound for the rulers in the small state of Shih Lo (later Chao) to appreciate fully. None of the activities, however, left a last impression on the Chinese Public Health System. The same is true for the Charitable apothecaries (hu-min- yao-chi) established by the state during the Sung period (960-1279) a scandal ridden and limited program that was never achieved more than a brief significance.

With the decline of Buddhism to a folk religion during subsequent centuries, official interest in such charitable organisation also seems to have died out. Not until the widespread of Christianity during the 19th century did the integration of missionary and medical activities by a foreign religion re-emerge in China, accompanies once again by the establishment of significant number of hospitals.

He, therefore, repeatedly demonstrated his knowledge and the value of his teachings through various magical and clairvoyant activities, including raising of the dead, rain spell and divination.

Medical concepts introduced by Buddhist literature followed a similar course. Tao Hung Chung (452-536), the renowned Taoist and author of medical works, wrote a supplementary to the prescription collection Chou-hou-fang of Ku Hung (281-341) entitled Chou-hou-pai-I-fang (Prescription handbook Enlarged by 101 prescriptions). In a preface-dated 500- the only portion of the work that has survived, the author acknowledges Buddhist influence. Additional evidence is provided by the Indian Titles in the bibliography of Sui dynasty (589-618). Even today Buddhist continue to pray for release from bodily suffering to the goddess Kuan–Yin the Chinese form adapted from the original male Bodhisattva Avalokitesvara, Buddhist oracular medicine is still prevalent wherever, Buddhist doctrine is able to develop unimpeded. Receptacles in the temple contain numbered wooden slips, which the faithful draw out after an appropriate prayer. The number drawn refers to a prescription-kept in the temple- that is to be followed as a direction of the Bodhisattva. Of the 6 part etiology, only illness caused by disharmony among the 4 elements, excessive meditation and improper conduct during a previous existence were completely new. While it is not difficult to understand that meditation and Karma etiology remained restricted almost exclusively to Buddhist writings. Sun-ssu-miao has repeatedly cited Buddhist influence on Chinese medicine in western secondary sources[4].

Buddhist writers were in fact deeply interested in a variety of medical approaches for the purposes of alleviating physical suffering, and they syncretically integrated Indian and Chinese medical knowledge into their major treatises. In many of the texts, it appears[5] that they embrace and advocate classical Chinese medical language involving *qi*(#l), *yin-yang* (p–}–), the Five Phases (*wu xing* "NL^), and the Five Viscera (*wu zang* "Nß□) alongside doctrines from an Indian milieu such as the Four Elements (*mahābhūta*), the Seven Bodily Substances (*dhātus*) and the Three Humors (*doca*). They also combine these medical models with prayer, repentance, exorcism, and other therapies drawn from Buddhist and Taoist practices.

The ways in which such divergent language and modes of thought were combined and systematized in Chinese Buddhist texts raises interesting theoretical questions. In the first place, although they did not use these words, Buddhist authors seem to have rather clearly recognized the distinctions between "medicine," "religion," and "magic," often thought to be the artefacts of modern theorizing. In reconciling diverse medical doctrines and practices, authors such as Tiantai Zhiyi (538–597 C. E.), for example, gave voice to three distinct medical logics. The first, the "physiological" approach, depended on an understanding of the organs, body fluids, and the inner workings of the material body. The second, the "karmic" approach, framed health and disease as the physical manifestations of karmic retribution. The third logic was at its core based on the "sympathetic response" (*gan-ying*) by which deities or other powerful beings could be called upon to intervene in the lives of mortals. This conceptual flexibility allowed Buddhist writers to easily absorb and incorporate ideas from competing medical traditions, such as classical Chinese medicine, Taoist therapy, and popular religious healing practices.

Another question that arises from the analysis of these texts concerns healing powers as cultural capital. Regardless of their origin, Buddhist writers invariably subsumed diverse Chinese and Indian therapies and doctrines within Buddhist philosophical frameworks and doctrinal rationales. Once they were incorporated into Buddhist texts, medical doctrines, practices, and narratives served the purpose of legitimizing the foreign religion in China. Healing disease was often a symbol of power and control over the seen and unseen realms, thus showcasing Buddhism's superiority over other religions. For example, in a discussion of healing in the hagiographies of Buddhist heroes, it appears[6] that stories of miraculous cures were central to Buddhism's proselytizing literature—part of the public face through which writers attempted to persuade audiences and influence converts.

A third area of theoretical interest is medicine as social practice. Buddhism's embrace of medicine allowed the foreign religion to more readily integrate into the sociopolitical landscape of medieval China. A number of extant texts demonstrate the importance of healing in cementing Buddhism's relationship with secular powers, as well as in establishing Buddhism as an institutional presence in towns and cities across China. Prescriptive texts on healing rituals, for example, were an important motivator of royal and elite patronage. Likewise, mass merit-making rituals for communal health and well-being must be counted among the chief services Buddhist institutions offered to patrons of even the lowest social classes. Thus[7] Buddhist discourses linking physical illness, karmic retribution, and divine intervention came to be internalized in the social practices and daily habitus of kings and commoners alike, while reinforcing the relevance and power of Buddhist monastic institutions at all levels of society.

In bringing into focus the theoretical questions raised by the ideology, practices, and rhetoric of Chinese Buddhist medicine, we hope to engage with several different historiographic traditions. However, in subsequent centuries, Buddhist concept of retribution appears only in discussion of medical- ethical problems. Perhaps[8] the cultural gap was too great or the attempts to bridge that gap too cursory; for to have genuine reception to have taken place. Sun–ssu-miao's text tends to support this conclusion. For historians of Chinese religion, centrality of medicine in Chinese Buddhism provides a new lens onto the relevance of religion in daily life in early medieval China and reveals one of the most important mechanisms by which Buddhism successfully gained prominence in new territories. For historians of medicine, it is amply demonstrated[9] that studying Buddhism as an option in the pluralistic medieval Chinese "medical marketplace" reveals important tensions and fissures between different types of healers and the role of religion in processes of social differentiation.

The transmission and reception of Indian medical knowledge in medieval China provides a focused historical case study for the investigation of the processes of syncretism and translation (both linguistic and cultural) that are currently research priorities for cultural theorists across a wide spectrum of the social sciences. Salguero[10] has analysed the multivalent quality of Buddhist healing knowledge, which was in China paradoxically both intimately familiar and radically foreign. Because of this, Buddhist medicine was valued both for the ways in which it perpetuated practices and ideas that were known since ancient times as well for its fresh conceptual approaches and technologies. It was Buddhist medicine's ability to appeal on these two levels—that is to say, its hybridity and biculturalism—that was instrumental in its success, and by extension the success of Buddhism itself, on Chinese soil. To summarize the arrival of Buddhism offered China through certain concepts of Indian Medicine an opportunity to become familiar with the analytic views of the body and the world that ultimately, in occident, led to the modern science.

Finally, it appears[11] that in crosscultural and transregional exchange, the body can become a critical site for the negotiation and reconciliation of divergent ideas about the individual, the state, and the cosmos as a whole. The prominence of discourses on medicine and the body in Chinese religious texts represents an attempt to render the abstract goals and benefits of the new religion in terms that were tangible and immediate, while naturalizing and making concrete complex foreign notions about ultimate reality using the most intimate referent possible: the human body. To appropriate Lévi-Strauss' famous dictum, medieval Chinese Buddhists knew well that "the body is good to think." While Buddhism is famous for its otherworldly emphasis on Emptiness and its goal of transcending the mundane world, the physical body, with all of its attendant ailments, remained squarely at the center of the Buddhist project in medieval China.

Buddhist Medicine in Mongolia

Traditional medical practices are enjoying a worldwide revival. Mongolian medicine, once criticized as unscientific, is now acknowledged to be highly effective. China and many Western countries are currently engaged in studying and promoting this ancient medical art.

History

Now a mere handful of former monks were left to keep the religion alive through secret meetings that, if discovered, would have meant almost certain death. And then, as all things must, Mongolia's fate came full circle when in 1987 Mikhail Gorbachev announced the withdrawal of the last Soviet troops stationed in the country.'

Mongolia has practised Tibetan Lamanistic Buddhism since the 16th century. At that time Shamanism was practised and absorbed into the Mongolian form of Buddhism as well as co-existing as a religion in its own right. Mongolia had been ruled by the Chinese for 200 years when, after a brief spell of independence, the Mongolian People's Republic was founded in 1924. The country's first leader was assassinated and Genden became Prime Minister. He increasingly came into conflict with Stalin and refused to carry out the Soviet's leader's demands to persecute the lamas and destroy the monasteries. In 1936 Genden was exiled to the Crimea and in 1937, he was executed.

During the 1930s, leader of the Mongolian Communists, Marshall Choibalsan, presided over the Stalinist purges in Mongolia when over 20,000 monks were murdered and more than 800 monasteries destroyed. [3] Genden's name was banned and not resurrected until 1990. In 1998, in his former home, his daughter Tserendulom opened the Memorial Museum of Victims of Political Persecutions to commemorate, not only her father but, the victims of political genocide - 14% of the population.

History of Mongolian Buddhist Medicine

Historical data shows that Mongolian doctors mastered pulse taking more than two thousand years ago. In 634, the Khan Soronzongombo of Tibet was gravely ill and summoned the best healers from many countries, including

India and China. After all had failed to diagnose the illness, a Mongolian healer arrived in khan's court and accurately discovered the cause of the problem using the pulse. In 789, Khan Tesrondevzun of Tibet arranged a competition among medics from India, China, Pakistan, Nepal, Persia, Khotan, and Mongolia. The winner was a Mongolian healer. As a result the khan issued an edict ordering the translation of the Mongolian medical treatises, Jadva zaril (An Analysis of the Pulse) and Sotvo shashdag jug (A Special Method Used by Mongolian Healers) into Tibetan.'[12]

Mongolian medical treatment traditionally uses a small amount of medicine to treat diseases. Costing less money, it is convenient and easy. Significantly, treatments are not traumatic. Today Mongolian medicine is frequently utilized for treating and preventing chronic and difficult diseases: stomach trouble, liver and gall disorder, coronary heart disease, gynaecological disease, and problems related to blood, skin and bone.

Until this century the history of traditional Mongolian medicine and its achievements were known only among Asians. An important foundation of Mongolian medicine rests with Indian ayurvedic philosophy. When the Mongol Huns travelled through India and Central Asia during the 5th century BC they made contact with the Indian subcontinent. Their travels, together with the spread of Buddhism into Mongolia, confirmed evidence of ancient Mongolian ties with Indian medicine. Much was lost or forgotten until recently but in the 1990s Mongolian doctors from both China and Outer Mongolia began disseminating their knowledge in an attempt to preserve this precious knowledge. Today scholars are translating old sutras written in the Mongolian, Tibetan and Sanskrit languages into English, German and Chinese.

Mongolian medical texts are rooted in history; some are more than 800 years old. Records indicate that sometime around the 11th century, Mongolians created many medical therapies based upon their environment, culture and lifestyle. By the early 13th century, ancient Mongolian medicine coalesced into a sound medical theory based on unique clinical experiences. From the 14th century onwards during the second spread of Buddhism in Mongolia, Mongolians again borrowed and learned from Indian ayurvedic medicine; they translated many Indian books at this time. By the 16th century, ancient Indian medicine and Tibetan medicine had thoroughly integrated into Mongolian medicine. treatments: diet therapy, traditional moxibustion therapy, acupuncture therapy, blood letting therapy, mineral bath therapy, hot-sand therapy and mud therapy, to the northern Chinese.

Since the People's Republic of China was founded it has heartily supported traditional Chinese and Mongolian medicine. In the 1950s Mongolian medicine added western scientific innovations to the vast body of traditional practices. The Chinese government has steadily promoted advances in Mongolian medical care, research and education. In 1958 the Department of Traditional Chinese and Mongolian Medicine at the Inner Mongolia Medical College opened its doors to students. This year it expanded, opening a brand new, state of the art campus just outside of Hohhot City. The Chinese government has also established scores of Mongolian medicine hospitals since 1999.

Mongolian doctors or *emchis* became so adept that they have been respected in Central Asia and China for centuries. During the Ming and Qing dynasties these *emchis* served the Chinese court. They also absorbed Chinese theories, thus propelling the profession again into a new stage of development. Many new principals based on the integration of the ideas of the three cultures were formulated and put in practice. They are still used today.

During the Qing Dynasty (1644-1911) not only *emchis* but also thirty bone-setting Mongolian doctors called *bariachis* waited upon Chinese nobility. These doctors introduced various treatments: diet therapy, traditional moxibustion therapy, acupuncture therapy, blood letting therapy, mineral bath therapy, hot-sand therapy and mud therapy, to the northern Chinese.

Since the People's Republic of China was founded it has heartily supported traditional Chinese and Mongolian medicine. In the 1950s Mongolian medicine added western scientific innovations to the vast body of traditional practices. The Chinese government has steadily promoted advances in Mongolian medical care, research and education. In 1958 the Department of Traditional Chinese and Mongolian Medicine at the Inner Mongolia Medical College opened its doors to students. This year it expanded, opening a brand new, state of the art campus just outside of Hohhot City. The Chinese government has also established scores of Mongolian medicine hospitals since 1999.

The Manba Datsan[13] clinic and training centre for Mongolian traditional medicine was originally set up in Mongolia in 1760 and is now reviving training for treatment by traditional medicine which was prohibited between 1937 and 1990. As part of the State policy to promote Mongolian national religion, culture, customs and historic tradition, the Manba Clinic has been licensed by the Government and is undertaking the following activities:

1. Religious services
2. Clinical and medical treatment
3. Small medicine producing factory
4. Training and research activities
5. Traditional Medical Institute

Religious services: The monks are mostly trained at the Buddhist University before going to the Centre. Further training in the practice of specific rituals and prayers relating to the medicine Buddha are then undertaken. This enables the monks to bestow blessings and perform meditation. They also make astrological calculations.

Clinical and medical treatment: Diagnoses using traditional methods are made and patients are treated with medicinal herbs, powder, pills, precious healing ointment. Treatments can involve non-medicinal therapy such as acupuncture, moxibustion, manipulation, massage, bloodletting, scarifying treatment, exorcism, mantra and meditation.

Small medicine producing factory: On the site of the Centre is a small medicine factory where over 100 traditional products are produced. these are made from imported and local ingredients, both animal and plant. Photography was not permitted in the factory because of the sterile conditions in which the work is undertaken.

Training and Research: The Centre is presently translating treatises on traditional medicine from Tibetan into Mongolian. It is also compiling data, for publication, of indigenous Mongolian herbs. Future plans involve training doctors to run MA and PhD courses in traditional medicine.

Traditional Medical Institute: The Institute's aim is to restore training in traditional medicine by training doctors, over a five-year period, in 70% traditional and 30% Western medicine. The teaching staff are medical doctors, scientists and Buddhist monks. Entry is competitive for students aged 18-24 who take entrance examinations in Mathematics, Chemistry and Physics. The Institute has international links with India, China, Japan, USA, Switzerland, Austria and Russia.

Between 1990 and 1997, 44,000 people attended the Centre for medical checks and treatment. 120,000 were prescribed either Mongolian or European medicines available from the hospital's pharmacy.

Originally a monastery for Chinese Buddhism, Geser Sum is now a working monastery, training young monks. It also practices traditional Buddhist medicine but is best known for astrology and fortune telling. From early morning there are queues of people waiting for 'counselling'. One lady, who came with her son, was born in Arhangai province and had lived in Ulaanbaatar for many years. She asked if she should return to Arhangai and the Lama said prayers and chanted. Dates and venues were asked, calculations made, the Lama consulted his scripts. The lady was told she should return to Arhangai; she paid the Lama and left. The next people who were already in the room waiting, sat down and asked their questions. The young woman who came with an older lady asked if she should go to Korea or Germany to study. After performing the same ritual as he had done with the previous people, the Lama told her to go to Korea. She then asked if her uncle should stay in America, again the calculations and scripts advised her that he should.

An Introduction to Traditional Thai Medicine

Based on Buddhist and Ayurvedic traditions from India, medical traditions from China, and local Hill-Tribe folk medicine, Thai medicine represents a colorful blend of cultural influences. With practitioners of Thai medicine still active in rural and urban Thailand, it remains a familiar tradition within the country of its origin.

Thai massage has become well known in recent years, and is now taught in many massage schools throughout the U.S., but the other branches of Thai medicine have not yet taken hold. Understanding the whole of the Thai medical tradition helps to place Thai massage in its holistic context.

History of Thai Medicine

Thai medicine, like most aspects of culture in Thailand, is based on indigenous tradition and a colorful blend of Indian, Chinese, and Khmer influences. The historical progenitor of Thai medicine, Jivaka Kumar Bhaccha (pronounced by Thais as "Shivago Komarpaj") is revered by almost all practitioners as the "Father Doctor" of Thai medicine. Jivaka was a historical figure, a contemporary of the Buddha, and personal physician to the Buddha's order of monks and nuns over 2,500 years ago. He was a renowned Ayurvedic doctor in his time, and is considered by Thais to be the original teacher of the Thai massage system as well as the source of Thailand's complex herb and mineral pharmacopoeia.

The Father Doctor plays a central role in the spiritual beliefs of Thai healers to this day. Most herbalists, masseurs, and traditional doctors maintain a shrine which includes statuettes of the Buddha and the Father Doctor side-by-side, and prayers such as the one at the beginning of this book

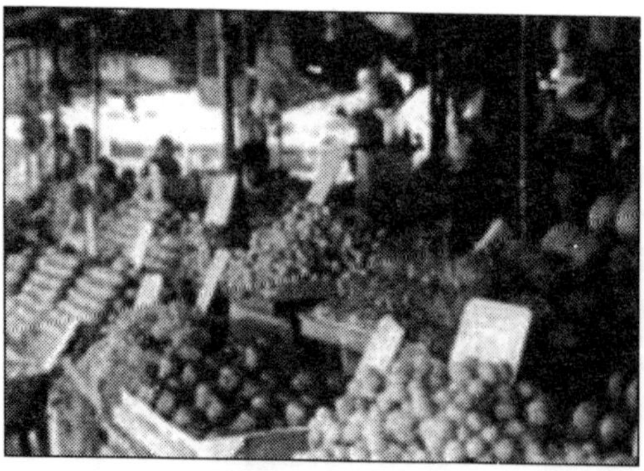

Herbal Medicine Starts with the Food we eat... a Fruit stand at Warorot Market, Chaing Mai

are chanted daily to invoke the spirit of the Father Doctor to assist in the healing of patients.

Legends aside, however, it is difficult to tell how much of the Thai medical traditions actually came from the Buddhist masters. Buddhist ideas are mentioned frequently in the herbal texts of Thailand. However, it is not exactly clear how pervasive this influence is, or at what point Indian ideas entered the Thai culture. According to Harald "Asokananda" Brust, the foremost Western writer on Thai massage, the historical origins of Thai Medicine are shrouded in mystery:

> *Despite what is known about Kumar Bhaccha, much of the origins of Thai massage and traditional Thai medicine still remain obscure. It is believed that the teachings of Kumar Bhaccha reached what is now Thailand at the same time as Buddhismýÿýÿýÿas early as the 3rd or 2nd century BC. It is unknown whether there was any indigenous form of [medicine] in the region before that time. Equally unknown is to what extent Chinese concepts of acupuncture and acupressure (as well as other aspects of traditional medicine) had any theoretical and practical influence.... Nowadays it is impossible to definitively answer such questions, since for centuries medical knowledge was transmitted almost entirely orally from teacher to student following a teaching traditional also common in India.*

It is clear, however, that—regardless of the ultimate dating of its arrival in Thailand—the Indian medical system has for at least 500 years been used as an explanatory model by the Thais, has served as the core theory around which other indigenous ideas have been organized or explained, and has contributed greatly to several important Thai medical practices. Many parallels to Ayurveda can be found in the Thai tradition, and some Thai concepts (such as tridosha and nadis) even share the same names as their Ayurvedic counterparts. Therefore, at least a cursory glance at the Indian traditions is unavoidable in any work on Thai medicinal traditions.

Rural and Royal Traditions

Scholars of Thai medicine have distinguished between the rural and the royal traditions, treating these two as distinct medical systems. There is much overlap between the two, as they share some terminology and herbal recipes. However, it is only the royal tradition that developed a formal theory of disease, symptoms, and treatment.

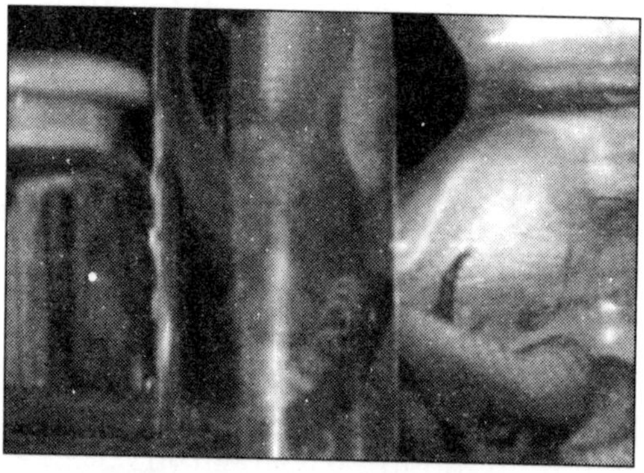

Traditional rural-tradition medicines made from venomous animals!

The Rural and Hill-Tribe Traditions The rural and Hill-Tribe traditions tend to be informal, varying considerably from village to village, tribe to tribe, and indeed from practitioner to practitioner. The livelihood of the rural tradition lies in the hands of uneducated, local male practitioners, famous in small circles for their healing "powers." Rural Thai and Hill-Tribe healers rarely attain the high levels of education that are prerequisite in the royal tradition. The medical knowledge is handed down largely orally, and through secret herbal manuscripts handed down from teacher to pupil. Whereas the royal medical practices have, in the past centuries, emphasized formal scientific treatises, rural Thai medicine has remained to this day more unorganized than centralized, more artistic than dogmatic, and more spiritual than scientific.

Because of the lack of formalized instruction, the local differences in practice, the language barrier, and the aura of secrecy which surrounds the tradition, rural herbal knowledge is difficult to collect, and even more difficult to study comprehensively. True to their secretive tradition, the herbal masters are not likely to give direct answers to theoretical questions, and will sometimes intentionally mislead anthropologists looking to study their healing systems. While this may seem frustrating to the modern scientific mind, it is important to realize that some of the most important practices in the rural tradition are difficult or impossible to explain verbally. Much of the rural and Hill-Tribe practice remains shrouded in spiritual tradition, and is difficult to translate to a modern context. Many of these healers are more properly shamans, and utilize a broad range of shamanic techniques such as exorcisms, amulet charming, and incantations of magic formulas.

It is not my intention to focus on the village traditions in this work. To my knowledge, there are no schools in Thailand that offer courses in rural medicine, and it is exceedingly difficult for Westerners to study under individual practitioners. To this day, there has not been very much written on the subject by either Thai or Western researchers. Of the few that have been written, one eloquent and interesting study (Brun and Schumacher, Traditional Medicine in Northern Thailand) is mentioned in the bibliography at the end of this book as an excellent introduction to this complicated field.

The Wat Po School of "Royal Medicine" At the same time that more informal traditions persisted for centuries in the countryside, temples and hospitals under royal patronage were establishing a consistent system of medical theory and practice. The royal tradition was based on traditional rural lore, but became organized and codified with the

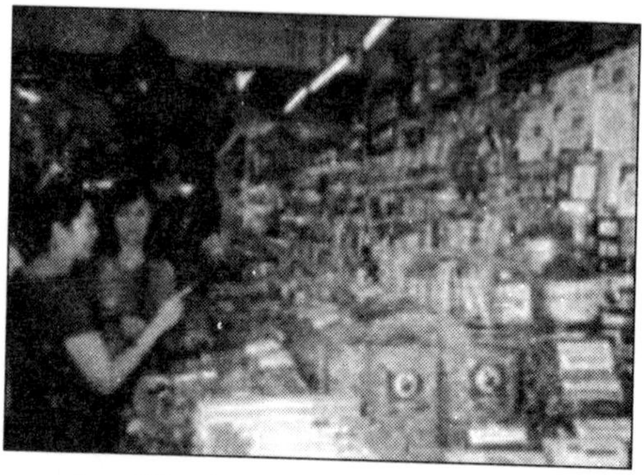

The royal tradition is now the standard form of herbalism in Thailand... An herb vendor at Warorot Market

introduction of Ayurvedic and Western concepts. Buddhism, and along with it many Indian ideas, arrived in the kingdom of Siam in several waves throughout antiquity. A constant flow of information came to the region along with Chinese, Arab, and Indian, merchants. European explorers arrived as early as 1504. The medical traditions picked up something from each of these groups as they came through.

According to Somchintana Ratarasarn, a traditional medicine researcher: *"by about 1600 AD the secular medical system of the Thai people had been established, and had attained maturity as a coherent and highly effective system of health care. It was sustained by... the king, his appointed officials, and the intellectual elite."*

The Wat Po temple was established in the late 1700s under the founder of the current Thai dynasty, Rama I. In 1836, Rama III ordered an extensive renovation of the grounds. At that time, 60 inscribed stone tablets bearing acupressure charts and 1100 herbal recipes were placed in the walls of the temple to preserve medical knowledge for future generations. Over 80 statues depicting massage techniques and yoga postures were erected throughout the grounds as well. These statues and stone tablets can still be seen by visitors to the temple today, and they still form the basis of the royal school of Thai medicine.

From 1895 to 1907, Wat Po's Traditional Medical School published several important herbal manuals to disseminate this valuable information throughout Thailand. These texts are a summary of the ancient traditional lore preserved at Wat Po, and are a useful font of information for Thai and Western scholars. Furthermore, these texts provide the basic curriculum for the school of traditional medicine that still operates on the grounds of the temple.

Unfortunately, to this day, the Wat Po manuals have not appeared in complete English translation. While tourists are able to take short courses on Thai massage in English, the herbalism classes are limited to the Thai language, and therefore remain relatively inaccessible to Westerners. However, enough information has become available to provide a clear picture of the medical practices of the royal school. The theories discussed in this book are based mainly in this royal tradition of Wat Po. Information that comes specifically from the Wat Po texts is noted, as is information that more properly pertains to the rural or Hill-Tribe traditions.

The Branches of Thai Medicine

Traditional medicine in Thailand is historically split into three disciplines: Spiritual healing, massage, and dietary regimens and herbal medicine.

Thai Massage: Thai massage is considered to be a therapy of energy. Masseurs apply acupressure to sensitive points on the body in order to impede or increase the flow of energy through the nadis, or sen lines (Thai energy meridians) as necessary to relieve symptoms and stimulate healing. While Thai massage has enjoyed increasing popularity in the West as of late, it is a field that, in Thailand,

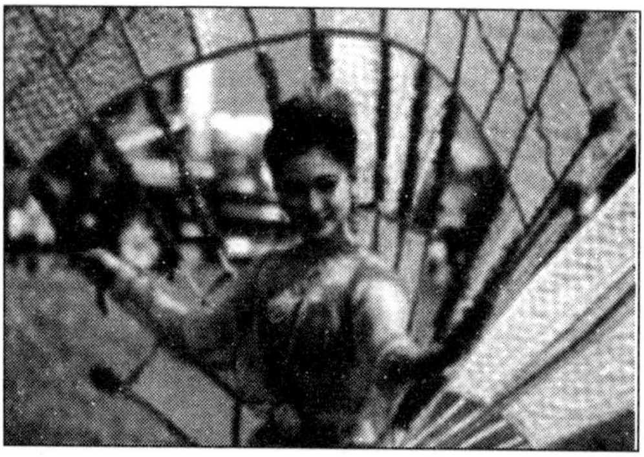

Thai dancer in traditional peacock dress

remains intimately tied to the other branches of traditional medicine.

Dietary regimens and herbal medicine: Herbs and food affect the human organism by causing physiological changes in body chemistry. This is expressed in traditional Thai medicine, like in the Buddhist medicine of India, by the idea of Four Elements. The constant interaction of the Four Elements gives rise to the processes of the body, and therefore is the impetus behind life. The Elements can become unbalanced due to a variety of reasons, including environment, food intake, age, and mental state. During the normal course of one's life, the Elements go in and out of balance in a continuously changing state of health or disease. The primary goal of traditional Thai dietary regimens and herbalism is to maintain balance of the Four Elements for optimum health.

Thai Spiritual healing: Thai medicine emphasizes the spiritual well being of the patient, and holds that many diseases flow from a troubled spirit. For this reason, even modern traditional Thai medicine is enveloped in a rich and intricate tradition of prayer, meditation, mantras, and mythology based around Buddhist and shamanic ideas, which are designed to heal the spirit in order to heal the body.

A Holistic Approach

In Thai philosophy, human life is holistically viewed as a combination of three essences: body, mind, and spirit. The three branches of medicine are each associated with one of these essences. The Thai medical tradition recognizes diseases caused by germs, allergies, environmental factors, heredity, and emotional or psychological imbalance. However, the root cause of any and all disease is the imbalance of the body, mind, and spirit. When the three essences are balanced, the human organism enjoys health and well-being. The imbalance of the three essences causes this natural health and immunity to break down, leaving the organism vulnerable to disease. Maintaining balance of the three essences is therefore the primary focus of traditional Thai medicine.

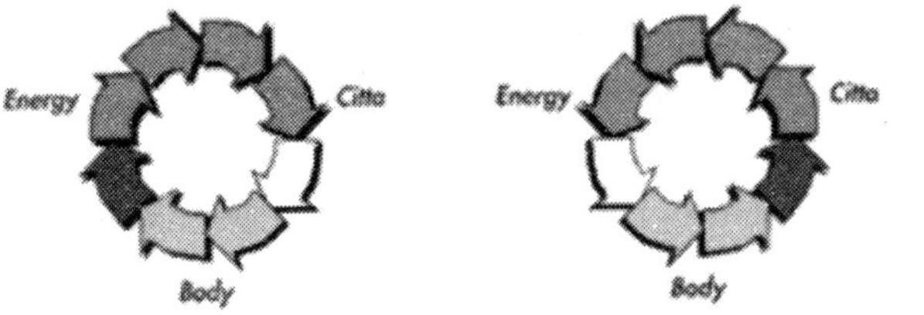

Any of the three traditional Thai therapies alone would work to some extent, but a holistic approach where all are undertaken in conjunction will prove to be much more effective. Thus, in the Thai tradition, all ailments are treated holistically. Holistic medicine follows a balanced approach to healing, treating the body, mind, and spirit together through a combination of therapies designed to strengthen the body's own defenses, instill a sense of mental and physical harmony, and eradicate disease from the root by promoting a naturally healthy lifestyle. A detailed discussion of these ideas, and of the history of Thai medicine, are presented in Pierce Salguero's book, A Thai Herbal.

Traditional Thai Medicine Today & in the Future

In recent years, holistic treatments for mind, body, and energy have slowly begun to gain acceptance by the Western world. While Western medicine still emphasizes body treatments such as prescription drugs, surgery, and so on, alternative or complementary therapies have lately gained much respect in the eyes of the public, and even are begrudgingly accepted in some medical circles. Techniques such as acupuncture and massage have become part of the modern hospital setting in many places, often even being covered under insurance plans.

Countries such as China, Japan, and a few European nations currently lead the way in the integration of modern and traditional practices. In modern Thailand, likewise, the state-of-the-art hospitals and the ancient traditions exist side by side in harmony. Most modern urban and rural Thais utilize the arts of massage, herbal healing, and spiritual healing in addition to modern medical technology from the West. The government of Thailand, in fact, is one of the biggest supporters of this blend of traditional and modern healing. In rural areas that remain far from Western hospitals, government-operated herbal clinics dispense tried and true traditional remedies alongside allopathic drugs with the support and blessing of the World Health Organization and UNICEF.

As East and West each become more familiar with the wisdom of the other, it is natural that the best of the ancient and the modern will come together in a new synthesis. It is the challenge of the modern era to create a new model of medicine, and this model will begin with a deeper understanding of the human as not merely a physical entity, but a complex interwoven system of body, mind and energy.

Herbal medicines are often thought to lack the effectiveness of over-the-counter and prescription allopathic medications, and are sometimes considered to be mere placebos. In fact, natural substances form the basis of many of today's synthetic drugs, including as aspirin, painkillers, and antibiotics. Many herbal medicines contain the same active ingredients as their allopathic counterparts, and can be just as effective.

Herbal remedies may not have the immediate effect of Western drugs in treating acute disease or discomfort, but this is because they tend to work on the body as a whole than on any specific group of symptoms. Because the impact of any particular herb on the body is ameliorated by that herb's natural bland of complementary alkaloids, herbal medicines have a subtler effect on the system. One who is desensitized to these subtle effects due to years of use of pharmaceuticals, alcohol, nicotine, and caffeine may not initially notice the impact of herbs. However, through persistent use of herbal remedies, generally improving the diet, exercising, meditating, and living in harmony with the body and with nature, one will soon find that the benefits of herbs are not only noticeable, but indispensable!

CHAPTER 5

TIBETAN MEDICINE
A "Science of Healing" Closely Related to Buddhism

The Tibetan culture is a magnificent culture, which started more than 4000 years ago in Shang Shung, the first kingdom of Tibet. Its deep knowledge and understanding has been kept alive through centuries. Knowledge in Tibetan culture is traditionally classified into five major fields: arts, crafts, linguistics and poetry, medicine and - most important - the so called "inner knowledge" which refers to the understanding of the relative and ultimate condition of the individual within his or her universe. It also includes a myriad of hidden and highly specialized esoteric instructions that can be considered as the real treasure of our planet. This treasure has been transmitted from generation to generation through all the centuries and is therefore still alive today.

The Tibetan medical system is one of the world's oldest known medical traditions. It is an integral part of Tibetan culture and has been developed through many centuries. We believe that the origin of the Tibetan medical tradition is as old as civilization itself.

It is interesting to note that east-to-east mutual technological exchanges among Asian nations were quite frequent in the past. The Silk Road must have played a significant role in the spread of early technologies. For example, the *Bower Manuscript* (mss) was found in 1890 in Kuchar, Turkistan in a Buddhist monastery on the great caravan route to China. The large medical treatise called *Navanitaka* forms the second part of the *Bower mss*. The date of that mss falls in the second half of the fourth century AD. It is believed that Buddhist monks played a significant role in the transmission of medicinal technologies among the Asian countries. Tibet was in a unique position to receive such knowledge both from China and India.

In the West, the field of Tibetan medicine has been a little known traditional medical system. Throughout Asia, however, for centuries it has been highly respected for its effectiveness. Tibetan medicine became known in the Western world with the exile of the Tibetan people from their homeland in Central Asia. With the Chinese invasion and occupation of the country of Tibet and the exile of more than 100,000 Tibetans to India in 1959, the Tibetan Medical Center in Dharamsala, India, was established by Tenzin Gyatso. Known as the 14th Dalai Lama of Tibet, the secular and religious leader of Tibetan Buddhists, he is perhaps more widely recognized as the Nobel Peace Prize winner of 1989. The medical center he created was meant to preserve the heritage of Tibetan medical practices and to maintain the ongoing study and practice of Tibetan medicine. The interest and practice of Tibetan medicine has also grown with the steady increase of interest in Eastern meditational, philosophical, and psychological methods and with their integration into Western culture. Despite these measures, the preservation of Tibetan medicine is imperiled by its inability to flourish in its own country as it had for centuries. Also, many Tibetan medical doctors were lost when "over one million Tibetans . . . died as a . . . result of the Chinese occupation"[14].

Among Asian traditional medicines based on a written corpus, Tibetan medicine was the latest to attain noticeable recognition outside its cultural area. Research on Tibetan "science of healing" (gso-ba rig-pa) in fact developed only from the middle of the 20th century, especially with the influx of refugees towards the South, escaping from the army of the young Chinese People's Republic, which had taken control of the Tibetan plateau. At the same time, teachings imparted throughout the world by religious leaders of the Diaspora, Tibetan defense groups' activism, promotion of alternative medicines, development of tourism in regions of Tibetan culture, and a certain craze for media coverage have publicized among the general public the existence and possibly the resources of this medicine to different extents.

Finally, since a few decades, Tibetan medicine has undergone an increasing institutionalization in many regions of its traditional geographic area, where it is now confronted everywhere with local avatars of the globalized biomedicine. NGOs implicated it in primary health or even environmental protection programs at the local level, and in some cases it was integrated into national health systems in different forms.

While we restrict our subject here to the scholarly system of Tibetan medicine, one should however emphasize that a majority of native health practices depended – and still depends in many remote areas – on ways that are not strictly medical: popular therapeutic practices, formal acts aiming to accumulate merits (donation to the poor or religious institutions, freeing an animal destined to be slaughtered, patronage of the recitation of religious texts for example), visits to sacred places and pilgrimages, blessings of great religious figures, wearing protective charms, resorting to divinatory and astrological calculations, rituals of exorcism, longevity or recovery, diagnostic or cure done by a medium possessed by a god.

History and Origins: Part 1, until 8th century

Design from a Tibetan medical text showing the three "rivers" of Indian, Chinese and Tibetan medicine flowing into one great lake of knowledge, from which arises the Arura, king of remedies.

The Tibetan medicine seems to be a creative combination of the Indian medical traditions, which it imported with Buddhism from India, and many forms of Chinese medicine. These multiple layers of medical knowledge and traditions merged with pre-Buddhist Shamanic traditions and have continued to develop up to the present as a thriving and highly effective indigenous medical system.

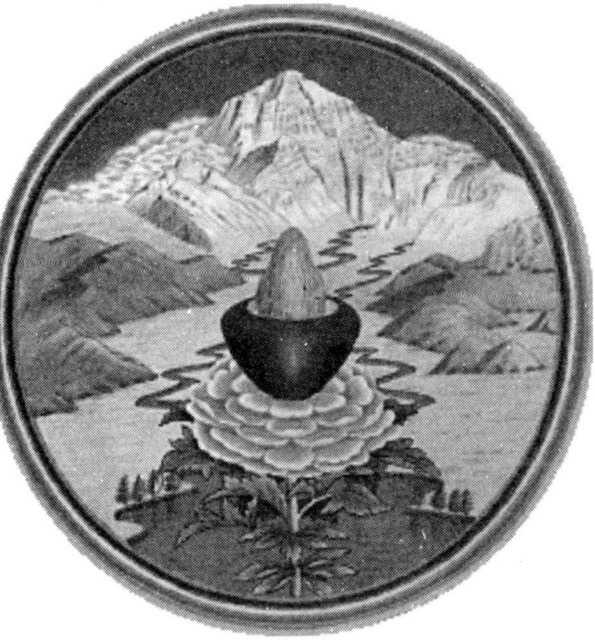

General: The main formation of what we know today as Traditional Tibetan Medicine (TTM) came in the 7th and 8th centuries C.E. Before this, Tibetans had a folk medicine and vetinary science, much other ethnic groups throughout the world, based upon experiential knowledge of the therapeutic qualities of local plants, salts, minerals and animal products. Before 7th Century: there were significant visits from foreign doctors, such as the physicians sent from India by the Buddhist King Asoka (3rd century BCE) to spread medical science through Asia. There was doubtless some intercourse with China through trading caravans. There are various accounts of early regional kings in whose biographies medicine is mentioned. Of note are the 5th century Lha-mtho-ri, who brought two eminent doctors (Vijay Gajay and Billa Gazema from Bodh Gaya, in Bihar) from India to teach diagnostic procedures to Tibetans, and the 6th century hBron-gnyan, whose son was successfully operated upon for cataracts using a couching method with a golden scalpel. A son of Vijay Gajay, Dungyi Tharchok, learnt the system from his father and became the first personal physician of the King.

7th Century: *King Srong-btsan* created the first unified Tibet and a Tibetan empire. He brought civilisation to his people by having scholars create an alphabet and grammar suited to the native tongue and by inviting scholars from the great civilisations of Asia.

To introduce the best of medical science, he brought knowledge from India, China and Persia.

This was facilitated by his two main queens being the result of royal marriage alliances with China and Nepal. Of note were: the translation and introduction of the "Great Medical Treatise", translated from Chinese by Ha-shang Mahadeva and Dharmakosha,

- the transmission of knowledge from the Chinese master physician Han-wang-Hang (Hsuan-Yuan Huang-ti)
- the transmission of knowledge from the Indian master physician Bharadaja (Rishi Bharadwaj)
- the transmission of knowledge from the Persian master physician Galenos (hard to tell whether he used this name himself or whether he acquired through constant reference to Galen).

These three eminent doctors set down severally the essentials of their healing arts in texts in the new language. More interestingly, they produced a seven-chapter treatise ("The Weapon of the Fearless") based upon their mutual discussions and interaction. The first two eventually returned to their homeland but Galenos remained as Court Physician, married and had three sons whom he trained as doctors and who subsequently *spread the medical science* in northern, central and southern Tibet. There was also a royal programme for training bright boys to become doctors.

8th Century: Many medical texts were translated into Tibetan (mostly from Chinese) in the first half of the 8th century and a first set of medical ethics were laid down for court and other physicians. The major event in Tibetan history, however, was the reign of *King Khri-srong-lde-btsan* during the latter half of the century. It was he who firmly established Buddhism in Tibet and under whose patronage hundreds of bright children were trained as translators to bring the best of Asian civilisation to the land. Of particular note was *Vairocana*, who mastered and translated the Fourfold Medical Treatise (*rgyud bzhi*), the extensive presentation of the Indian Buddhist medical system which was to become the very foundation stone of the Tibetan medical system. However, the main spiritual figure in Tibet at the time - Padmasambhava - judged it to be too early to introduce so complete and profound a system [there was considerable religious tension at the time as the ancient animist religion and healers were holding out with much resistance; their numbers included influential government ministers]. It was decided to conceal the translations and instructions in a chalice-shaped pillar on the rooftop of the great Samye monastery, with prayers that the right person would discover and propagate this complete medical science at the right time.

Nevertheless, King Khri-srong was determined to establish an excellent medical system. Knowing that the full system - based upon the Fourfold Treatise - would come later, he brought eminent physicians from neighbouring lands and had them translate from medical sources of the great countries of Asia. During this period a great wealth of Asian medicine came to Tibet. Later, with the unveiling of the Fourfold Treatise, all these strands of wisdom would be drawn together under a great and unifying light, benefiting from the rigour of Buddhist logic and the already 1,300-year old psychological and psychiatric knowledge developed through Buddhism's thorough analysis of mind, body and their interrelation, not to mention its direct investigation of these through meditation. The king had a number of intelligent young men trained in the techniques embodied in these translations. Nine of them became most learned and were appointed Court Physicians. Of particular note was the first gYu.THog.Yon.Tan.Gon.po. (pronounced Yutok Yeunten Gonpo), probably the most famous Tibetan physician of all. The more extraordinary stories about him make him almost the incarnation of the healing art itself and contain all the wonder and vastness of the discovery of that art by humankind. He is seen by Tibetans as remanifesting (one may consider this as reincarnating) some centuries later to become the guardian and expounder of the Fourfold Treatise teachings hidden at Samye.

Philosophy of Tibetan Medicine System

The Tibetan medicine system is essentially based on the Buddhist philosophy. According to them the universe is composed of four basic elements: *sa* (*prithivi-mahabhuta*), *chu* (*jala mahabhuta*), *me* (*agni mahabhuta*), and *rlun* (*vayu mahabhuta*). But in Ayurveda the fifth element *akasa* is also present. The Tibetans also believed that the individual is an exact replica of the macrocosm.

Note 1: Some commentators talk of Indian ayurveda as being one of the sources of Tibetan medicine. This point needs some clarification, otherwise one might understand it to have its roots in Hindu medicine, which is not the case. "Ayurveda" - as its name suggests - is the term used these days for the medical science of India which started with the ancient Hindu scriptures, the *Veda*. One must bear in mind, however, the fact that Hindu and Buddhist medicine nourished and cross-fertilised each other for almost 1,700 years after the modest medical beginnings of the Vedic period and became similar in their material application, if different in their world-vision and healing rituals. Around the 12th-13th century, Buddhism was virtually eradicated from India by foreign invasions. The multi-sourced Indian medical science, however, continued under Hinduism with the Hindu name of *ayurveda*. As mentioned above, Tibetan Medicine has one of its main roots in the Indian *Buddhist* medicine of the 8th-12th centuries, which somewhat resembles the *ayurveda* of India today.

Note 2: Another aspect of Indian Buddhist medicine at the time was *siddha medicine*. The *siddha* were highly-accomplished meditators and quite extraordinary beings, with a great deal of knowledge of chemistry. They had elaborate techniques for detoxifying metals and minerals used in complex medical formulae employing metals, precious stones, minerals, plants and sometimes animal products. They also had superlative knowledge of using the mind to benefit the body. Their skills were handed down in a very discrete and secretive way. This tradition went to Tibet under the influence of the great Indian masters of the 8th-12th centuries and has persisted in an unbroken tradition until this day. However, in India, due to the virtual disappearance of Buddhist siddhas, this form of medicine has deteriorated considerably from its high origins but nevertheless continues, in a diminished and sometimes even quite corrupt form, mainly in southern India. One should not confuse the ancient and mostly secret techniques preserved carefully over a millennium by Tibetan master physicians with the *siddha medicine* of southern India today.

Development 8th Century on

General: Part One took us to the end of the 8th century, by which time many of the elements of Tibetan Medicine had been introduced into Tibet but were not yet well established. Some had been kept secret and hidden for future times, especially those related to the Fourfold Treatise. From the 9th century until the present day, those initial elements have become firmly rooted, enhanced and practised in a widespread way. 9th Century: There was period of violent reaction to the new wave of Buddhist and foreign culture introduced by King Khri-Srong, under his successor King Langdarma and his animist priests and ministers. Most vestiges of the Buddhist religion were destroyed. During and after his reign, the empire crumbled, there was considerable anarchy and a low period in Tibetan history.

Some medical historians say that although Buddhism suffered terribly, the medical tradition continued unaffected. This is very doubtful. It probably continued but in a diminished form, as many of the best physicians had been based in the Buddhist monasteries destroyed and the whole ethos of modernising Tibetan knowledge had suffered through reactionaries trying to restore the old order. Although so much was translated, very few manuscripts remain from this early period.

It was in the latter half of the 10th century that Tibetan medicine took its the next significant step forward. A wave of diligent and heroic people of both lands plied between India and Tibet, working hard to restore culture in Tibet and bring it the best that India had to offer. They were known as *lotsawa*, which literally means translators. These were not mere linguists but great scholars end enlightened beings in their own right, 'translating' in the very broadest sense the jewels of one culture into another. From the 10th-12th century, they not merely restore Buddhism and medicine in Tibet but considerably augmented them, broadening their bases and firmly implanting a culture which was to last until the late 20th century. Among other things, they translated one of the most important early medical texts, the *yan-lag brgyad-pa'i snying-po bsdus-pa* ("Quintessence of the Eight Branches of Medicine), in 120 chapters, and its commentary, *bZl.ba'i 'od.Zer* ("Moonbeams").

11th Century : Probably the most influential of the translators was *Rin.chen bZang.po* (958-1055). He studied in general under 75 great masters of India and spent much time mastering the medical teachings of Janadarna, especially the Quintessence of the Eight Branches text and its commentary. He taught, established and spread these medical teachings in Tibet. *The lineages arising from his students* gave a major uplift to, and considerably increased, the practice of TTM.

In all, 158 texts were translated and edited under his guidance.

During this century, profound notions of the psychosomatic nature of the human being and his/her interdependence with the immediate and more distant universe in which s/he lives were adopted, through the teachings of the *Kalachakra tantra*. These study, among many other things, the influence of time of day, season of the year etc. on human biology and temperament: as Professor Meyer puts it: *inherited ... Indian concepts pertaining to the structure of the body, conception, physiopathology and therapy.*

History makes particular mention of nine master physicians of Rin.chen bZang.po's lineage towards the end of the 11th century. Two of them brought new developments. *Shang-ston gZi Brjid-'bar* went to India and studied the Eightfold Quitessence extensively in Nalanda under the great doctor Chadravi. He returned to Tibet with many teachings, which he translated. *sTod-ston dKonchog Skyabs* also went to India and studied these same works under Master Shintipa. sTod ston is best known for instructing the Later Yuthog (see below) in the *Moonbeams* commentary on the Eightfold Quintessence. During the last half of the century, *gTer-ston Gra-pa mNon-shes* (1012-1090), is believed to have revealed the Fourfold Treatise hidden three centuries previously in the pillar of Samye monastery by Vairocana. Some Tibetans see him as the reincarnation of Vairocana because of this.

12th Century: This brings us to the most famous of Tibetan physicans - the *2nd Yuthog* (1112-1203) - and the most famous medical work - the Fourfold Treatise. The latter work draws together in a masterly way all the elements that had entered Tibetan medicine up to that time. About its origins, Professor Meyer says, in "Oriental Medicine":

The origin and history of the Four Tantras remain obscure and were the subjects of heated dispute among Tibetan scholars. Some accepted it for what it claims to be: the authentic teachings of the Buddha 'Master of Remedies' (*Bhaisajyaguru*), translated from Sanskrit, whereas others saw it as a treatise of dubious authorship. Some even went as far as to deny a Sanskrit original and believe it to be the work of a Tibetan author - one or the other Yuthog - observing quite correctly that it contains notions foreign to India, notably those which appear to be Chinese. However, the opinion that the Four Tantras were the authentic word of the Buddha prevailed under the political authority of the Fifth Dalai Lama and his regent Sangye Gyamtso, who firmly upheld this view. They believed the Four Tantras were first taught in India by the historical Buddha when he first manifested as the 'Master of Remedies'. Later, in the eighth century, Vairocana is said to have translated and offered the text to his master Padmasambhava, who then concealed it in the monastery of Samye. In the second half of the leventh century it was supposedly rediscovered by Drapa Ngonshe (1012-90) and the following century it ended up in the hands of Yuthog the Younger, who completed the Treatise by adapting it to the local conditions of Tibet. This would explain how it came to contain non-Indian elements. This is a reasonable exoteric explanation. The view of one of (if not the) greatest contemporary TTM physician, Professor Khenpo Troru Tsenam, resolves any controversy by pointing out the way the Buddha is envisaged in Northern Buddhism, i.e. not just as an historical Indian figure but also as a constant inspirational presence (*sambhogakaya*) to this world during the five millennia following his enlightenment and, more generally, as the guiding presence of the absolute, anywhere and in anyone. If this 'pure mind' had appeared to Yuthog and guided his brilliant work of the Four Tantras, then the text becomes at one and the same time the authentic teaching of the Buddha and a contemporary edition. This does not preclude the possibility of it being also a revision and update of an ancient text-authentically from the Buddha - made suitable to its times by the Buddha's own, later, influence on Yuthog.

Whatever the origins of the Fourfold Treatise, it is certainly *the* text of TTM and a brilliant one at that. So much of TTM literature is composed of commentaries to the Fourfold Treatise and, like many great works, it always seems to stand above and beyond its commentaries in a pristine and commanding position.

Yuthog himself is surrounded by legend and was doubtless an extraordinary figure, who visited India many times and whose clear and all-encompassing mind was able to possess and present an overview of all the various components present in the medical science of Tibet at the time. His work is not merely the fruit of a clear mind but also that of a wide-ranging medical experience and considerable travel.

12th-15th Centuries: the main recorded medical tradition over this period was that of Yuthog, in Central Tibet. Other similar traditions flourished in Western Tibet and the Sakya area and all over Tibet medicine continued in a simple and domestic way as father-to-son transmission.

15th-17th Centuries: the two famous traditions of BYANG and ZUR In the early to mid 15th century, these two important systems of TTM developed, in Northern and Southern Tibet respectively, each based upon the Fourfold Treatise but with a different view to its nature, some slight differences of interpretation and some variance in plant recognition. The latter is not surprising and evokes a problem we have often encountered in preparing our database of TTM *materia medica* here at Tara Rokpa. Whereas in the West botanical recognition is based primarily upon plant shape and colour, which define whole species and subspecies, in TTM the prime importance lies in the medicinal properties. Often several quite different plants bear the same name in TTM.

Not all plants grow in all countries. Even when the same species is found in different places, its medicinal properties can vary enormously depending upon the altitude, climate and geographical conditions of its situation. As medicine spread from other countries to Tibet and from one region of Tibet to another, local substitutes had sometimes to be found for the *materia medica* prescribed in the Fourfold Treatise and other authoritative texts but not found locally. These substitutes frequently took on the name of the original remedy. It happened that sometimes local substitutes even turned out to have properties surpassing those of the original.

The Byang and Zur systems developed independently in the 15th century, cross-fertilised each other in the 16th century and virtually merged into one during the late 17th century, under the powerful influence of *Regent Desi Sangye.*

The BYANG system originated with Jangdagpa (*byang.bdag rnam.rgyal grags.bzang*) (1395-1475). He and his followers composed many medical treatises, especially commentaries on the Fourfold Tantra. Their system flourished in the north of Tibet. They held the Fourfold Treatise to be a teaching given directly by the Buddha.

The ZUR system started some 50 years later, in Southern Tibet, through Zurkhapa (*zur.mkar mnyam.nyid rdo.rje*) (1439-1475). A child prodigy, he was strongly influenced by the Yuthog Nyintik esoteric medical tradition stemming from the Second Yuthog. In a powerful dream, he received instruction that the extant versions of the Fourfold Treatise and other related texts had become corrupted over the centuries, through additions and alterations, and that he should revise them. This he did meticulously, returning to Indian source documents and convening conferences of doctors from all parts of Tibet. His brief but important life gave a great renewal to TTM and launched one of its most famous traditions.

17th Centuries: the influence of the Vth Dalai Lama and Regent Desi Sangye Gyamtso The Vth Dalai Lama (1617-16820 gained power over many Tibetan areas and became a powerful monarch. He *founded several medical schools,* away from the new capital Lhasa. His main disciple and future Regent, Desi Sangye (*sde.srid sangs.rgyas rgya.mtsho*) (1563-1705) was a brilliant scholar. Under his direction, a team of doctors and scholars studied the various commentaries of the Byang and Zur traditions on the Fourfold Treatise and reported back to him on differences, discrepancies and moot points. From all this research, a major commentary, the 'Blue Vaidurya Treatise' was composed. It has many great qualities and is very highly respected today. The shortcoming of the work is that Desi Sangye was not a practising physician but a medical theoretician. He had a busy political, academic and religious life. It is for this reason that we have - for many years now at Tara - have used a wide range of commentaries, especially those based on deep practical experience, for our researches even though the Blue Vaiduya has received much attention in the West in recent years and is thought of by many as being *the* commentary on the Fourfold Treatise. This is not really at all the case.

The Vth Dalai Lama was not completely happy with his medical colleges and asked Desi Sangye to find a suitable location near Lhasa to found one. It was thus that (some years later, after the Dalai Lama's passing and during Desi Sangye's regency) the Iron Hill (lcags.po.ri) Medical College was established. It was ordained that each monastery, i.e.

each district, would receive a doctor trained in the College and thus it represented the beginnings of a public health system in Tibet. The political power of Desi Sangye's tradition - the Gelugpa school - at the time meant that this medical movement soon came to dominate a great part of the Tibetan plateau. It effectively drew the Byang and Zur traditions into one (although it was more the case that the Byang was absorbed into the Zur) and launched a new wave of TTM.

18th Centuries: The Iron Hill Medical school became a model that was copied in Eastern Tibet, at Kumbum in 1757, at Labrang in 1784, in Beijing at the Yonghegong around 1750 and also in Mongolia and Transbaikalia.

There was a flowering of TTM in Eastern Tibet during this century, under the influence of Dilmar Geshe, whose catalogue of *materia medica* became the widely accepted reference. Eastern Tibet is far less barren than Central Tibet and is one of the main sources for many of the herbs, plants and trees used in TTM. Dilmar Geshe's famous disciple was the 8th Situpa, Choji Jungnay (*chos.kyi byung.gnas*) (1700-1774) a religious figure, grammarian, poet, scientist and doctor of incomparable skills. He founded a medical school at Palpung, in the Tibetan kingdom of De-Ge in far Eastern Tibet, which also showed a great open mindedness to the great wealth of classical Chinese knowledge of art, medicine and science.

Tibetan Medical System

The development of Tibet's scholarly medical system was intimately linked to its culture, and therefore to Buddhism that has strongly influenced all its aspects. Buddhism in fact shows close affinities to medicine at several levels. As a doctrine and path to salvation, recovery from illnesses has quite naturally imposed itself as a metaphor for the ultimate liberation from being enslaved to the endless cycle of re-births. Besides, and more fundamentally, the problem of suffering has always remained at the heart of its Soteriology. Finally, this affinity of Buddhism to medicine was further strengthened, in the beginning of our era, with the doctrinal development of Mahayana and its new idea of Bodhisattva, "Being dedicated to Enlightenment", for which healing of the battered bodies is both the opportunity for cultivating the perfections of compassion and generosity, and a skilful means of converting the beings. Medical science itself was from then on open to being part of the syllabus for Buddhist studies, especially in the monasteries. Around the same time, the Buddhist pantheon developed with figures having therapeutic connotation. Among these, the Buddha, Master of Medicine, (Bhaisajyaguru) was worshipped with great devotion in Central Asia, then in the Far-East, and later in Tibet.

Classical Tibetan historiography places the origins of the medical tradition in the 7th century, when Tibet, at the time unified for the first time to the extent of being an empire, came in contact with ancient neighboring civilizations: India, China, Central Asia and the Iranian world. Having acquired a style of writing borrowed from India, it could gradually assimilate a great many texts (especially Buddhist), including medical books. The variety of influences, particularly Indian and Chinese, probably even Greco-Arab, which according to the Tibetan historiographers would have marked the origins of their medicine, is corroborated by ancient Tibetan documents and by traces of these influences that can be found in the medical treatises that are still used today. Through the centuries, some of these influences were abandoned, while others were integrated, with the heritage of native therapies, into a coherent whole of knowledge and specialized practices. The treatise called The Fourfold Tantra (rGyud-bzhi) became the corpus of reference for all the Tibetan practitioners, in a vast medical literature that is still little known.

Medical teaching, texts as well as oral instructions and practical techniques, was imparted for centuries, often together with religious teachings, not in specific institutions, but from master to disciple, often in a monastic setting, or from father to son along family lineages. Traditionally, this teaching was not sanctioned by formal degrees, and the medical practice did not require any recognition, by any civil or religious authority, which would have required a standard level of theoretical knowledge or technical expertise. Moreover, the Tibetan practitioners have never constituted a well-defined socio-professional group, and many had other main functions, particularly religious. It's only at the end of the 17th century that the first monastic establishment especially devoted to medical teaching was founded, on the Iron Hill (Lcags-po-ri) near Lhasa. Later it served as a model for establishing some other similar establishments in Eastern Tibet, at Beijing and in Mongolia. Finally, Tibetan medical science gained a renewed impetus when the Tibetan Astro-Medical Institute (sMan-rtsis-khang) was founded by the Thirteenth Dalaï Lama in 1916, with a lesser clerical orientation, in the very heart of Lhasa. Nevertheless, parallel to these centers of institutionalized medical teachings, sanctioned by examinations, medical tradition continued to be imparted, like in the past, outside all official control, by individual practitioners, in family lineages or not, at inevitably very varied levels of knowledge and practices. Some women had thus access to medical teaching, generally with their father.

Tibetan science of healing, as it is presented in its reference treatise, The Fourfold Tantra supposed to have been taught by the Buddha Master of Medicine, has nothing of an empiric medicine. On the contrary it was consciously developed as a sophisticated system of which all the parts, whether they come under empirical experience or theoretical speculation, are integrated into a coherent whole subjected to epistemological rules and formal logic, based on a limited number of natural laws.

Tibetan Buddhist Medicine is a fascinating and complex interweaving of religion, mysticism, psychology, and rational medicine . . . . It is the product of an ancient culture very different from our own . . . and at first may seem . . . incomprehensible, especially to [one] unacquainted with Buddhism, with which it is so inseparably linked. The tradition includes a vast body of medical literature . . . enormous pharmacopoeia . . . and unusual methods of diagnosis and treatment.

Its practice contains in-depth philosophical and psychological bases for diagnosis and treatment of illness, including physical, mental, and spiritual imbalances. Numerous ideas and concepts are combined to affect the healing process, and various medications and treatments are also used. Using a humanistic framework to treat the client with dignity and to assist in the alleviation of suffering, the profound wisdom embodied in the development of this medicine is seen clearly through the practical application of its deeper theories and its functional ability to effect cures. To a Tibetan medicine practitioner, removing symptoms without treating the whole being is to miss the opportunity to assist the client in true healing and would be considered neglect.

One important aspect of Buddhism is its psychological belief system that addresses the many concerns of one who is seeking a deeper meaning in life. Its aim is to bring out the true self beyond the mask of personality, leading to meaningful life objectives and personal growth. Viewing personality as the learned complex of characteristics with which we identify our individuality, the purpose of Buddhist psychology and meditation is to go beyond these traits and recognize one's true nature or wholeness. Called "the truth body" or the unobstructed mind of enlightenment, one's true nature is considered to be "free of all coverings" (i.e., personality) (Landaw, 1987, p. 167). The Tibetan concept of personality is drawn from the two major branches of Buddhist texts. The first, the Maha Anuttara Yoga Tantra (Highest Yoga Tantra), deals with spiritual and emotional aspects of the mind in relationship with the body's various psychic energies. The second, the Abhidharma texts, contains a psychological theory derived from the study of observations of the mind's workings. Different levels within the branches can be studied, according to the level of mind and the ability of the student.

Three distinct disciplines of practice lie within Tibetan medicine: dharmic, tantric, and somatic medicines[16]. As Rapgay (1985) explains, "the Tibetan tradition contains a comprehensive theory of personality, a diagnostic system and theory of pathology derived from Tibetan medicine, systems of classification of psychopathology and a cosmology that allows for the intervention of non-human (or transpersonal) entities" (p. 52). As in contemporary holistic health practices, the essence of health in Tibetan medicine is holistic harmony. Yet theirs is a harmony of formless, subtle and manifest worlds, of mental, emotional and physical bodies, of spiritual, psychological and organic developments, of self, others and total environment. In the view of Tibetan medicine the microcosm of the body and the macrocosm of the universe are constantly dancing with each other. When they are out of step with each other or when they are out of tune with the spiritual reality that sets them moving, disease results. (Clifford, 1984, p. 89).

As in contemporary holistic health practices, personal responsibility, co participation between client and practitioner, and prevention are stressed in Tibetan medicine. The need to assist in removing physical symptoms so that true healing can occur is accepted, and complementary therapies are often prescribed. Suggestions by the practitioner may be given as a means for helping a client effect positive changes in lifestyle behaviors. Caring, an attitude of kindness and compassion, is seen as an essential ingredient in assisting clients to mobilize their resources toward a state of wellness, and causative factors, the deeper meanings of illness, are explored with clients. The depth of the healer's wisdom and compassion is believed to be directly related to the ability to effect a cure. The Tibetan medical doctor aspires to emulate the Medicine Buddha, the form of Buddha nature that embodies the healing aspects to cure spiritual, psychological and physical disease. It is believed that "through the practice of meditation on the Medicine Buddha, one can generate enormous powers for self-healing and the healing of others" (Clifford, 1984, p. 33). This art of healing involves maintaining balance within the body and its functions, as well as between the person and the outer environment. Illness, therefore, is considered a lack of harmony within the mind-body complex or between it and the world at large.

Dharmic Medicine

As the mind-to-body relationship is considered of foremost importance, control of the mind is the main key to this balance. Mind creates matter and therefore also illness and wellness. Meditation and yoga are used as therapeutic modalities to balance the mind-body complex. This is the realm of dharmic medicine[17]. Dharma, from the Sanskrit literally meaning "that which holds one back from suffering," is the spiritual teaching of Buddhism (Landaw, 1987, p. 160). Meditation and the mind training practices commonly called the practice of dharma) taught in dharmic medicine are considered means of learning how to control one's mind so that it can be trained to function in a balanced fashion with the body. The integration of this philosophy into daily life is an important element in the development of general health and well-being. This is akin to the holistic health model in nursing in which "in work, goals, relationships, the nexus of the body, mind-spirit connections [are] made and the search of these patterns and processes becomes a way of existence" (Dossey, 1981, pp. 37-38). The dharma is considered the "best medicine," and the purpose of dharma is "to cut the root of the mind's delusion," which is viewed from the Buddhist perspective as the true or ultimate cause of suffering.

The primary aim of Buddhism is to understand the nature of mind and to develop compassion and greater awareness in one's life. Illness can encourage us to examine our lives and to learn what supports good health and what aspects and behaviors of our lives generate disease and suffering. Emotional, spiritual, and physical suffering that helps one develop compassion for oneself also provides a meaningful link with the outside world. All beings desire happiness and peace of mind. "Feeling somehow incomplete, insecure and unfulfilled, we look outside ourselves for something or someone that will make us feel whole," which we try to possess. When that attractive object does not fulfill our desires, we grasp after yet another object. As Landaw describes, "in this way we continue to circle around and around, changing this and that in our lives but never really getting any closer to our desired happiness and peace of mind" (pp. 35-37). Because all people are alike in wanting happiness and avoiding suffering, this awareness then becomes one of the primary bases for choosing compassion and compassionate action as "one wing of the bird" of personal growth. The other is skillful means or wisdom, the insight into emptiness (shunyata in Sanskrit meaning the absence of all false ideas about how things exist — specifically, the lack of apparent independent self-existence of phenomena [Landaw, 1987, p. 161]). The opposite of emptiness is subject-object dualism.

This dualistic view is considered an ignorant view characteristic of the unenlightened mind in which all things are falsely conceived to have concrete self-existence; to such a view, the appearance of an object is mixed with the false image of its being independent or self-existent thereby leading to further dualistic views concerning subject and object, self and other, this and that, etc. (Landaw, 1987, p. 161).

Karma, the workings of cause and effect whereby positive actions produce happiness and negative actions produce suffering, are considered latent predispositions that exist at the subconscious level of the mind. When internal or external causes and conditions arise, an experience of positive or negative factors is activated. These factors are considered one significant cause of disease. An awareness of karma and the law of impermanence (a recognition that all things change) are essential to understanding suffering. Renunciation is the attitude of wishing to leave behind the suffering of life and death and their causes, and to attain instead the peace of full enlightenment of Buddhahood. The view of renunciation, the attitude of compassion, and the correct view of emptiness make up the three principle aspects of the path of dharma. Realization of Buddhahood, which all can attain, is the ultimate goal of Tibetan Buddhism and Tibetan medicine. Physical medicine can help the body but ultimately will not affect a spiritual disease. Spiritual diseases when diagnosed must be addressed by a qualified teacher, and the student guided in the appropriate dharmic or tantric healing practices.

Tantric Medicine and Healing

In Tibetan Buddhism, religion and medicine are never truly separated from one another, and this blend in relation to health is called tantric healing or medicine[18]. "A highly sophisticated and complex system, a sort of para-science of psychic and spiritual reality, and in terms of medicine, of psychic and spiritual healing" (Clifford, 1984, p. 66), this science of healing, similar to some forms of Oriental medicine, includes seasonal effects, astrological aspects, and spirit influences in addition to other measures.

In tantric healing, visualization practices are performed during which one transforms oneself and the world around one into the body, speech, and mind of the Buddha, a completely whole, integrated being or deity. "These three bodies of the Buddha," Clifford (1984) explains, "represent the sacred trinity of the three levels of expression of the reality of Buddha nature" (p. 31). As in using positive affirmations, it is believed that what one focuses on is more readily created in one's life. Also, as is taught to practitioners of various forms of energetic healing modalities, the quality of intention and attention greatly affects the outcome of the session. In these tantric meditation practices, three aspects are held as most important: (a) to have the intention of doing the practice for the benefit of all beings and to assist in their liberation from suffering, (b) to remain unattached to the results of the meditation experience, and (c) to dedicate the benefit one may gain from the practice (which can include heightened awareness and other positive results) to the enlightenment of all beings. In this form of meditation, the "desirous energy that ordinarily propels us from one unsatisfactory situation to another is transmuted through the alchemy of tantra, into a transcendental experience of bliss and wisdom." This blissful wisdom is intensely focused so that it "cuts. . . through the false projections of this and that and pierces the very heart of reality. . . It destroys the very cause of our dissatisfaction: our fundamental ignorance of the nature of reality" (Landaw, 1987, p. 37).

As in various healing modalities (e.g., acupuncture, Therapeutic Touch, etc.), in tantric healing, health and disease as well as mental disorders are often related to disruptions or blockages of the system's vital force or energy flow. Tantric medicine provides in-depth descriptions of the complex patterning of this energy and its movement. The energy is related with the breath, air, wind, or creative life force, and the channels and pathways through which it moves is the concern of much of Tibetan psychiatry and medicine, its diagnosis and treatment. It is said that the mind, or more correctly consciousness, requires a physical source for its base and rides on this flow of energy. Consciousness is defined as "that which cognizes objects and is by nature clarity itself and does not have a form" (Rapgay, 1985, p. 14). Simply expressed, if the body's subtle energies are in balance, the mind's balance will follow more readily, and vice versa.

Somatic Medicine

The third discipline of Tibetan medicine is somatic medicine[19]. The historical Buddha, Shakyamuni or Gautama Buddha (563 BCE), called "the Fully Awakened One," cited two reasons for disease. The first was the spiritual factors, or those brought from past life karma, and was called the distant cause. This included the three delusions of the mind: desire or attachment; close mindedness or ignorance; and hatred, anger, or aversion.

These were the objects of the mind to be abandoned through the healing practices. The second reason for disease was the factors from this life and was called the proximate cause. Somatic medicine generally attends to the proximate causation of disease and ascribes to the humoral theory. This theory speaks in terms of the three humors of the body—wind, bile, and phlegm. Humor (nyes-pa in Tibetan; doshas in Sanskrit literally meaning "fault") generally means a "subtle principle of life energies." Although available, a literal translation of each humor is an in-depth undertaking, too lengthy for the scope of this article. In the Tibetan tradition, it is said that the 84,000 delusions cause 84,000 different disorders that lead to 404 diseases. Four main categories of proximate causes are seasonal changes, habitual tendencies and behaviors, poisons, and negative spirits.

Although considered physical in nature, the three humors originate on a spiritual plane from the basic mental confusion that produces the subject-object dualism discussed earlier in this article. From this view comes the karmic force to manifest life and the universe. This subject-object dualism refers to the idea of holding to a permanent "self."

Attachment to one's ego, or self, is the main cause of all three delusions. This is the main cause of suffering and the idea to be refuted to obtain a state of enlightenment and freedom from suffering. As Clifford has written, "the delusions, ignorance, desire and aversion evolve into the humors phlegm, wind, and bile respectively" (p. 90). Each delusion can cause the disturbance or imbalance of the three humors, and these imbalances cause physical disorders that lead to disease. They also affect one another: if one humor is imbalanced, the other two are affected as well. The main point of physical health is the balance of these three humors and their relationship to one another Each person has a primary humor relating to the individual's body type, personality, and so forth. The humoral theory and principles can be used as a guide for preventative care and for promoting wellness. One is encouraged to observe the effects of seasons, seasonal activities, diet, and environment, and behavior modification in these areas and numerous other treatments are often prescribed to attain optimal health (Clifford, 1984).

Psychosomatic Medicine

It is known as the earliest form of mind-body medicine and can lend much of its wisdom to holistic and psychosomatic medicine and nursing, as well as the emerging field of psycho-neuro-immunology. The psychosomatic approaches in India have been of a very ancient origin. The evolution of these approaches started with Hindu medicine 1500 B.C. ago and was expanded and spread to other parts of Asia like China. Korea, Indochina, Thailand and eventually Japan by Buddhist medicine in 510 B.C.[20] The Buddhist medicine as originated from the teaching of Lord Buddha and completed by Jivaka spread to the whole of Asia by Buddhist monks and with the spread of Buddhist religion. Philosophy, science, religion, spiritualism and culture merged through the time and greatness of people to make Hindu Buddhist medicine a holistic one, yet based on bio-psycho-social and ecological concept. In this paper non-pharmacological approaches of Hindu Buddhist medicine is described which could be of significant therapeutic benefit in the management of psychosomatic diseases. Hindu Buddhist approaches impart information and knowledge concerning the measurable structure and powers of psyche. Hindu approaches clarify the processes by which experiences are apprehended, assimilated, interpreted, and comprehended while Buddhist approaches eradicate the cause of sickly spells, dream of ignorance, and thus to make possible the attainment of serene awakened perfection. The combined approaches of two ancient religions help us to assimilate the foundation of our being without which everything remains stressful and empty. The combined and cohesive approaches produce the state of utter consciousness super-rationally and open the door of self, which is composed of spiritual, physical and emotional joy. Psychosomatic diseases are pathological expressions of biological, psychic and social parameters of health and illness whereas Hindu Buddhist approaches show the way to bind closely the normal interrelationship of the above. The increasing uses of Yoga, Morita, Zen, Monko, Mo-he-zhi-guan, Nai Kan and Kenpo therapies in psychosomatic disorders are consistent and successful examples. Vyasa, Patanjali, Bodhidhara, Chih-i. Morita with their teachings have harmonized the physical, spiritual and emotional parameters of human life.

The Buddhist medical system is also based on the five elements principle. According to this principle, all beings are composed of five elements—earth, air, fire, water, and space. The humors are also related to the elements: phlegm is composed of the earth and water elements; bile, the fire element; and wind, the element of air. Although the above explanations may appear theoretical and philosophical, one can find in medical texts very clear explanations with great detail of the processes by which these principles function. For example, the digestion of food products and their eventual breakdown into the regenerative fluids that nourish the physical body and support health are explained by the three humors and five elements principle.

Herbal preparations made from a variety of herbs that grow naturally in Tibet are uniquely combined to provide desired therapeutic effects. It is said that over a thousand natural substances were available to the Tibetan physicians in their homeland. Besides herbs, rocks and minerals, earths and salts, fruits, twigs, roots, saps, and animals are included in the medicaments. As in the Native American tradition, the method of gathering and the state of the preparer's mind are very important to the medication's beneficial outcome. All the preparations of medicines begin with a prayer. Besides oral ingestion, substances are burned as incense and inhaled, and herbal baths are prescribed. Dietary patterns, cleansing procedures, massage, exercise, and activities including physical yoga, meditation, and breath work are considered common treatments. Acupuncture, moxibustion, and lancing are viewed as stronger methods, and minor surgeries and cauterizations are rarely used and only when absolutely necessary.

Based on the discussion thus far and judged by Western medical standards, Tibetan medicine may indeed appear to be a folk medicine based on cultural practices and religion. When studied in more depth, however, it is learned that it is a highly structured system of clinical medicine with 15 divisions of Clinical Pathology. They are: three pathophysiological processes (three humors), internal diseases, fever, diseases of head and neck, diseases of solid and hollow organs, venereology, urology, miscellaneous diseases, hereditary diseases, pediatrics, gynecology, toxicology and sexology. (Rapgay, 1985, p. 8).

In somatic medicine, the methods of diagnosis include 1,200 ways of examining disease. The three basic methods, however, are interrogation, sight, and touch. First, an in-depth interview is conducted about the client's life on all levels. Sight is then used for assessment, including urine and tongue diagnoses, and finally, touch is used for a pulse diagnosis. It is an analysis of 12 pulses on the fingers. Again, astrological and seasonal aspects are connected with the elements; therefore, they are also considered in the diagnosis.

For Tibetan medicine, like for the Indian ayurvedic medicine, from which it has borrowed the basic theoretical essentials concerning physiology, pathology and therapy, the living body is made up of an organic substrate on which three humoral fluids, pneuma, bile and phlegm ensure the different vital functions. These humours, blood and other organic fluids flow through the body in channels forming a network. While the humours endow the body with life and health as long as they remain in harmony, the state of the illness is nothing but the pathological symptoms of these very humours in an imbalanced state, under the influence of food, lifestyle, seasons etc.

Medical diagnosis is conceived as the outcome of a process of logical inference during which the doctor should ideally compare clinical signs obtained by questioning, palpation of pulses and visual examination, especially of the tongue and urine. In fact, diagnostic examination is often limited to taking the pulses, according to a technique that was, obviously, borrowed from China.

The treatment requires four types of therapies supposed to get more and more drastic in the following order: healthy lifestyle, dietetics, remedies and external therapeutic procedures. Generally it involves setting excessive humours against qualities that are opposite to them and if the need arises to discharge them from the body. Among the tangible qualities attributed to food items and drugs, their flavors and their hot or cold nature are particularly taken into account. The remedies combine the elements of a very rich materia medica, in varied preparations (mainly powders, decoctions or pills) where products of plant origin predominate to a great extent. The external therapeutic procedures include moxibustion with relatively frequent use, possibly fomentations and medicinal baths, unction, bleeding and small surgery.

Since three decades, Tibetan medicine has experienced major transformations in all the settings where it was traditionally practiced, as much in the Tibetan regions of China, as in the Himalayan regions or in the diaspora. In China, it was a victim of major upheavals that followed the Dalaï Lama's escape into exile, in 1959, then of extreme political violence of the Cultural Revolution. With the period of relative liberalization that started around 1980, Tibetan medicine however appeared as one of the cultural heritage elements to have best survived, in spite of everything. It owes this no doubt to several factors: traditional medicine having recognition in China itself, its availability at a low cost locally, its pragmatic orientation with a rational side set to be encouraged at the expense of its religious aspects, and its aptitude, easily controllable, to serve as an emblematic image of a Chinese politics wanting to be anxious in promoting both the well-being and cultural heritage of the Tibetans. Tibetan medicine has thus been integrated into the health system of the Tibetan regions of China at the expense of an evolution that has borrowed some traits from biomedical model: institutional education sanctioned by degrees, - and therefore, evolution towards a relative standardization of knowledge and practices -, secularization, professionalization, more exclusive focus on the somatic nature of illnesses to the detriment of their psycho-affective or social aspects, more impersonal consultation of patients in a formal context of a small clinic, a dispensary or hospital, re-evaluation of some notions or practices with reference to modern science, practitioners giving up on preparing medicines to make way for pharmaceutical companies with more and more commercial goals, recourse to certain diagnostic or therapeutic biomedical techniques. Some of these tendencies also mark, in varying degrees, the evolution of Tibetan medicine outside Chinese borders under the influence of so-called development programs, local process for government integration, or even at the behest of the exile community. Finally, Tibetan medicine, which is also being subjected to identity issues, is present today on the globalized market of alternative medicines. The concerned practitioners have found a way of adjusting themselves to this by shifts in their statements and practices and which is are in turn echoed in their native settings.

Because humankind has depended on nature for sustenance and survival, the instinctive urge to health and accumulated knowledge has guided us to discover certain remedies for common ailments from natural sources. For example, applying residual barley from chang (Tibetan wine) on swollen body parts, drinking hot water for indigestion, and using melted butter for bleeding are some of the therapies that arose from practical experience and gradually formed the basis for the art of healing in Tibet. The Tibetan medical heritage is based on the book of the Four Tantras (rgyud-bzhi), which remains the fundamental medical text even today. There is some evidence to suggest that several forms of medical practice existed at that time.

SOWA-RIGPA OR THE TIBETAN MEDICINE IN INDIA

"Sowa-Rigpa", commonly known as Tibetan or Amchi medicine, is the traditional medicine of many parts of the Himalayan region. *Sowa-Rigpa* means 'science of healing' and the practitioners of this medicine are known as *Amchi* (superior to all).

In India, this system of medicine has been popularly practiced in Ladakh and Paddar-Pangay regions of Jammu and Kashmir, Himachal Pradesh, Arunachal Pradesh, Sikkim, Darjeeling-Kalingpong (WB) and now in Tibetan settlements all over India and abroad. *Sowa-Rigpa* originated from India.

The fundamental text book "*Chatush-Tantra*" of this medicine was delivered by *Bhagwan Buddha* 2500 years ago, and it was further developed by eminent Indian scholars like Jivaka, Nagarjuna, Vaghbhatt and Chandranandan etc. *Chatush-Tantra* (rGud-bZi) was translated into the Tibetan language around the 8th century AD by Kashmiri Acharya Chandranandan and Tibetan Translator *Verochana*, but before introducing this medicine in Tibet.

It was amended and enriched with other medical traditions like Chinese, Persian and Tibetan folk medicine to make it most effective and more suitable to the socio-climatic conditions of Tibet. From Tibet, the impact of *Sowa-Rigpa* along with Buddhism and other Tibetan art and sciences spread to the neighboring Himalayan regions like Mongolia, Bhutan, Nepal, China and some parts of former Soviet Union etc. and to this day, *Sowa-Rigpa* is very popular in these regions. Besides *Chatush-Tantra*, around two dozen Indian Medical texts are translated into Tibetan from Sanskrit, followed by thousands of commentaries and texts written by Tibetan scholars.

Tibetan medicine is an ancient synthesis of the art of healing, drawing on the knowledge of medical systems existing in a wide region of Southeast and Central Asia. Through the process of this synthesis, Tibetan medicine was established during the 7th to the 12th centuries A.D. The fundamental theoretical concepts are based primarily on the Indian Buddhist system of medicine. The Buddha himself developed this system of medicine 2500 years ago. Tibetan cultural notions and the Buddhist belief system underline the socio-ecology of Ladakh. Ladakh is one of the few remaining Himalayan area where the Tibetan system of medicine remains undisturbed. This indigenous health care system plays a major part in the health care of Ladakhi communities. Tibetan medicine known in Ladakh as 'Amchi' medicine has usually been passed down from fathers to son or daughter within the village. This is known as the rGYUTPA lineage. New 'Amchis' have to take their passing out examination orally in front of the whole village. Thereby they are examined by a panel of respected senior Amchis from surrounding villages. In every village, there is usually one or sometimes two amchi families.

Most of the Amchis are the sixth generation of unbroken family lineages. They provide health care in the villages. No charge is made for treatment, but Amchis are helped by the villagers with farm work particularly with spring ploughing and autumn harvest. Occasionally, the villagers collect barley during the harvest and offer it to the Amchi family. The Amchi doctor holds a high position in Ladakhi society. They are often not only the medical doctors but also very strong community leaders. Often they hold the position of the 'Goba', the head of the village.

Many Amchis practise Buddhist astrology and astronomy. These subjects play an important role within Amchi medical practise as they do within Ladakhi society in general. In fact, there is very strong relationship between Buddhist astrology and Tibetan medicine.

As well as its curative role, Tibetan medicine has played crucial part in preventive health care within the villages, emphasising water and spring cleanliness, good diet and healthy lifestyle practices. In present day, Ladakhi Amchi practice still plays a crucial role within Ladakhi communities.

Basic Principles of Tibetan Medicine

Tibetan medicine is a science, art and philosophy that provides a holistic approach to health care. It is a science because its principles are enumerated in a systematic and logical framework based on an understanding of the body and its relationship to the environment. It is an art because it uses diagnostic techniques based on the creativity, insight, subtlety and compassion of the medical practitioner. And it is a philosophy because it embraces the key Buddhist principles of altruism, karma and ethics.

Imagine a medical tradition, highly effective, using medicines that produce no lasting negative side effects, sustainably harvesting resources of the natural environment, and respecting basic sanity and compassion as the essential basis of health and well being. Classical Asian medicine, in general, and in particular Tibetan medicine, as practiced throughout a vast area of central Asia for many hundreds of years, was just such a tradition.

Beginning in about the fourth century, A.D., the Tibetan people began expanding their own medical knowledge with information drawn from other cultures. Eventually the process became quite formal, with government sponsored conferences bringing together doctors from other lands and medical traditions, for theoretical debate and clinical demonstrations of methods for dealing with health problems of all sorts. Physicians who demonstrated superior skill and understanding were invited to stay and work with the best Tibetan doctors. Eventually, this combined medical understanding, refined, systematized and highly effective, led to Tibet's reputation, throughout the entire region, as the Land of Medicine.

Perhaps it's time to do that again — bring together all the various surviving medical traditions and let the sparks fly. Indeed, many people are now working to preserve, as much as possible, what remains of Tibetan medicine, and to give people all over the world access to this unique insight into human well being.

Buddhist philosophy states that everything in the universe is in a constant state of flux - that all phenomena are characterised by impermanence, and that the only permanent feature is impermanence itself. As Buddha said, "No matter whether perfect beings arise or not, it remains a fact, and a hard necessity of existence, that all creations are transitory." It is this impermanence that causes each and every being to suffer at one stage or another. Suffering is thus not accidental but springs from a specific cause, whether from this life or a previous life. Only through proper learning and the genuine practice of Dharma can liberate from the vicious cycle of suffering.

Tibetan medical theory states that everything in the universe is made up of the five proto-elements:

1. sa (Earth)
2. chu (Water)
3. me (Fire)
4. rLung (Wind)
5. Nam-mkha (Space)

Although all five proto-elements are responsible for the formation of each tissue cell, each element has a specific influence:

1. sa exerts a greater influence over the formation of muscle cells, bones, the nose and the sense of smell
2. chu is responsible for the formation of blood, body fluids, tongue and the sense of taste
3. me is responsible for body temperature, complexion, the eyes and the sense of sight
4. rLung is responsible for breathing, skin and the sense of touch and
5. nam-mkha is responsible for body cavities, the ears and the sense of hearing

The Three Principle Energy

1. *rLung* (wind) is one of the three principle energies of the body which manifests the the nature of Air element. It is characterised by rough, light, cold, subtle, hard and mobile. It is responsible for the physical and mental activities, respiration, expulsion of urine, faces, fetus, menstruation, spitting, burping, speech, gives clarity to sense organs, sustains life by means of acting as a medium between mind and body.
2. *mKhris-pa* (Bile)basically has the nature of fire. It is characterised by oily, sharp, hot, light, fetid, purgative and fluidity. mKhris-pa is responsible for hunger, thirst, digestion and assimilation, promotes bodily heat, gives lustre to body complexion and provides courage and determination.
3. *Bad-kan* (Phlegm) is cold in nature and is characterised by oily, cool, heavy, blunt, smCTAh, firm and sticky. Bad-kan is responsible for firmness of the body, stability of mind, induces sleep, connects bodily joints, generates tolerance and lubricates the body.

A Healthy Body

Sowa rigpa (the art and science of healing or traditional Tibetan medicine, astronomy and astrology) involves the proper alignment of these divisions i.e. the 3 humors, 7 bodily constituents and 3 excretions, into a state of equilibrium. If this is accomplished, then the body is said to be in a state of health or free from psycho-physiological disorders; whereas a disequilibrium in any of these energies constitutes a state of disorder or ill-health.

Like the phenomena of conditioned existence, diseases are also the product of causes and conditions. There are two main causes of the disease: a long term cause and short cause. Ignorance or unawareness is the ultimate cause of all diseases. Because of ignorance or delusion, one cannot see the reality of the phenomena and thereby clings to personal self or ego which in turn give rise to the three mental poisons: desire. hatred and stupidity. So ignorance and three mental poisons constitute the long term cause of disease. Secondly the short term causes of disease are the three humours: wind energy (Tib. rlung), bile energy (Tib. mkhris pa) and phlegm (Tib. bad kan). They are in fact produced by the three mental poisons: desire gives rise to wind, hatred to bile and stupidity to phlegm. These three humours constitute the basic energy system in the body. They are interrelated to all vital functions of the body, organs, seven constituents and three excretions. Seven constituents of the body are: food (nutrition), blood, flesh, fat, bone, marrow, semen. The three excrements are: sweat, urine and faeces.

When the three humours, seven body constituents and the three excrements are balanced one is healthy, when they are unbalanced one becomes sick. There are four factors responsible for the imbalance, they are: improper climate, influence of demons, improper diet and improper behaviour. Since everything is interrelated, imbalance in one organ or one of the humours effects the rest of the organism. Because of the interdependence of humours and body constituents etc., their imbalance can be diagnosed by the methods specially used by Tibetan doctors.

Health Care in Tibetan Medical System

Tibetan Medical System is one of the world's largest and oldest known medical traditions. With the beginning of civilization in Tibet and being situated at the highest plateau in the world, the Tibetan Medicine has evolved and refined with the time to combat the disorders arises from the imbalance of three principle energies. Even animals like

Cervus albirostris Przewalski (deer) seeks the herb called *Soroseris hookeriana* to revive their wounds, *an avian (Alanda gulgula)* applies *Coriandrum sativum* to bind the crack of their egg's shell. Similarly, as in the case of human being applying of apricot kernel oil to smooth the skin, & use of *Melandrium glandulorium* as a perfume, mixture of washing soda and *Ulmus punila* as a detergent. Paste of honey, mineral exudates, *Asparagus racemosus and Acacia catechu* to protect the skin damage from the harsh and cold weather applying Chang (Tibetan beer made by brewing barley) to reduce swelling, using melted butter to stem bleeding, pig fat to restore the crack, mixture of goat's fat and *Arnebia sp.* for the treatment of freckles, mustard seed and butter to moisturize the skin etc. these and such traditions are basic foundation for the evolution of Tibetan medicine. Generally, the skin is considered as the largest and most sensitive organ of the body. As in the text, the more we plaster cement on the brick of house, the better will it project its physical appearance and prevents from damage. Similarly, the more we render to care our skin the better the health of our skin and protect it from damage. It also elevates sensory power. However, it is also important that the sole external application doesn't result to the health of the skin. Proper life style and balance diet also play a key role besides one needs to keep the positive mental attitude. This is the basic principle applied in Tibetan Medicine as a remedy for the treatment of physical and mental disorders. The suffering and mental stress does affect the condition of physical appearance like the luster and glory of skin. Therefore, imbalance and fluctuation of the physical energies (Loong or rlung) which helps to function our inner systems and the energies which provide smoothness to our skin results to aging prolong sickness, mental and physical stress, distortion of body, appearance of wrinkles, graying of hair and beard, weakening of sensory organ are some feature of the ageing. The external factors that affect the condition of our bodies are pollutions, toxic gases, and evil spirit. The pollutants and agents which cause the disease get penetrate from the surrounding to the body system and other connective tissues like blood and muscle through the skin and get carried away by the serous fluid and result to the skin disorders like mole, freckles, wart, wrinkle, rough & dry skin, and weak skin are some of the features of the ill health skin. Sorig Products not only does it helps for the health of outer body but also supports the inner mental state. Sorig products are prepared from the herbs which are grown at the Tibet and Himalayan regions located at about 3000 meters above the sea level. Such herbs are collected with the utmost care and respect to the surrounding environment. For instances, herbs like *Medicago lupulina* helps to revive the dry and rough skin and improves the skin texture, *Asparagus racemosus* strengthens the body by improving the hemoglobin count and promotes the skin texture by treating pimples and freckles. *Hibiscus moschatus* has the potencies of anti-wrinkle & anti-ageing and also act as an antiseptic. *Holarrhena antidysenterica* improves the glory and luster of the skin. *Areca catchu* helps to treat wound, itch and burns. *Curcuma longa* helps to soothe the skin, erase the scares, and treat the inflammation. Terminalia belerica treats serous fluid disorders, and strengthen the condition of skin and also has a blood clotting properties. *Irs sp.* improves the skin texture by promoting the blood circulation, *Embelica ribes* act as an antiseptic and elevate the blood circulation, *Butea monosperma* has an anti-microbial property and purifies the blood. *Myristica fragans* balances the body loon (rlung), thereby strengthen the body, promote the blood circulations and retains the mental stability. *Carum carvi* helps to combat the nerves & muscle constriction, also help for the loong disorders aggravated due to obese. *Zingeber officinalis* help to promote the blood circulation and relief the muscle restrains & Helianthus annus helps to promote the body heat. Prunus aamemica (apricot oil) dries up the serous fluid, purify the blood & help to grow the healthy hair. Embilica officinalis helps to dispel the blood febrile, relief the itch and strengthen the hair growth. Terminalia chebula alleviates all kins of disorders like elevated the blood and loong circulation,clear up the nervous route, strengthen the muscle and make the skin supple. Oxytropis microphylla relief the inflammation, swelling, binds the detach nerve and act as an antiseptic also. Cinnamomum camphora dispel all kinds of febrile, & Gymnadennis conopsea strengthens the body, promotes kidney heat, alleviates all kinds of cold disorders and has property of rejuvenation. Elettaria cardamomum promotes kidney heat, and alleviated all kinds of cold disorders. Withania somnifera also alleviates all kinds of cold disorder, promotes kidney heat and also act as abhrodiasc,& carthamus tinctorius cures all kind the Tripa and hepatic disorders, strengthen the body,& restore the body hemoglobin level. Rubussp. Combat pulmonary disorder like different kinds of fevers such as epicemic febrile, fever aggravated due to loong (wind) and baeken (phlegm) disorders & fever due to cold, Syzigium aromaticum helps to relieve loong disorders and promote the body heat, Sesemum indicum (Til) strengthen the body and act as aphrodiacse, Symplococcus paniculate is used as a mouth freshener and relief the fever. Rosa combats the bile and rlung disorders, Amebia sp. relieves the fever and purify the blood, Rhododenron sp. promotes the body heat, strengthen the weak body & relieves the baeken disorders. Cinnamomum zeylinicum promotes the digestive heat and food appetite, Punica granatum cures all kinds of baeken disorders especially for the cold disorders and also promotes digestion heat, illinium vernium promotes digestive heat and blood circulation, & also alleviates cold and loong disorder, Amomum sabulatum promotes food appetite and digestive heat, also alleviate gastro-pancreatic disorders, Kaemferia (wild ginger) also promotes digestive heat and food appetite, and also cure both the loong and baeken disorders. These are the application of some of the herbs which are used in the production of the Sorig product. The main objective of any of medical system is of to free from suffering and prevents from getting diseases. Tibetan Medicine for the past thousands of years has accumulated substantial recipes. Based on those recipes and integrated with the modern scientific method, Herbal Product Research Department comes out with the varieties of Sorig products. To assure the highest possible quality to retain the products at its highest potency, this department is consulting various experts within and outside the institute. For instance products like Gaay-Pa-Sowae- Chudlen, Loong tea, Chee-Nyii Tea and Trakshey Tea are used to restore and strengthen the weak body. For beautifying the physical appearance for the health of skin, products like Shasoe Paekar Zaesel (Beauty Cream), Nyerdak Gamoli (Anti –Wrinkle cream), Jukpa-Agar Dhether (Massage oil) and Ta-Nuum are applied. If these product are continuously used it also help to relieve the mental stress and strain, free the wrinkle,and making the skin soft and supple to touch.

Diagnosis in Tibetan Medicine

The general methods of diagnosis and therapeutics used by Tibetan doctors follow the Indian tridosha system; that is, being based on three humors (see Table 1).

The imbalances in an individual are revealed by a combination of reported symptoms, pulse diagnosis, tongue diagnosis, and urine analysis. The overall physical

Table 1
The System of Three Humors Adopted into Tibetan Medicine from India

English	*Tibetan*	*Pinyin*	*Indian*	*Basic Concept*
wind	rLung	long	vayu	movement, breath, cold
bile	mKrhispa	chiba	pitta	metabolism, digestion, fire
phlegm	Badkan	peigen	kapha	restraint, lubrication, moistness

appearance of the person and information about their daily habits, and consideration of seasonal influences also contribute to the analysis. The Tibetan pulse diagnosis appears to be derived from the Chinese system, and is taken at the same artery of each wrist, but the method of feeling the pulse and the interpretations differ. Tongue diagnosis is simplified compared to the Chinese system (long disorders are characterized by red and dry tongue; chiba disorders by a yellowish tongue coating; and peigen disorders by a greyish and sticky coating with a smooth and moist texture). Urine analysis is unique to the Tibetan system and may have been introduced from Persia. Physicians inspect the color, amount of vapor, sediment, smell, and characteristics of the foam generated upon stirring, relying on the first urine excreted in the morning.

Traditional Tibetan formulas are described mainly in terms of the diseases and symptoms that they treat, rather than their properties and influences on the humors. For example, in this article, several formulas that treat lung diseases are presented and their description mainly involves characteristic symptoms (cough, coloration of sputum, fever, involvement of the throat). In order to select among various possible remedies, it is important to know if the lung disease is hot or cold in nature, and to know the disturbances of the three humors that form the background to the disease in an individual patient. The humors may either be insufficient and require supplementation (invigoration) or they may be excessive and require pacification. In an attempt to correlate Tibetan and Chinese concepts, it has been suggested (3) that long corresponds roughly to concepts of qi and wind, chiba corresponds to fire or gallbladder, and peigen corresponds to moisture, the earth element, and phlegm.

The modern Materia Medica of Tibet is derived from the book *Jingzhu Bencao* (The Pearl Herbs), published in 1835 by Dumar Danzhenpengcuo (7). This text has been compared to the famous Chinese herbal *Bencao Gangmu*. Its format includes two sections, one being in the style of the Buddhist sutra with praise of the medicines, and the other being a detailed classification of each substance, giving the material's origin, environmental conditions where it is found, quality, parts used, and properties. The text included 2,294 materials, of which 1,006 are of plant origin, 448 of animal origin, and 840 minerals. The heavier reliance on minerals and animals than on plants-compared to other traditional medical traditions-can readily be understood for a country at such high altitude that is very rocky and supports only small areas of plant growth over much of the terrain.

About one-third of the medicinal materials used in Tibetan formulas are unique to the Tibetan region (including the Himalayan area in bordering countries), while the other two-thirds of the materials are obtained from India and China. The Tibetan population that had access to the medicines was relatively small until this century, so the total amount of pills produced were correspondingly small. Bringing herbs from India and China to Tibet has always been difficult and has limited the production of herbal formulas. Today, it is relatively easy to get Chinese herbs into Tibet, and China cultivates most of the herbs indigenous to India that might be needed.

Although Tibetan herbal medicine includes the use of decoctions and powders, for the most part, Tibetan doctors utilize pills that are usually made from a large number of herbs (typically 8-25 ingredients). Pills have the advantage of being easy to use and they can be prepared in advance at a medical facility where all the ingredients are gathered together. Due to the vast distances, rough terrain, and limited development of Tibet, it was not possible to have the broad range of ingredients available to individual doctors who might compound formulas for decoction, as was often done in China. Instead, the doctors to their patients would carry a relatively small variety of pills prepared at central facilities. For many doctors, a collection of about two dozen principal formulas would have to suffice. In Lhasa, where there was a centralized population, the doctors have had access to about 200 kinds of pills.

The traditional Tibetan pills were often large and hard and time consuming to prepare. Dr. Lobsang Dolma Khangkar (8) explained that each herb had to first be processed meticulously and then had to be mixed and preserved properly:

> *If we are using cardamom, we have to use only the inside, because the outside has no value and then we have to peel each one. There is no machine that can do this, it has to be done by hand. After treating each of the ingredients like this, we will mix maybe three, thirteen, or twenty-five ingredients to make one pill. The first step is to mix all of these ingredients together. If this is not done properly, then each of these ingredients will maintain their own potency without combining with the rest. So, first they have to be completely mixed and this takes a long time of grinding and mixing. After that, it has to be left at rest for a whole day. After the rest, the person who is preparing the medicines has to clean his hands and then begin again with mixing and grinding that medicine. After this, we make the pills. The pills can be made with machines....Then the pills are put into a very long bag made of cotton cloth. Two men hold the cloth from each side and move it back and forth so that the pills roll from one side to the other. This is done for a whole day. This last procedure is what is responsible for making Tibetan*

medicine pills so hard. This procedure takes out all the air that is still in the pills. If air remains in the pill, then it is prone to bacteria getting in, and for the pills to go bad.

In order to make Tibetan medicines available to more people, modern factories have worked out new methods of blending, grinding, and making the pills as well as producing other forms of the finished materials to make them easier to consume. There are regulations on the production of pills made in Tibet, with 97 different formulas formally recognized; of these 25 are covered under State medical insurance.

Many of the formulations that are still in use were established many centuries ago. The principles of herbal combining to yield a traditional formula are not clearly defined in the Tibetan system. There are complex methods of analyzing the qualities of medicinal materials: 6 tastes, 8 properties, and 17 effects (see Table 2), but the precise organizational principles for compounding numerous ingredients into the formulas is lost to history.

Categorically speaking, the diagnostic techniques in Tibetan Health System include visual observation, touch and interrogation.

Visual Observation

This involves checking a patient's skin complexion, the colour and texture of his/her blood, nails, sputum, faeces, and other general conditions. Special attention is paid to the condition of the patient's tongue and urine.

Disorders of Tongue

In wind disorder, the tongue will red, dry and rough. In bile disorder, the tongue will be covered by a thick, pale yellow coating of phlegm. In phlegm disorder, the tongue will have a pale, thick coating of phlegm and dull, smCTAh and moist texture.

Urine Disorder

The doctor advises the patient, how and when to collect the urine sample. It is essential that patient avoid taking too much of tea, buttermilk or wine etc. which otherwise would cause discoloration of the urine sample. They are also suggested to have a sound and sufficient sleep, refrain from mental and emotional stress and desist irregular activities. It is best to satisfy these conditions a night before the examination. The urine in Wind disorder looks like water and has large bubbles when stirred. In Bile, the urine is reddish yellow and malodorous with much steam. In Phlegm, the urine is whitish with little odour or steam.

The first urine passed at dawn is suitable for examination, since its colour is not affected by digestion and by the colour the doctor can detect diseases. The colour, steam and sediment should be tested. The urine should be kept in a plain container, so that the colour is not affected, and either a stick or straw of white colour must be used for stirring it during examination.

Touch

Pulse reading forms the most important touching method employed in Tibetan medicine. Only after ensuring an important set of preconditions, the physician proceeds with a pulse diagnosis.

This involves placing the index finger, middle finger and ring finger of a doctor at patient's radial arteries. The fingers must be held in a line close to one another yet not touching each other. The index finger must not put too much pressure on the skin; more pressure should be applied by the middle and ring fingers.

Left hand of patient examined by the right hand of the doctor a. the tip of the index finger on the right side detects heart diseases and on the left intestinal diseases b. the tip of the middle finger on the right side detects diseases affecting the spleen, and on the left stomach diseases c. the tip of the ring finger on the right side detects kidney diseases and on the left diseases affecting the seminal vessel.

Right hand of patient examined by the left hand of the doctor d. the right tip of the index finger detects lung diseases, the left tip diseases affecting the guts; e. the right tip of the middle finger detects liver diseases, the left tip diseases due to unbalanced bile; f. the right tip of the ring finger detects kidney diseases, and the left tip diseases affecting the urinary bladder The right hand pulse should be examined first in the case of female patients, and the left hand one in the case of males. The reason for this is that the tip of the female heart is tilted towards the right and vice versa with males.

Interrogation

Interrogation forms the most important clinical aspect of the diagnosis. There are three main elements to a medical interrogation: g. determining the causative factors; h. determining the site of the illness; i. studying the signs and symptoms - this involves the doctor asking the patient about the sort of food and drink s/he has been consuming, and what kind of physical and mental behaviour s/he has been experiencing.

Traditional Tibetan Medical Treatments

Dietary and Lifestyle Factors

At an immediate level, a disorder is primarily caused by an improper diet and/or lifestyle. In fact, a majority of health problems, both in developing and developed countries, can be either directly or indirectly traced to poor diet or lifestyle. Examples of this include alcoholism, hypertension and heart disease. The first form of treatment in Tibetan medicine is thus not medicines but changing a patient's diet and/or lifestyle. Only if this fails to remedy an ailment is the use of medicines considered.

Tibetan Medicines

Tibetan medicines take various forms, from decoctions, powders, general pills, precious pills, and syrups, and are prescribed in small doses — a fact that reflects the emphasis Tibetan medicine places on gentle treatment.

Moxibustion and Other Treatments

Many disorders, caused by proliferation of bad blood and mKhris-pa are also treated by blood-letting at one of the body's seventy seven blood-letting points. For cold disorders, nerve malfunction and non-malignant tumors, moxibustion, golden-needle therapy may be used to stimulate the energy channels of the body. Many diseases of the nerves and muscles, as well as pain and insomnia related to rLung, are treated with gentle massage using various medicinal oils. Medicinal bath and natural spring baths are used to treat an assortment of skin disorders as well as chronic arthritis, gout and cold types of rheumatism, and rigid and stiffness of the extremities.

Tibetan Herbal Medicine

Tibetan medicine[21] has a rich heritage and is currently practiced not only in Tibet, but also in the adjacent Chinese provinces of Qinghai, Gansu, Sichuan, and Yunnan, and in the neighboring kingdoms of Bhutan, Nepal, Ladakh, and Sikkim, where communities of Tibetan people have long been established. Many non-Tibetans also seek out treatment by this traditional system because of its good reputation. As a result of the flood of refugees from the Chinese military occupation of Tibet, Tibetan medicine extended to India, and, from there, to many countries of the world (especially in Europe and North America) under the guidance of a small number of refugee physicians. One of the most famous of the refugee doctors is Dr. Yeshe Donden, who was the personal physician of the Dalai Lama in exile from 1961-1969. Dr. Donden has spent much time in the U.S., where he has diagnosed and treated patients, given teachings to doctors and laypersons, written books and articles, and answered numerous questions about the Tibetan system of health care. Tibetan medicine has also been popularized by a lineage of the Badmajev family that originated in Russia, near Mongolia; members of the family traveled West during the 20th century. Tibetan herbal formulas they brought with them have been available as pharmaceutical products in Europe since 1980.

Tibetan medicine originated with the local folk tradition (known as Bon) that dates back to about 300 B.C. and was formally recorded by Xiepu Chixi, the physician to the Tibetan King Niechi Zanpu, in 126 B.C. Aspects of both the traditional Chinese and Indian (Ayurvedic) medical systems were added later; Ayurveda has had the most profound influence on Tibetan medicine. The medicine of India was introduced to Tibet as early as 254 A.D., with the visit of two Indian physicians. During the following century several physicians from India reinforced the teachings.

The greatest influence from India came about when Buddhism was adopted in Tibet as the state religion. This occurred as Tibet was unified under King Songzan Ganbu (618-652 A.D.). Buddhism had great implications for the practice of the Indian approach to medicine that evolved separately in Tibet. The Ayurvedic principles, especially the concept of tridosha, or three faults (in Buddhism, the three poisons) provided the basis for analyzing physical disorders and designing treatments, while Buddhism provided a strong spiritual component.

The legend of how Tibetan medicine was introduced to Tibet is relayed in the story *The Life of the Great Physician Yuthog Yonten Gonpo* [pinyin: *Yutuo Yuandan Gongbu*] which has been translated and presented in the book *Tibetan Medicine* by Rechung Rinpoche (1). The following is the command by Tara (the Buddhist god of compassion, which is identified in the Chinese tradition as the goddess Guan Yin) to two famous physicians of India who are said to have become immortals (now living in the sandalwood jungles of India):

> *It has been prophesied by the Buddha about the country of Tibet; and all the Buddhas have discoursed on Tibet, and Avalokitesvara [also called Chenrezi; a champion of Buddhism: a boddhisatva] was made the special protector of Tibet. Avalokitesvara is the chief protector and I am helping him. When you go to Tibet, you will teach the people medicine, in the way the Buddha comes with his teaching. There is no doubt of success. Go quickly, and I shall look after you with my merciful eyes. And you will have the blessing of Avalokitesvara and great results. By the strength of your former prayers, the teaching of medicine will be kept up by the lineage of your families. Be of good cheer and go to Tibet!*

The lineage spoken of here involved the birth in Tibet of Yuthog Yonten Gonpo (708-833 A.D.), who studied medicine since an early age and was exposed to Buddhism during his teen years. Yuthog made three trips to India and studied with the great masters of Buddhist and Ayurvedic medicine there, and he eventually wrote 30 classic medical works integrating the local, Indian and Chinese medical traditions (2, 3). The involvement of Chinese medicine came about in 641 A.D. when a Tang Dynasty princess, Wen Cheng, was married to the Tibetan leader Songzan Ganbu (who was also married to a Nepalese princess that introduced him to Buddhism). Wen Cheng brought with her many Chinese books, including the medical books, as well as herbal formulas and medical instruments. Seventy years later, during Yuthog's life, another Chinese princess, Jin Cheng, brought additional medical books, as well as several Chinese physicians, to Tibet.

Yuthog is viewed as the father of Tibetan medicine. He became a royal court physician and established the first Tibetan medical school at Congpo Menlong; he also became a monk at the Samye Monastery. A great medical conference was held at Samye during this time, bringing together Indian, Chinese, Persian, and Greek medical experts. Yuthog received the forerunner of the Four Medical Tantras (*Sibuyidian*; in Tibetan: *rGyud-bzhi*, ca. 770 A.D.) that serve as the basis of Tibetan medical practice. The original version is thought to have been written in Sanskrit around the 4th Century A.D. and then translated into Tibetan and given to the royal court (4). Yuthog's work in reorganizing and clarifying these books, as well as adding supplemental material (including that from other traditions described at the Samye conference) made him the true author of the Tibetan traditional text. Because of the vast contributions he made, he is considered a reincarnation of the Medicine Buddha, venerated as "the second Medicine Buddha."

The Four Medical Tantras were revised (1573 A.D.) by the "younger Yuthog" who was a 14th generation descendent of the original Yuthog, now referred to as the "elder Yuthog." Additional revisions were made during the 17th century to bring forth the current version. The first two medical tantras (called the "root tantra" and the "explanatory tantra") have been translated and annotated by Dr. Yeshi Donden (5) and translated again in expanded form by Dr. Barry Clark (6). These first two tantras make only brief mention of herbal medicine, and focus instead on behavior, diet, diagnostics, disease categories, and other aspects of traditional medicine. The third tantra ("instructions") details the cause and treatment of each major category of disease, and the fourth tantra ("concluding text") is devoted to the details of diagnosis, herbs, moxibustion, and other techniques. One major obstacle to translating the section on herbs is that the identification of the original materials in this 1,200 year old text is quite difficult.

Classification of Tibetan Herbal Medicine[22]

Table 2

Grouping	*Characteristics*
Six tastes	**sweet** (e.g., bamboo, grapes, saffron; pacifies *long* and *chiba*; increases *peigen*); **sour** (e.g., pomegranate, hippophae, crataegus; pacifies *long* and *peigen*; increases *chiba*); **salty** (e.g., salt and several minerals; pacifies long and peigen; increases *chihba*); **bitter** (e.g., gentiana, aconite, berberis; pacifies *chiba*, increases *long* and *peigen*); **acrid** (e.g., piper, ginger, garlic; pacifies *long* and *peigen*, increases chiba); and **astringent** (e.g., sandalwood, terminalia, aquilegia; pacifies *peigen*, increases *long* and *peigen*)
Eight properties	**heavy, smooth** (these two treat combat *long*); **cool, soft** (these two combat *chiba*); **light, rough, acrid,** and **sharp** (these four combat *peigen*). To increase *long*, rough and cool medicines are used; to increase *chiba*, warm, sharp, and smooth medicines are used; to increase *peigen*, heavy, smooth, cool, and soft medicines are used.
Seventeen effects	**cold, hot, warm, cool, thick, thin, moist, rough, light, heavy, steady, motive, blunt, sharp, tender, dry,** and **soft**. Disease is treated by the opposing effect; a hot disease by a cold effect, stagnant diseases by a motive effect, an accumulation by a sharp effect, a moist condition by a dry effect, etc. *Long* disorders tend to be dry, light, cool, mobile, subtle, and hard; *chiba* disorders tend to be oily, sharp, malodorous, purging, hot, flowing, and light; *peigen* disorders tend to be cold, heavy, blunt, smooth, oily, stable, and sticky.

In general, Tibetan remedies emphasize the use of spicy (acrid), aromatic, and warming herbs. The climate has a substantial influence on these choices: the high altitude of Tibet means that cold and windy conditions prevail. The warm, spicy, aromatic herbs help to compensate for this condition. Ayurvedic medicine relies heavily on spicy herbs for stimulating the digestive system functions, which is understood to be the key to health. Thus, among the commonly used Tibetan herbs are those derived mainly from the Ayurvedic system, such as the peppers, cumins, cardamom, clove, ginger, and other hot spices, complemented by the local aromatics such as saussurea and musk. Also, the Tibetan system emphasizes astringent herbs, possibly representing an attempt to conserve body fluids and alleviate any inflammation of the mucous membranes. The "king" herb of Tibetan medicine is the chebulic myrobalan (*Terminalia chebula*), which is an astringent herb, but is said to possess all the tastes (different parts of the fruit have different tastes), properties, and effects. Despite this emphasis on herbs with properties that are generally needed for the Tibetan climate, cooling and bitter herbs are often required to treat the disease manifestation, as inflammatory processes finally result if the pathogenic influences are not conquered or expelled.

Tibetan medicines are today prescribed by several thousand Tibetan doctors that have been trained in recent decades in Tibet, Qinghai, Gansu, and Sichuan. Ten cities in China have set-up Tibetan medical facilities (teaching and clinical units), including a large one in Lhasa and an even larger one in Beijing. There are also 57 hospitals of Tibetan medicine throughout China and 30 Tibetan medicine factories. The refugee community in Dharamsala has a medical college and there are several small manufacturers of Tibetan herb products throughout India and Nepal.

Tibetan medicine, like other traditional medical systems, is highly complex, and represents a comprehensive effort at dealing with health and disease. Some modern pharmacologists, herb enthusiasts, and product developers have focused on certain herbs that can be used in a general way, thus making them accessible to the world population without having to transmit the medical system itself. Two such herbs are rhodiola and hippophae.

RHODIOLA

Rhodiola is mainly found on rocky slopes at 3,500-5,000 meters (11,000-16,000 feet). The Chinese name *hongjingtian* refers to the red flowers of the stonecrop-the common name given in the West (hong = red, jingtian = view of heaven or heavenly view, probably referring to its growth on high altitude stone faces). This herb is in the family Crassulaceae, which yields a small number of genera of medicinal plants, mainly rhodiola and sedum. The root of the plant is used in the current medicinal applications. The outer peel of the root has a light golden color, so that the herb is sometimes referred to as golden root; the inside of the root is pink. There are several species of rhodiola collected, with the main ones being Rhodiola rosea and Rhodiola kirilowii; others are being investigated, including R. eoccinca, R. crentinii, R. krifida, and R. atropurpurea.

Tibetan rhodiola has become so popular in recent years that, according to a survey by the Tibet Institute of Biology, 10,000 tons of it are collected annually and six factories make products that have rhodiola as a key ingredient (or sole ingredient). Rather than relying on its traditional applications, rhodiola is presented as a health product of general benefit, described as an adaptogen.

The concept of an adaptogen has been attributed to the Russian pharmacologist N.V. Lazarev from his work during the period 1958-1959. Basically, he defined an adaptogen as a substance that has no toxicity or side effects at normal dosages and that non-specifically increases the resistance to disease and to physical and chemical stresses. Put another way, use of an adaptogenic herb will safely assist the body in maintaining its homeostatic balance and recovering from the effects of adverse weather, emotions, and disease influences. The leading advocates of developing natural resources as adaptogens were the Russian researchers I.I. Brekhman and I.V. Dardymov. They reviewed the status of research into adaptogenic agents in the seminal article "*New substances of plant origin which increase non-specific resistance,*" published in 1969 (9).

The leading adaptogens identified at that time were eleutherococcus (*Eleutherococcus senticosus*), ginseng (*Panax ginseng*), rhaponticum (*Rhaponticum carthamoides*), and rhodiola (*Rhodiola rosea*). The Russians went on to develop eleutherococcus (usually simplified to eleuthero) as a major health product, used locally and exported to Western countries. The Chinese developed their own resources of this herb (which grows in abundance in northeast China), eventually becoming the world's main supplier. Ginseng had long been used in the Orient and revered as a health tonic; the Koreans developed the world market for this herb, promoting research into its pharmacology and clinical effects and cultivating huge quantities of the roots. China and the U.S. (providing an American species, *P. quinquefolium*) eventually became major suppliers as well. Rhaponticum is still being investigated in China and Russia; it is mainly studied in relation to antioxidant activity, but is also reputed to improve circulation and mental acuity. Rhodiola has been researched in Russia and China and has become a common health food product which has been promoted in the West in recent years. The development of rhodiola as an adaptogen represents one aspect of Chinese efforts to promote Tibetan medicine (as one of the Chinese indigenous medical systems).

As an adaptogen, rhodiola is considered to be like ginseng (*renshen*) and eleuthero (*ciwujia*) in terms of effects and applications; adaptogens from numerous different plant species have the same basic actions (25). Modern promoters of rhodiola have dubbed the herb "Tibetan ginseng." Though some herbalists object to this off hand use of the term ginseng (similarly, ashwaganda is called Indian ginseng, eleuthero is called Siberian ginseng or eleuthero ginseng), it may well represent the current intended use of the herb for consumers who are already familiar with ginseng as a general health tonic. One of the adaptogenic applications of rhodiola that has received considerable research attention recently is for aiding adaptation to high altitudes, thus, as a preventive and treatment for mountain sickness (23, 24, 25).

Information about traditional uses of rhodiola remains somewhat limited; it was used for treatment of dysentery, back pain, lung inflammation with expectoration of bloody mucus, painful and irregular menstruation, leukorrhea, and traumatic injuries (25). Based on the indications for use, rhodiola appears to be cooling and detoxifying, and vitalizes blood circulation.

By including the related genus *Sedum* in the discussion, one can get a better understanding of the herb since the two are nearly interchangeable. Some of the Chinese and Tibetan species of *Sedum* go by the name *jingtian* that is used for rhodiola: *Sedum erythrostictum*, is the main species known by this name. Sedum was described (10) during the Song Dynasty as "being sweet in taste, cold and slightly toxic in nature, the plant crawls on stones of the southern side of a mountain and it is tender and lustrous...." *Sedum erythrostictum* was described in the *Bencao Gangmu* of the Ming Dynasty (11) as having the reputation of protecting from fire. It was grown in pots on housetops to protect the house (i.e., protecting thatched roofs), and the herb would be used to treat people burned by fire or scalded by hot water, or who suffered from the burning sensation of insect bites. It is used topically much the way we currently use *Aloe vera*, which has a similar mucilaginous quality to the leaves. Some Chinese species of *Sedum* are administered as hemostatics; this especially applies to *Sedum aizoon*, which is known as *tushanqi*, being named the same as the famous hemostatic notoginseng (*sanqi; tu* means local variety). The traditional Tibetan use of both sedum and rhodiola is for lung diseases, specifically, lung heat (generally meaning a lung infection). In fact, the two herbs are combined in a simple decoction with licorice and lacca (*zicaorong*) for treating lung heat (12).

In recent years, sedum extracts have been shown to protect the liver from damage due to chemicals and the herb has been used in treatment of viral hepatitis. The most commonly used species for this purpose in China is *Sedum sarmentosum* (*chuipencao*). The whole plant is applied in cases of damp-heat and to counteract toxic-heat (13). A tablet made from this herb, containing 8 mg of the glycoside component was used to treat chronic hepatitis at a dosage of 9 tablets per day (72 mg of glycoside). Its main effect was to lower transaminase levels within two weeks (23). In addition to tablets, rhodiola is produced in the form of a wine, oral liquid (that includes other Chinese herbs), capsule, and tea bag.

Much of the research on rhodiola has been carried out in Lhasa. The Tibet Institute of High Altitude Biology has done research with rhodiola and confirmed that it is of benefit as an adaptogen, including use against mountain sickness. A capsule with rhodiola and hippophae (plus lycium fruit) is produced by one factory and is promoted as a treatment for altitude sickness. In Chengdu, the West China University of Medical Sciences undertook a review of the research on this herb, which was published in 1988, evaluating 90 reports on the botany, chemistry, pharmacology, toxicology, and clinical effects. They reported that *hongjingtian* was obtained from the root and rhizome of several species of *Rhodiola*, with studies conducted on the constituents of 20 of China's 70 species. The active constituents include numerous flavonoids (such as quercetin, rutin, and kaempferol), condensed flavonoids (polyphenols, mainly gallic acid and epigallocatechin), cyanoglycosides (which have histamine-inhibiting activity), and salidroside, which is deemed one of the main active constituents of interest by virtually all authorities. In concentrated extracts of rhodiola, salidroside makes up about 1-2% of the content. Salidroside is comprised of tyrosol linked to glucose; tyrosol is one of the major flavors and aroma ingredients of the olive which confers notable antioxidant activity to olive oil. Rhodiola also contains sterols, notably daucosterol and sitosterol.

According to mouse experiments conducted in China, rhodiola extract has a central stimulant action and increases the tolerance to anoxia, fatigue, microwave irradiation, poisoning by strychnine, tetanin, and other toxins; it regulates brain functions, leukocyte count, blood glucose, and promotes protein hydrolysis; and it enhances the functions of the thyroid gland, adrenals, and ovaries. According to the reports from recent clinical research efforts conducted mainly in Russia, rhodiola may prove helpful in treating depression and its use may result in improvements in mental performance and alleviation of fatigue. All reports suggest that the toxicity of rhodiola is very low and that there are no significant side effects (24).

As can be seen, the modern research (both laboratory and clinical) is aimed at the potential of rhodiola as an adaptogen rather than its traditional function as a treatment for lung diseases.

HIPPOPHAE

Hippophae (Chinese: *shaji,* literally: sand thorn, the English common name is sea buckthorn) is a member of the Elaeagnaceae family, a family that has very few medicinal herbs, mainly *Hippophae, Eleaegnus,* and *Elaeocarpus.* There is one dominant species of *Hippophae* used in China and Russia: *H. rhamnoides.* Hippophae is usually found at an altitude of 1,200-2,000 meters (4,000-6,500 feet) in cold climates, though it can grow at both higher and lower altitudes, in sandy soil. It has recently been planted in temperate zones worldwide to prevent soil erosion and to serve as a source of food and medicine (15). Hippophae has been developed into a major resource for China, with numerous organizations devoted to the project, including the following three that have sponsored a journal, *Hippophae,* that has been published (in Chinese) since 1988:

- China Research and Training Centre on Sea Buckthorn
- Sea Buckthorn Office of the Yellow River Water Commission
- Shaanxi Sea Buckthorn Development Office

The fruit is the main part used as food and medicine. It is one of the richest sources of vitamin C, with about 6 mg/gram in the fruit and about 5 mg per ml of fruit juice (16), so the juice has been made into a health beverage on that basis. Medicinally, the flavonoids of the fruit and the oil of the seed are deemed the main active constituents. The flavonoid are present in the range of 1-10 mg/gram of fresh fruit.

Injected into laboratory animals (17) at a dose in the range of 2-5 mg/kg, they improve non-specific immunity (one of the actions of an adaptogen). In addition, the flavonoids promote bone marrow production of red blood cells, and reduce allergy reactions (26). Both the vitamin C and flavonoids are thought to help protect against carcinogenesis when ingesting food contaminated with carcinogens (18). In a double-blind clinical trial (19) 128 patients with ischemic heart disease were given total flavonoids of hippophae at 10 mg each time, three times daily, for 6 weeks. The patients had a decrease in cholesterol level and improved cardiac function; also they had less angina than those receiving the control drug isosorbide dinitrate. No harmful effect of hippophae flavonoids was noted in renal functions or hepatic functions.

Hippophae seed oil is rich in vitamin E and essential fatty acids, including several that inhibit inflammation. One ingredient, palmitoleic acid, is a component of skin that is considered very valuable in treating burns and healing wounds. The oil is used alone or in various preparations topically applied for a wide range of skin ailments, including burns, scalds, ulcerations, infections, and as an aid in promoting regeneration of tissues and protectant in sunblocks (hippophae oil itself has UV-blocking activity). The seed oil and the bark of the plant have been found to possess anti-tumor effects in preliminary laboratory studies (15). For internal use, the oil is put into soft gelatin capsules, which are used for treating gastric and duodenal ulcers, liver inflammation, and skin disorders, such as atopic dermatitis. Both the seed oil and flavonoids have been used in laboratory animal studies aimed at revealing adaptogenic properties, such as protection against harmful effects of radiation, cold, fatigue from excessive activity demands, and oxygen deficits (26).

In the Indian Materia Medica, hippophae is mentioned briefly, the fruit being used for lung diseases (20). In Thousand Formulas and Thousand Herbs of Traditional Chinese Medicine (21), hippophae fruit is described as sour, astringent, and warm in nature, and used to eliminate phlegm, stop cough, improve digestion and remove accumulations, and to move blood and remove blood stasis. Examples of uses are:

cough with profuse sputum;
abdominal pain due to accumulation of food and indigestion;
amenorrhea due to blood stasis; and
swelling and stagnation in trauma.

These functions and applications are similar to those described in Tibetan medicine, where hippophae is used for lung-heat disorders and stomach-intestine disorders with bleeding. However, the emphasis of modern research and product development is on its nutritional and general health benefits rather than the traditional medical applications. Some simple formulas with more specific applications have been developed recently; for example, there is a liquid preparation of hippophae, carthamus, and licorice intended for use in treatment coronary heart disease and sequelae of heart attack and stroke, based on improving blood circulation.

Traditional Tibetan Formulae with Rhodiola and Hippophae

T. J. Tsarong outlined 175 important Tibetan formulas in his Handbook of Traditional Tibetan Drugs (22). In the next two tables, formulas with rhodiola and/or hippophae are mentioned; other herbs commonly included in these formulas are: sandalwood, saussurea, carthamus, bamboo, terminalia, licorice; geranium, emblica, gentiana, inula, and grapes (see also Tables 5 & 6). Of these, all are used in

Chinese medicine except emblica and grapes, both used extensively in Indian medicine. Tsarong included 12 formulas that utilize rhodiola, all of which are used for lung disorders (see Tables 3 & 4).

Table 3
Traditional Tibetan Formulas with Rhodiola. The Number of Herbs in the Formula is Indicated in the Formula Name or Added in Parenthesis After the Formula Name

Formula	*Main Uses in Tibetan Tradition*
Blue Garuda Bird (9)	acute inflammation of the lungs and throat, as well as fever and dysentery
Bamboo 9	coughing, infections, fever and diarrhea (this formula is usually used for pediatric cases)
Pulmonary Medicine of Death Healing Nectar (15)	acute and chronic cough and sputum streaked with pus (formula includes hippophae)
Eliminator of Lung Inflammation (13)	inflammation of the lungs, cough, chest congestion
Eliminator of All Lung Imbalances (11)	chronic cough with expectoration of phlegm, and fever
Blood Gentian Pill (18)	antipyretic and expectorant for inflammation of the lungs and cough
Gentiana 15	cough, shortness of breath, hoarseness, blood in sputum
Sandalwood 8	inflammation of the lungs, blood and pus in the sputum
Sandalwood 9 (add cinnamon to above)	inflammation of the lungs, pus in the sputum, fever
Yuthog's Bamboo 25	pain and inflammation of the lungs, blood in the sputum, inflammation of the respiratory tract (formula includes hippophae)
Copper Calcine 25	all types of lung inflammation; difficulty breathing, coughing

A representative rhodiola formula is the Eliminator of Lung Inflammation. Its ingredients, in addition to rhodiola, are bamboo, carthamus, clove, white and red sandalwoods, geranium, terminalia, aconite, myrrh, musk, saussurea, and cinnabar (vermilion). Though this is considered a valuable remedy by the Tibetans, it is not a suitable preparation for use in the West, as it contains raw aconite (a toxic substance, though used in small amounts), musk (obtained from the musk deer, an endangered species), saussurea (collected from wild sources; it is an endangered species), and cinnabar (contains mercury). The main characteristic of the formula is that it is very fragrant, mainly due to the clove, saussurea, sandalwood, geranium, myrrh, and musk; it has a bitter, acrid, astringent taste (sandalwood, saussurea, and terminalia are the main astringents); and the overall action is cooling. When interpreting its effects and uses, it must be understood that the classification of the herbs are often different in the Tibetan system compared to the Chinese system. As examples, both carthamus and sandalwood are deemed warming in the Chinese system but cooling in the Tibetan system; sandalwood is used to regulate qi in the Chinese system, but is applied as an astringent in the Tibetan system; carthamus is used in the Chinese system to vitalize blood circulation, but it is used to stop bleeding and nourish blood in the Tibetan system. In this formulation, phlegm-fire (chiba; bile) is controlled by ingredients such as white sandalwood, carthamus, and bamboo, while phlegm-damp (peigen) is controlled by aconite and penetrated by the fragrant herbs. This formula is suited to treating lung diseases in which there is considerable difficulty breathing due to sticky phlegm.

Two of the formulas in Table 3 include hippophae; there are also 6 formulas with hippophae that do not include rhodiola (see Table 4). Most of these are also used for lung diseases and phlegm accumulation problems, but hippophae is also included in formulas for treating blood-heat disorders (these usually manifest as bleeding disorders).

Table 4
Traditional Tibetan Formulas with Hippophae
(see Table 3 for two Additional Formulas)

Formula	*Main Uses in Tibetan Tradition*
Blue Poppy 8	to control excess blood from the liver into the stomach lining (hematemesis)
Balancing Comforter (17)	for all types of phlegm accumulation with lack of stomach heat (symptoms of anorexia, indigestion, stomach tumors), discomfort of stomach and liver, hematamesis, lymphatic disorders, skin disorders (including itching)
Reed of Comfort (17)	for phlegm accumulation, pain along with emesis of sour and watery vomitus, inflammation of the stomach, indigestion, hematemesis, irregular menstruation, painful menstruation
White Nectar Pill (5)	to promote digestion (increases stomach fire), disintegrates stomach tumors and mucus, removes phlegm accumulations, acts like a nectar for colic and cold parasites
Amla 25	removes bad blood, reduces blood pressure, treats dryness of throat and mouth, and redness of eyes
Hippophae 5	for chronic inflammation of the lungs, with discharge of pus and blood; it suppresses coughing and treats hidden fever

A representative formula with hippophae is Hippophae 5; which also contains licorice, grape, emblica, and saussurea. This is a formula compatible with Western requirements in terms of safety of the herbal materials, though the main Tibetan source for saussurea, *S. lappa*, is on the endangered species list (cultivated sources and a related herb used as a common substitute, *Vladimiria souliei*, can resolve this problem). Hippophae 5 has the characteristic of being sweet (mainly due to licorice and grape) and sour (mainly due to the hippophae and emblica) with only modest fragrance (mainly contributed by saussurea) and a cooling quality (not compensated by spicy warm herbs). Sweet herbs are considered useful for controlling *chiba* (phlegm-fire), while *peigen* (phlegm) is controlled both by sour herbs and those that are coarse (hippophae). This formula is given for lung disorders with accompanying fever, and with free flowing mucus. Comparing the two formulas-Eliminator of Lung Inflammation and Hippophae 5-the former is more suited for lung disorders dominated by stuffiness and the latter is more suited for lung problems associated with fever and infection (which can lead to discharge of copious mucus including pus and blood), while both are good for the most general category of lung inflammation.

Tibetan Herbs Commonly Combined with Rhodiola and Hippophae

In traditional Tibetan formulas, rhodiola and hippophae are combined in complex formulas, as depicted above, for treatment of lung diseases. Table 5 presents these two key herbs along with several of the other herbs commonly included in the formulas. Table 6 presents information about the inclusion of these herbs in the same formulas that are listed in Table 3 and Table 4. Other herbs, that are in some of these formulas but mentioned less frequently, include geranium, emblica, gentiana, inula, and grapes.

Tibetan medicine is a derivative of the Indian and Chinese medical systems, with a dominant Buddhist influence, especially that carried over as a translation and revision of the Four Medical Tantras during the 8th Century

Table 5
Tibetan Herbs Commonly used in Formulas for Treating Lung Diseases. The Tibetan Name is Presented According to the Transliteration System used in the Quintessence Tantras of Tibetan Medicine (6), and the Indian Name is Presented According to Indian Materia Medica (20)

Herb (common name); (botanical name)	*Tibetan name; Part used*	*Sanskrit name; Bengal name*	*Chinese name; Category*
Bamboo resin *Bambusa sp. or Phyllostachys sp.*	chu-gan gresin	vansa bans	*tianzhuhuang* resolve phlegm
Carthamus* *Carthamus tinctorius*	gur-kum flower	kamalottera; kusumbakajireh	*honghua* vitalize blood
Hippophae *Hippophae rhamnoides*	star-bufruit	dhurchuk (Hindi) dhurchuk	*shaji* resolve phlegm
Licorice *Glycyrrhiza glabra* or *G. uralensis*	shing-mngar root	madhuka, yashti-madhuyashto -madhu	*gancao* tonify qi
Rhodiola *Rhodiola sp.*	sro-lo whole plant	Not included	*hongjingtian* tonify qi
Sandalwood (red) *Pterocarpus santalinus*	tsan-dan dmar-poheart wood	rakta chandana pit-sal	*hongtanxiang* regulate qi
Sandalwood (white) *Santalum alba*	tsan-dan dkar-po heart wood	chandanam; srigandha sada-chandan	*tanxiang* regulate qi
Saussurea *Saussurea lappa*	ru-rta root	puskara, kushta kashmirjagada pachak	*guangmuxiang* regulate qi
Terminalia *Terminalia chebula*	a-ru-ra fruit	haritaki, abhaya, pathya, etc. hirda	*hezi* astringent

*common substitute for saffron, the originally-specified ingredient

Table 6
The Inclusion of Common Tibetan Herbs in the Formulas with Rhodiola and/or Hippophae

Formula	*Rhodiola*	*Hippophae*	*Sandalwood*	*Saussurea*	*Carthamus*	*Bamboo*	*Terminalia*	*Licorice*
Blue Garuda Bird	•						•	
Bamboo 9	•		•		•	•		
Pulmonary Medicine of Death Healing Nectar	•	•	•	•	•	•		•
Eliminator of Lung Inflammation	•		•	•	•	•	•	
Eliminator of All Lung Imbalances	•		•				•	
Blood Gentiana Pill	•		•	•		•	•	•
Gentiana 15	•			•		•	•	•
Sandalwood 8 & 9	•		•		•	•		•
Yuthog's Bamboo 25	•	•	•	•	•	•	•	•
Copper Calcine 25	•		•		•	•		•
Blue Poppy 8		•			•	•		•
Balancing Comforter		•	•		•	•		
Reed of Comfort		•		•	•	•	•	
White Nectar Pill		•						
Amla 25		•	•	•	•		•	
Hippophae 5		•		•				•

A.D. Tibetan herbal medicine represents a complex system that involves a large number of medicinal substances, about a third of which are high altitude plants (especially those that grow in dry sandy or rocky areas). The classical Tibetan Materia Medica was developed in the 19th Century, and remains the primary source of pre-scientific herb information. Rhodiola and hippophae are examples of herbs frequently included in traditional Tibetan formulas, especially for treatment of lung diseases. They have been developed into health products apart from the Tibetan tradition, with rhodiola promoted as an adaptogenic agent, and hippophae as a nutritious beverage, a treatment for circulatory disorders, and as a skin protectant and healer.

Tibetan medicine has been promoted and further developed in recent years both by China and by Tibetan refugee physicians. The main Tibetan texts are being translated into other languages (mainly Chinese and English) and scholars are investigating archeological sites and lost texts. The Tibetan medical system is experiencing a revival as the growing world population seeks solutions for difficult medical problems for which the modern system lacks adequate remedies. However, there are not enough trained physicians to support the demand. It is likely that more of the individual Tibetan herbs will be taken from this tradition and developed as health products as further research is undertaken. These general health products may stimulate interest in the preservation and further development of this unique medical tradition.

Concludingly, Tibetan medical philosophy is a holistic philosophy involving the harmonious operation and balance of all the energies that constitute the human psycho-physical being. These energies are the psychologically originating three "NYES-PA", or humours, which correspond to the three mental poisons, and the five cosmo-physical energies that are at the basis of all phenomena. If all the factors that influence these energies (seasonal factors, diet and nutrition, life style and mental attitudes) are positively disposed, then these energies remain in balanced operation and health is experienced. It is the objective of Tibetan medicine that the balance in these energies should be maintained.

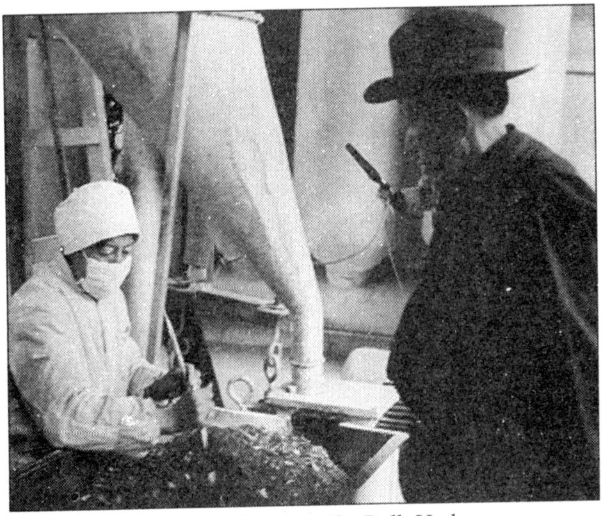

Figure 1: Blending the Bulk Herbs

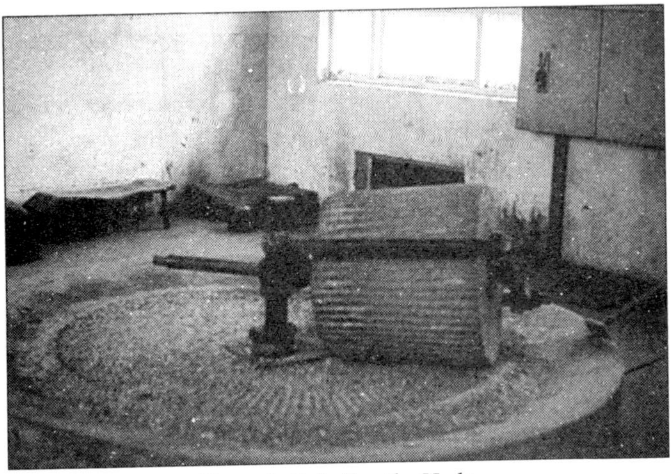

Figure 2: Grinding the Herbs

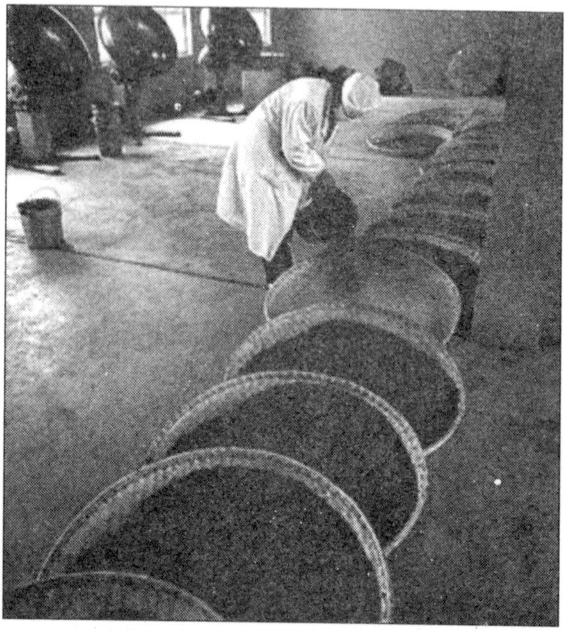

Figure 3: Setting the Pills out to Dry; note Pill Rolling Machines in Background

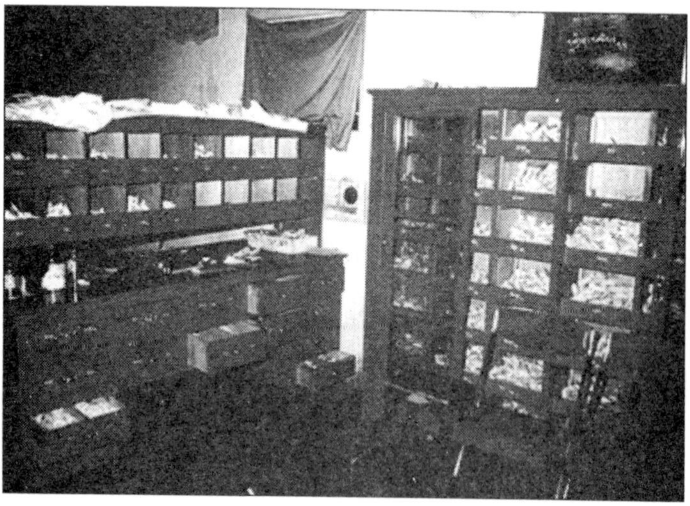

Figure 4: Tibetan Dispensary; White Bundles are Pre-packaged Pills

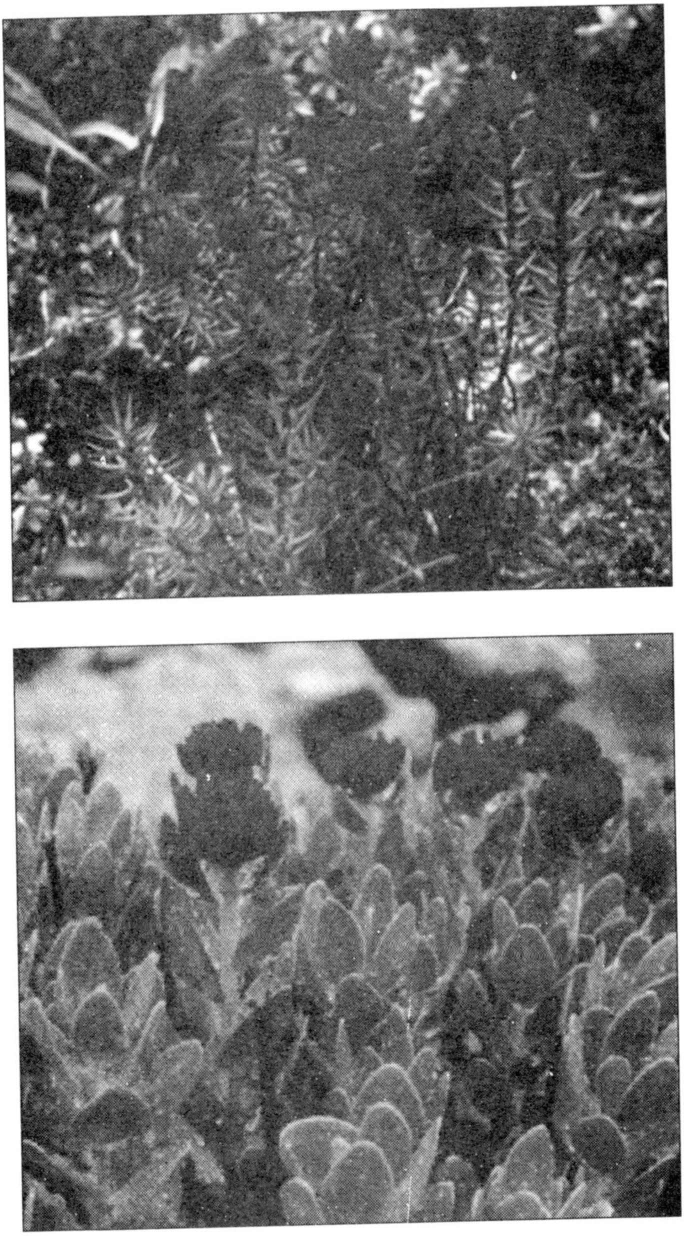

Figure 5: Two Views of Rhodiola (Different Species)

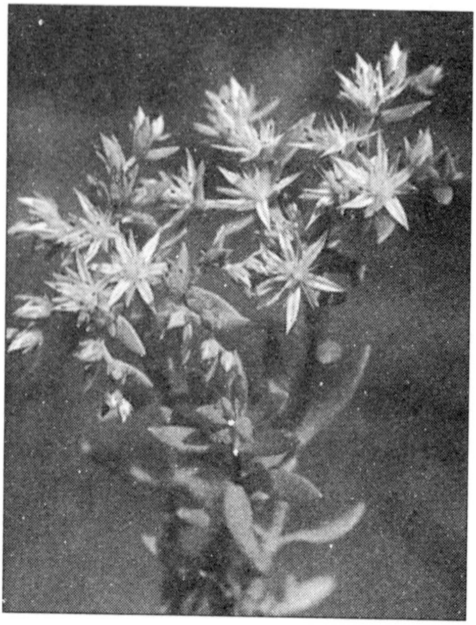

Figure 6: Sedum Sarmentosum

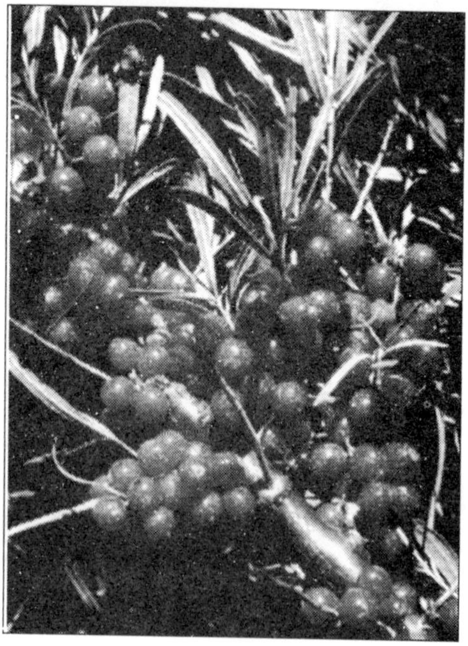

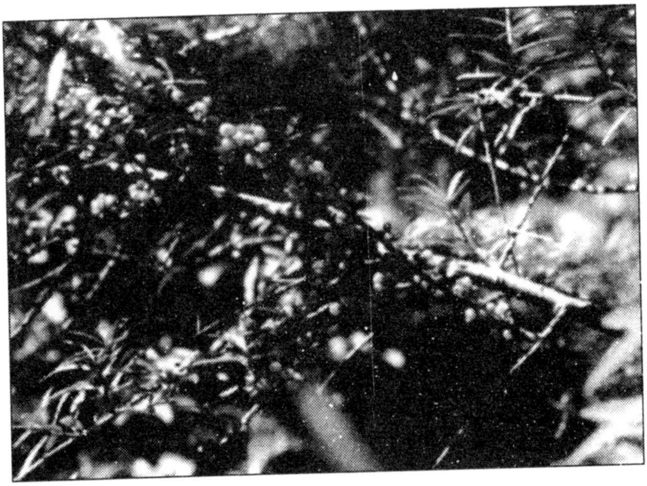

Figure 7: Two Views of Hippophae

HERBAL SOURCES AND TIBETAN MEDICINE

Tibetan medicine is celebrated as a source of sustainable and affordable healing preparations that are effective without lasting negative side effects. Our goal is to give people all over the world access to this unique insight into human well being.

Along with the need to provide training for a new generation of physicians and herbal pharmacists, and to translate the Tibetan medical so that students can begin their training without first having to learn to read Classical Tibetan, the main obstacle to wider use of Tibetan medicine is the limited supply of many herbs used in compounding the medications, some of which are already endangered by excessive non-professional harvesting.

His Holiness The Dalai Lama has warned that the health of the billions of people in the world cannot be sustained by medicines made with rare and endangered Himalayan plants. Even now, when Tibetan medicine has hardly begun to be practiced in Western countries, the herbs needed for making many of the medicines are in short supply. For example, the Men-Tse-Khang pharmacy in Dharamsala, India — the most respected source of Tibetan medicines — turns away all requests for medications except those accompanied by a prescription written by one of their own doctors. They will not accommodate even orders from their own graduates, those who have emigrated from India to other countries, explaining that to do so would deplete the supply of medicines needed in their branch clinics in India and Nepal.

Three different approaches to this scarcity of medicines are being explored. The most obvious and the most urgent is to preserve whenever possible the plants and animals currently used in Tibetan medicines, by protecting the ecologies that support those organisms, planting some species to increase the supply, and developing resources like seed banks to insure these species against extinction.

A second strategy is to extend the area where the herbs grow by planting in the wild and by finding ways of cultivating some species, as a way of preserving those that cannot be preserved in the wild, and as a way of increasing supplies.

The third is to evaluate the medicinal qualities of plants in other areas. Tibetan doctors have always used many imported materials in making their medicines, and believe that using substitute materials with similar therapeutic action is entirely appropriate when the ingredients of choice are unavailable. Tibetan physicians can identify plants indigenous to other areas that are suitable for use as substitutes for ingredients in traditional formulas and in developing new preparations.

Herbal medicine systems from other cultures will be useful in identifying promising species. Especially promising are two other systems which have ancient connections with Tibetan medicine and are still practiced: Indian Ayurvedic medicine and Chinese herbal medicine. Many of the herbs used in these systems are already used in Tibetan medicine.

The research needed for effort seems endless. The newsletter of the Chakpori Tibetan Medical Institute in Darjeeling, India, comments on some of the main issues: "To know which plants are vulnerable, endangered, or close to extinction, detailed studies have to be made. Also, the cause of rarity should be investigated (e.g., environmental causes, over exploitation by non-expert gathering, etc.). An important decision has to be made to replant not only the economically valuable plants but also the plants that are environmentally valuable and supportive of the total environment.

"Replanting sites should have the same characteristics as the original habitat. In traditional Tibetan medical texts, the side of the mountain, altitude, climatic condition, soil composition, etc. are mentioned [as important influences on the properties and potency of the herbs] .... research findings are essential guidelines for replanting the herbs in their natural environment. The size of the replanting area is also crucial because of genetic diversity and the problems of insular ecology. Monocultures, like the usual big plantations, should be avoided: mass plantations of certain species will not have the desired quality or power."

Medical Research Tibetan Style

Tibetan medicine is celebrated as a source of sustainable and affordable healing preparations that are effective without lasting negative side effects. Our goal is to give people all over the world access to this unique insight into human well being.

Along with the need to provide training for a new generation of physicians and herbal pharmacists, and to translate the Tibetan medical so that students can begin their training without first having to learn to read Classical Tibetan, the main obstacle to wider use of Tibetan medicine is the limited supply of many herbs used in compounding the medications, some of which are already endangered by excessive non-professional harvesting.

His Holiness The Dalai Lama has warned that the health of the billions of people in the world cannot be sustained by medicines made with rare and endangered Himalayan plants. Even now, when Tibetan medicine has hardly begun to be practiced in Western countries, the herbs needed for making many of the medicines are in short supply. For example, the Men-Tse-Khang pharmacy in Dharamsala, India — the most respected source of Tibetan medicines — turns away all requests for medications except those accompanied by a prescription written by one of their own doctors. They will not accommodate even orders from their own graduates, those who have emigrated from India to other countries, explaining that to do so would deplete the supply of medicines needed in their branch clinics in India and Nepal.

Three different approaches to this scarcity of medicines are being explored. The most obvious and the most urgent is to preserve whenever possible the plants and animals currently used in Tibetan medicines, by protecting the ecologies that support those organisms, planting some species to increase the supply, and developing resources like seed banks to insure these species against extinction.

A second strategy is to extend the area where the herbs grow by planting in the wild and by finding ways of cultivating some species, as a way of preserving those that cannot be preserved in the wild, and as a way of increasing supplies.

The third is to evaluate the medicinal qualities of plants in other areas. Tibetan doctors have always used many imported materials in making their medicines, and believe that using substitute materials with similar therapeutic action is entirely appropriate when the ingredients of choice are unavailable. Tibetan physicians can identify plants indigenous to other areas that are suitable for use as substitutes for ingredients in traditional formulas and in developing new preparations.

Herbal medicine systems from other cultures will be useful in identifying promising species. Especially promising are two other systems which have ancient connections with Tibetan medicine and are still practiced: Indian Ayurvedic medicine and Chinese herbal medicine. Many of the herbs used in these systems are already used in Tibetan medicine.

The research needed for effort seems endless. The newsletter of the Chakpori Tibetan Medical Institute in Darjeeling, India, comments on some of the main issues: "To know which plants are vulnerable, endangered, or close to extinction, detailed studies have to be made. Also, the cause of rarity should be investigated (e.g., environmental causes, over exploitation by non-expert gathering, etc.). An important decision has to be made to replant not only the economically valuable plants but also the plants that are environmentally valuable and supportive of the total environment.

"Replanting sites should have the same characteristics as the original habitat. In traditional Tibetan medical texts, the side of the mountain, altitude, climatic condition, soil composition, etc. are mentioned [as important influences on the properties and potency of the herbs] .... research findings are essential guidelines for replanting the herbs in their natural environment. The size of the replanting area is also crucial because of genetic diversity and the problems of insular ecology. Monocultures, like the usual big plantations, should be avoided: mass plantations of certain species will not have the desired quality or power."

Evaluation research can explore whether Tibetan physicians, using traditional methods of diagnosis and treatment, are successfull in treating various health problems, or in helping to prevent them. However, designing studies that will truly and fairly address that question presents a real challenge.

Furthermore, even research that involve Tibetan doctors may fail to fairly assess the full potential of the traditional Tibetan medical system, unless the Tibetan physicians are allowed to practice medicine in whatever ways they consider most appropriate. Many studies have imposed restrictions on various aspects of the Tibetan doctor's work.

Our goal here is to design a research project that could truly show whether the Tibetan system of medicine, as defined by the preferred diagnostic and therapeutic practices of respected Tibetan physicians, is truly effective, using Western standards of evaluation.

To fairly assess, scientifically, the full potential of Tibetan medicine, we must make sure that the treatments we are evaluating are the best available — and for this we must rely on Tibetan doctors. However, we can assume that the treatments they are using are the best that Tibetan medicine has to offer only if our research design does not interfere in the relationship between the Tibetan doctors and their patients.

Tibetan doctors naturally strive to give their patients the best possible treatment, so any restraints we place on the Tibetan doctors choice of medicines, or any other interference we impose in the relationship between the doctors and their patients, will mean that the treatment we are evaluating is not the best that Tibetan medicine has to offer.

In this type of research the Tibetan physicians would have to be entirely in charge of how their diagnosis and treatment is done. Western scientists would be in charge of the evaluation statistics, and Western doctors would provide medical diagnosis before and after the treatment of each patient, so the results will make sense to us. Including Western diagnosis will also allow us to begin to study traditional Tibetan medical diagnosis, by comparing Tibetan diagnosis and Western diagnosis of the same patients.

The overall outline of such a study is simple; however, working out the details of how to make such a study truly informative presents some real challenges.

The first challenge we face comes from our presumption that we already basically understand what is important in Tibetan medicine and what can be safely discarded. If a traditional medical system, combining spiritual, psychological and material practices, actually works to improve some serious health problem, we easily assume that it must have been the material elements of the system, the medicines or physical manipulations of the body, or perhaps the physiological consequences of changes in behavior or diet, that caused the improvement. Accordingly, with passionate faith in scientific materialism, we further assume that there is no need to include spiritual aspects of the system in a test of it's efficacy, since they can't really be making any difference.

This does presume too much, however, as I think you can see. If we are trying to enter into a dialog with the Tibetan physicians, then it is not enough to translate their terms into our language. We need to add Western diagnosis to the study, in order for it to make sense to us as evaluating treatments for diseases that we recognize; but we also need to include whatever the Tibetan doctors want to include in order for them to accept it as a scientific study of the full potential of Tibetan medicine. For example, if the doctor wants to prescribe mantras to the Medicine Buddha, and the patient wants to say them, who are we to insist that they must be irrelevant? We can study compliance in saying the mantras in the same way that we study compliance in taking the medicines, without much extra effort.

If we do find that Tibetan medicine is effective for certain types of illnesses, then interested people could certainly perform follow-up studies to see if it might be just as effective without the mantras (or without the herbal medicines). At first, though, we can avoid possible confusion about whether we have really done a fair test of the Tibetan system of healing, by respecting the Tibetan doctors as experts on issues of how Tibetan medicine is practiced.

A commitment to respecting the Tibetan doctors' standards of practice will challenge our ingenuity. For example, if our research design is to impose no restrictions on the doctors' choices of herbal medicines, that might require waiting to do the study until the FDA has approved all the tibetan medicinal formulas that our doctors would like to be able to use; or it might mean that the study would have to be done in India or some other country that allows Tibetan physicians the full use of their traditional pharmacopoeia.

We also will need to develop a way to provide Western diagnostic services for the patients, including interviews and lab work, under the direction of Western physicians. These services will be needed before treatment, to establish the type, severity and complications of the patients problem (from the Western perspective), and after treatment, to determine whatever improvement may have occurred.

We can deal with these challenges; not easily, perhaps, but straightforwardly. However, one major challenge remains: If the Tibetan physicians are to be entirely in charge of how their diagnosis and treatment is done, we obviously cannot require them to merely pretend to treat half of their patients. Thus we will have to set aside the generally accepted standards for clinical evaluation studies: Specifically, we cannot use a randomized double-blind placebo-controlled clinical trial.

We will need to review the reasons for the various aspects of the standard research protocol, to see if we can come up with an alternative design — one that would preserve the validity of the study without interfering in the relationship between the Tibetan doctors and their patients.

In the next section we will discuss the detailed logic of a research plan that seems to meet both those criteria.

Research Design for Evaluating Tibetan Medicine

Randomized double-blind clinical trials are a powerful tool for assessing whether a certain medicine, or some other treatment, is effective. However, several characteristics of this particular design make it less appropriate for an initial exploration of a traditional medical system.

Specifically, for this purpose randomized double-blind clinical trials are overly expensive, overly focused, and overly disruptive of normal clinical practice, when compared a less disruptive design that we will discuss in some detail. However, before we would want to seriously consider adopting such a design, whatever its virtues, we would need to be assured that it would provide valid evidence of the effectiveness, or lack of effectiveness, of the medical system we intend to study. So we will need to consider some of the specific characteristics of the standard clinical trial, to see what criteria any alternative design must meet.

In a typical randomized double-blind clinical trial, patients who present with a particular condition, e.g., people with the symptoms of diabetes mellitus, are randomly assigned to either of two groups. Those assigned to the "treatment" or "experimental" group are given the medicine or other treatment that is being evaluated, and those assigned to the "control" or "comparison" group, are given a placebo treatment — a sham treatment administered in the same way, by the same personnel, as the test treatment, but having no physiological effect. If possible the study is double blinded, so that neither the physician nor the patient knows what treatment the patient is receiving, although both are aware of other aspects of the study. In research governed by modern Western ethical standards for medical research, the patient and the physician must both understand that they are participating in a clinical trial that may randomly deny treatment to the patient.

In randomized double-blind clinical trials, the procedure for obtaining informed consent for participation in the study is just the first of many disruptions in the normal operation of the clinic and the normal relationship between patient and doctor. Uncertainty about whether the patient is receiving real treatment or a placebo can undermine the atmosphere of healing generated by the environment of the clinic and the psychological and spiritual bond between the patient and the physician. The more serious the illness, the more this aspect of the study may tend to make the patient anxious, and undermine the doctor's confidence that she is doing her best to help the patient. Taken together, we might think of these influences as a Negative Placebo Effect, produced by the requirements of the randomized double-blind research plan.

The design we are proposing eliminates the control condition. All patients will be given whatever treatment the physician considers appropriate. There are no placebo treatments and no procedures for withholding information from patients or physicians. No physician is asked to pretend to treat some of her patients. With each patient she does the best she can to provide appropriate treatment, and both she and the patient understand that.

If we want to eliminate the control condition from the design of a clinical trial, we need to consider why the randomized double-blind design has become the standard for research of this type, and whether we can find other ways of accomplishing the objectives that led to its adoption.

Randomized: Random Assignment of Patients to Treatment and Non-treatment Conditions

Controled experiments are so common in scientific work in almost all fields that many people erroneously believe that all scientific research involves them. Actually, non-experimental observation is an equally valuable method, which is especially useful in beginning to explore a subject. Most likely an observational study would be more appropriate than the standard experimental clinical trial in the initial phases of studying Tibetan medicine.

In a standard clinical trial the control condition makes it possible to determine whether it is the treatment we are studying that caused whatever improvement we may see. People's medical problems can improve for all sorts of reasons — a change in the season, a change in diet or behavior, or simply the passing of time, which works quite well in resolving the common cold and many other medical problems. If we randomly assign patients with a particular diagnosis to either a group that will be given the treatment we are studying, or a group that will not be given the treatment, we can compare the two groups to see if the patients who were given the treatment improve more than the untreated patients.

In the study we are proposing, we do not need a control condition to determine whether patients have improved.

Assessing whether any given patient has improved during the period of the study can be accomplished by comparing the results of the standard Western diagnostic measures that will be taken before and after treatment.

However, in our study, just as in other clinical trials, it will take more than improvement in a patient's condition to demonstrate that the medicine we are studying has helped them. Including a non-treatment control condition would have allowed us to determine whether it is the Tibetan doctor's treatment that causes whatever improvement we may see. However, since we want to avoid the control condition and the Negative Placebo Effect it may cause, we have to come up with some other way of determining whether Tibetan medical treatment is contributing to whatever improvement we may see in the patients.

There is a way to do that: We can determine statistically whether the Tibetan medical treatments were an effective curative agent by comparing the results from patients in the study with historical evidence of what would be expected in people with that particular diagnosis. What percentage of people with that illness would recover, what percentage would continue to suffer the condition chronically, and for what percentage the problem would be fatal or have other undesirable consequences — we would need to find such statistics in the medical records for various regions. The records may show what outcomes can be expected both without treatment and with standard Western medical intervention.

This is not a new idea. It is what is normally done when placebo- controlled studies are considered ethically inappropriate, for example in research on life-threatening diseases where a somewhat effective treatment is already available, and researchers are testing alternatives that might be more effective.

In preparation for a study evaluating the Tibetan medical system, Western medical consultants would have to determine, for each type of health problem, how much improvement on the diagnostic indicators would be required to demonstrate that the Tibetan treatment had indeed produced a therapeutic effect. For example, Western physicians might consider it quite unlikely for a particular type of tumor to disappear from a patient's x-ray without effective treatment. So if a group of patients are given Tibetan medical treatment, and in a large percentage of them the tumor shrinks or vanishes, we can safely conclude that the treatment caused the improvement in most of them, since only a very small percentage of these tumors would normally disappear spontaneously. In contrast, for an illness that will normally clear up without treatment, we might have to see an improvement that was clearly faster than normal, or which left fewer lasting negative effects such as loss of function or disfigurement, before concluding that the treatment had a real therapeutic effect.

The main disadvantage of the base-rate comparison we are proposing is that it is less sensitive than the standard randomized treatment / non-treatment comparison. However, the proposed design offers a way to make a very cost effective preliminary evaluation of the traditional Tibetan treatments for a wide range of medical problems. Any results that are dramatic enough to inspire further study can be followed up with more sensitive experimental studies.

Placebo (Sham Treatment) Control

Patients assigned to the control condition in clinical trials used to be simply given no treatment, but this is no longer generally considered appropriate. To control for the effects of a phenomenon known as the "placebo effect" patients in the control group are given fake treatment which is as similar as possible to the real treatment except for omission of the therapeutic agent being studied: sugar pills, injections of slightly salty water, whatever will most resemble the actual trealment without having any physiological effect is given to the patients in the placebo control condition in the same way that the active medicine is administered to the patients who are receiving the real treatment.

"Placebo Effect" is the term commonly used for improvement that results from the psychological effects of *believing* that one is being given an effective treatment. The Placebo Effect was believed to result in measured improvement on various physiological indicators, and it even makes sense in light of evidence showing that improvements in a person's mood can have a positive effect on the immune system. However, some people have raised the question of whether a placebo effect exists at all.

Before deciding to use a placebo-controlled randomized experimental design in a clinical trial we should be clear about exactly what we intend to study. If we are focusing solely on the therapeutic value of a particular medication or other treatment, then radomly assigning half of the patients in the study to a placebo control condition may be a straightforward way to isolate the effects of the treatment from other known and unknown factors that could lead to improvement in a patient's condition. However, if what we intend to study is an entire medical system, one that we don't understand, then we have to study the system as is is traditionally practiced, at least at first.

Specifically, if the system we intend to study is traditional Tibetan medicine, in which psychological and spiritual influences are intentionally included for their synergistic enhancement of the therapeutic effects of medications and other treatments, then the Placebo effect, or something very much like it, is part of the therapeutic process, and is not in any sense something we should be trying to control for. In an initial study of the Tibetan medical system, subjecting all the participants in the study to the Negative Placebo Effect we discussed earlier is clearly inappropriate.

If a preliminary survey of the effectiveness of the Tibetan medical system, in treating each of the different medical conditions that it is commonly used for, finds that it does actually offer some benefit for patients afflicted with one or more of these conditions, we will of course want to know how it works. For each particular medical problem, we can ask which of the many elements of traditional Tibetan medical practice actually make some positive contribution to the therapeutic effect demonstrated in the preliminary studies.

In research aimed at answering those questions, placebo controls may have some role to play. However, the design used in standard clinical trials will not allow us to answer the question of whether something like a placebo effect mught be synergistically enhancing the effects of other aspects of Tibetan medical treatment. Do do that would require a design with four different groups: Treatment, No Treatment, Placebo, and a group that is given the treatment withiout being aware that they are participating in a randomized clinical trial in which some of the other patients will be given no treatment or placebos. This design would also allow us to determine whether the standard design does in fact produce what I have called here a 'Negative Placebo Effect."

Double-Blind

Another issue is the absence of double blinding in our study. Since there is no untreated control group there is no need for keeping the patients and the doctors ignorant about what is going on. However, double blinding also avoids any bias on the part of the physician in evaluating the results of treatment. In our pre-test / post-test design such biases are prevented from affecting the results by the fact that the Tibetan physician is not involved in the Western diagnostic assessments, except in one way — deciding when the patient has been cured or has improved sufficiently so that the post test diagnosis should be given.

In addition, it would be fairly straightforward to make sure the technicians in the lab or x-ray facility are not even aware that the procedures are part of a research project. However, the possibility of bias influencing results is present whenever people perform diagnostic procedures involving contact with the patient and direct assessment of relevant variables, for example temperature and blood pressure readings, vision tests, neuropsychological assessments and any of a host of other procedures. These people, along with physicians making overall assessments of patients clinical status, could be made aware that the work they were doing was part of a research project and that their findings would not be involved in the treatment of the patients, but they and those running the statistical tests could remain unaware of the nature of the study until it is completed.

In later follow-up studies which may appropriately involve control groups, it may be impossible to blind the subjects regarding certain aspects of the treatment such as dietary and behavioral changes, performance of prayers to the Medicine Buddha, exercises, etc. Furthermore, although it will be possible, in general, to ensure that the people evaluating the outcome from the perspetive of Westarn medicine are unaware of the treatment, it will be difficult if not impossible to blind the Tibetan physician as to whether the patient is recieving real medicine or placebos. Traditional practice includes re-examining the patient after a few weeks to assess the effect of the medicine and adjust the prescription if necessary — and to reexamine the patient and consider readjusting the prescription whenever there is a notable change in symptoms. Tibetan physicians believe that they can tell by pulse analysis what effect the medicine is having, and that would of course include telling if the medicine is having no effect at all.

Medical Statistics

Comparing the results from patients in the study with historical evidence of what would be expected when people with a particular diagnosis are not treated, and when they receive standard Western medical treatment, will allow a survey of the relative effectiveness of Tibetan medicine for a wide range of different medical problems. Tibetan medicine might come to be considered the prefered treatment for a particular condition because it is more effective than the available Western treatments, or because it is less expensive than equally effective Western treatments, or because it is less likely to result in serious negative side effects. All of these possible outcomes can be considered for each type of medical problem that is included in the study. However, even though this design would be much more cost effective than standard clinical trials, the expense of the Western diagnostics will require some care in selecting the specific maladies to be included in the study.

We can easily gain a rough estimate of the types of medical problems where Tibetan medicine is most likely to make a real contribution to modern medical practice by looking at what is happening in the few places where both Western and Tibetan medicine are available, places like the town of Dharamsala in India. In general, Western medicine tends to be the treatment of choice for acute illness and emergency problems, whereas Tibetan medicine is preferred for longer-term and chronic problems — but what we need is a list of the specific conditions for which Tibetan medicine is considered the treatment of choice when both systems are available.

After selecting a list of medical conditions to be studied, historical data can be consulted for the particular regions that will be included in the research. For each disease or other problem which is found to be included in the appropriate databases, statistical consultants can determine what size the sample of patients would have to be to show a statistically significant improvement over base rate outcomes, given the estimated average effectiveness of the Tibetan treatment for that particular problem.

Potential Sampling Problems

Since patients will not be randomly selected for treatment, the research team must take care to minimize biases in sample of patients that are included in the study. For example, in areas such as Europe and America, patients who come to a Tibetan clinic are certainly not representative of the population as a whole, but are generally more affluent and better educated, and have better nutritional resources and better access to sophisticated Western medical care. For this reason, it might be better to begin the research in an area where Tibetan medicine is available to the entire population — like some of the Tibetan refugee settlements in India.

Even in such a community, sampling biases can easily arise. For example, if patients are expected to pay for their own medicine, as is often the case in these settlements, relatively affluent people are more likely to appear at the clinic as patients. For this reason, it might be best if the funding for the research project could include resources for providing medicine free of charge to all the patients in the study. If that is not possible, at the very least such biasing factors as are likely to have influenced the inclusion of patients in the study should be carefully reported.

TIBETAN MEDICAL CENTRES IN INDIA

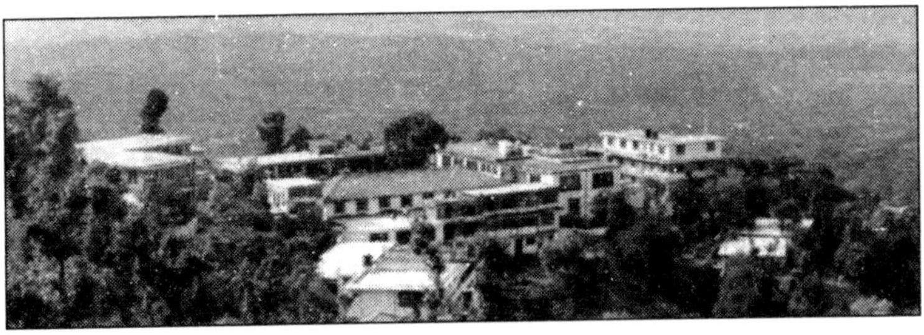

Men-Tsee-Khang
(Formerly the Tibetan Medical and Astrological Institute)
Gangchen Kyishong, Dharamsala, 176215 Distt. Kangra (H.P.) INDIA

In 1961, a small clinic providing traditional Tibetan medical care opened in the main encampment for Tibetan refugees in India. Men-Tsee-Khang is now a large complex in a spacious compound where traditional medical theory and practice are taught to over fifty students per year. Identifying, gathering and preparing ingredients for medicines, and preparing the hundreds of different medicines is just as important as diagnosis and the various aspects of treatment.

Men-Tsee-Khang has a pharmacy, an in-patient unit and a surgical ward; along with Tibetan refugees, non-Tibetans from nearby areas and patients from all over the world are treated. Also, an astrological department provides training and services in traditional Tibetan medical astrology.

Chakpori Tibetan Medical Institute
Trogawa House, North Point, Darjeeling 734104, West Bengal, India

Tibetan Medical School, Central Institute of Higher Tibetan Studies, Sarnath, Varanasi, India

Traditional Ladakhi Amchi Course
Central Institute of Buddhist Studies
Choglamser, Leh, 194101, Ladakh, India

Schools teaching Tibetan medicine in "China"
Lhasa Tibetan Medical School
and
Qinghai Tibetan Medical School

Notes

1. C Pierce Salguero, Johns Hopkins University, Institute of the History of Medicine, USA.
2. C Pierce Salguero, Johns Hopkins University, Institute of the History of Medicine, USA.
3. *Medicine In China,* Paul Ulrich Unschuld, Munich University.
4. *Medicine In China,* Paul Ulrich Unschuld, Munich University.
5. *Buddhism and Medicine,* C Pierce Salguero, Johns Hopkins University, Institute of the History of Medicine, USA.
6. *Buddhism and Medicine,* C Pierce Salguero, Johns Hopkins University, Institute of the History of Medicine, USA.
7. *Buddhism and Medicine,* C Pierce Salguero, Johns Hopkins University, Institute of the History of Medicine, USA.
8. *Medicine In China,* Paul Ulrich Unschuld, Munich University
9. *Buddhism and Medicine,* C Pierce Salguero, Johns Hopkins University, Institute of the History of Medicine, USA.
10. *Ibid.*
11. *Ibid.*
12. *The ancient healing powers of traditional Mongolian medicine* . The Mongol Messenger 13 May 1998. p. 8.
13. Leaflet on Manba Datsan, Clinic and Training Centre for Mongolian Traditional Medicine.

14. Piburn, 1993, p. 12.
15. S. S. Begley,J Holist Nurs, *Tibetan Buddhist Medicine: A Transcultural Nursing experience*, Vol. 12 No. 3, Sep. 1994, Pp. 323-42.
16. S. S. Begley,J Holist Nurs, *Tibetan Buddhist Medicine: A Transcultural Nursing experience*, Vol. 12, No. 3, Sep. 1994, Pp. 323-42.
17. S. S. Begley, J. Holist Nurs, *Tibetan Buddhist Medicine: A Transcultural Nursing experience*, Vol. 12, No. 3, Sep. 1994, Pp. 323-42.
18. S. S. Begley, J. Holist Nurs, *Tibetan Buddhist Medicine: A Transcultural Nursing experience*, Vol. 12, No. 3, Sep. 1994, Pp. 323-42
19. S. S. Begley,J Holist Nurs, *Tibetan Buddhist Medicine: A Transcultural Nursing experience*, Vol. 12, No. 3, Sep. 1994, Pp. 323-42.
20. Amarendra N. Singh FRCP. (C) W.H.O. & A.C.P.M. Professor in Psychosomatic Medicine & Psychopharmacology Programme Director, Hamilton Psychiatric Hospital, McMaster University.
21. *Tibetan Herbal Medicine*, Subhuti Dharmananda, Ph.D., Director, Institute for Traditional Medicine, Portland, Oregon.
22. Compiled by Subhuti Dharmananda, Ph.D., Director, Institute for Traditional Medicine, Portland, Oregon.
23. Explained by the Venerable Master Hua in 1983 at Gold Wheel Monastery in Los Angeles.

BIBLIOGRAPHY

Primary Brahmanical Sources

(A) Atharva Veda, Rig Veda, Sama Veda, Caraka Samhita, Susruta Samhita, Hastyayurveda (Veterinary Medicinal Text), *Rasaratnasamuchaya (Vagbhata), Ashtanga Sangraha (Vagbhat),* - all in Sanskrit. There are also texts in regional langauges such as the *Siddha Vaidya* in Tamil, as well as texts with diagrams of manufacturing processes in Persian and Urdu.

Sushruta Samhita Translated by K.L. Bhishagratna English translation, Three Volumes

Charaka Samhita Translated by P.V.Shrama , English translation, Four Volumes.

Ashtanga Samgraha Vagbhata, Translated by Prof. K.R. Srikantha Murthy devinagri, English translation, Three Volumes.

Ashtanga Hridyama agbhata, Translated by Prof. K.R. Srikantha Murthy Devanagari, and English translation, Three Volumes.

Bhavaprakasha Bhavamishra, Translated by Prof. K.R. Srikantha Murthy Devinagri, and English translation, TwoVolumes.

*Sarngadhara Samhita Sharangadhara,*Translated by Prof. K. R. Srikantha Murthy devinagri, and English translation.

Primary Buddhist Sources

Medical Treatises

Sūtra on Embryology: T . 310.13, T. 317.

Great Treasure Trove Sûtra (section on Four Elements): T. 310.16.

Sūtra on the Baths and Saunas of the SaCgha (and Commentaries): T. 701, T. 1793, T. 2780.

Sūtra on Buddhist Medicine: T. 793.

Medical Deities

Medicine Buddha Sūtra: T. 450, T. 451, T. 1331.

Sūtra on the Bodhisattva Medicine King and the Bodhisattva Supreme Medicine: T. 1161.

Medical Dhāraī

Spell for the Protection of Children (and ritual manual): T. 1028A-B.

Spell to Rid all Diseases: T. 1323.

Spell to Clear all Eye Diseases: T. 1324.

Spell to Cure Piles: T. 1325.

Spell for Illnesses of Seasonal Qi: T. 1326.

Spell for the Teeth: T. 1327.

Spell for the Eyes: T. 1328.

Spell for Children: T. 1329.

Consecration Sûtra: T. 1331.

Collection of Spells: T. 1336.

Philosophical Texts

Yogācārabhūmi Sūtra: T. 606.

Oral explanation of the twelve karmic links in the Âgamas (section on four elements): T. 1508

Ritual Texts

Sūtra on Perfect Wisdom for Benevolent Kings: T. 245.

Sūtra of Golden Light (with commentaries): T. 663, T. 664, T. 665, T. 1785, T. 1787.

Texts on Monastic Discipline

Various *Vinaya* texts and commentaries with medical content: T. 1421, T. 1425, T. 1428, T. 1433, T .1435, T. 1463.

Meditation Treatises

Secret Essentials for Curing the Diseases of Meditation: T. 620.

Śamatha and Vipaśyanā: T. 1911 and T. 1915.

Hagiographies

Amrapāli and Jivaka Sūtra: T. 553, T. 2121: 166-170.

Lives of Eminent Monks: T. 2059.

Continued Lives of Eminent Monks: T. 2060.

Lives of the Nuns: T. 2063.

Collection of Notices on the Translation of the Tripitaka: T. 2145.

B. Collectanea

Forest of Gems in the Garden of the Dharma: T. 2122: 984-989.

Buddhist Monastic Traditions of Southern Asia: T. 2125, Ch. 27-29.

Outline of the History of the SaCgha in the Great Song Dynasty T. 2127: 306.

C. Others

1. *Atharva Veda* translated by Maurice Bloomfield [1897] (Sacred Books of the East, Vol. 42).
2. *The Rig Veda*, Ralph T.H. Griffith, Translator. (1896).

Secondary Sources

A. *Printed*

1. B. Dossey,. (1981, May). *Holistic nursing: What is it? Texas Nursing*, pp. 37-38.

2. Debiprasad Chattopadhyaya, *In Defence of Materialism in Ancient India.*
3. R. C. Dutt, *A History of Civilization in Ancient India.*
4. *Studies in the History of Science in India* (Anthology edited by Debiprasad Chattopadhyaya).
5. T. Clifford, (1984). *Tibetan Buddhist medicine and psychiatry: The diamond healing*. York Beach, ME: Samuel Weisner.
6. J. Landaw, (1987). *Introduction to Tantra,* Lama Yeshe. London: Wisdom.
7. M. Leininger, (1988). *Leininger's theory of nursing: Cultural care diversity and universality*. Nursing Science Quarterly, 1, 156-160.
8. Bose, Sen, Subarayappa: *Concise History of Science in India,* (Indian National Science Academy).
9. Chin Keh-Mu: India and China: Scientific Exchange *(History of Science in India Vol 2.)*
10. N. K. Sinha's *Economic History of Bengal* (Published in Calcutta, 1956).
11. S. Piburn, (1993). *The Dalai Lama: A policy of kindness.* Ithaca, NY: Snow Lion.
12. L. Rapgay, (1985). *Tibetan medicine—A holistic approach to better health.*Dharamsala, India: Author.
13. Robert A. F. Thurman, *Essential Tibetan Buddhism* (1995).
14. Denise Patry Leidy and Robert A. F. Thurman, *Mandala: The Architecture of Enlightenment* (1997).
15. Marilyn M. Rhie and Robert A. F. Thurman, *Wisdom and Compassion: The Sacred Art of Tibet* (1991).
16. Barbara Lipton and Nima Dorjee Ragnubs, *Treasures of Tibetan Art: Collections of the Jacques Marchais Museum of Tibetan Art* (1996).
17. P. V. Sharma (Ed). 1992. Medicine in Buddhist and Jaina traditions. In *History of Medicine in India.* New Delhi: INSA.
18. Paul Ulrich Unschuld, *Medicine In China,* University of California, 1988.

Tertiary Sources

1. Lama Shakya Zangpo. (1993). *Psychospiritual healing.* Unpublished manuscript.
2. Rechung Rinpoche, *Tibetan Medicine,* 1976 University of California Press, Berkeley, California.
3. TJ Tsarong (translator and editor), *Fundamentals of Tibetan Medicine,* 1981 Tibetan Medical Center, Dharamsala, India.
4. Y. Donden (annotator) and Keisang J (translator), *The Ambrosia Heart Tantra,* 1977 Library of Tibetan Works and Archives, Dharamsala, India.
5. Raoul Birnbaum. *The Healing Buddha.* Boulder: Shambhala Publications, Inc., 1979.
6. Theodore Burang. *The Tibetan Art of Healing.*London: Robinson & Watkins Books Ltd., 1974.
7. Theodore Burang. *The Tibetan Art of Healing.*London: Robinson & Watkins Books Ltd., 1974.
8. Yeshi Donden, *Health Through Balance: An Introduction to Tibetan Medicine.* Ithaca: Snow Lion Publications, 1986.
9. Tom. Dummer, *Tibetan Medicine: And Other Holistic Health-Care Systems.* New York: Routledge, 1988.
10. Peter Gold,. *Tibetan Pilgrimage.* Ithaca: Snow Lion Publications, 1988.
11. Lobsang Rapgay, *Tibetan Medicine: A Holistic Approach to Better Health.* India: Indraprastha Press, 1985.
12. Tulku Thondup, *The Healing Power of Mind.* Boston: Shambhala Publications, Inc., 1996.
13. T. J. Tsarong, *Fundamentals of Tibetan Medicine.* New Delhi: Tibetan Medical Centre, 1981.
14. David P. and Janice A. Jackson. *Tibetan Thangka Painting: Methods and Materials.* (London: Serindia Publications, 1984),p. 15.
15. Tibetan Medical Institute of H. H. Dalai Lama, New Delhi, India. August 28, 2006. "Medicine Buddha and Tibetan Medicine,".

16. S. W. Changbhar, 1993. Brief introduction of Tibetan traditional medicine. In *Traditional Medicine.* (Ed.) B. Mukherjee. New Delhi: Oxford-IBH.

17. A. Jayasuriya, 1997. *The Future of Complementary Medicines.* Colombo: Medicina Alternativa International.

18. Charles Leslie, 1998. *Asian Medical systems: a Comparative Study.* Delhi: Motilal Banarasidas.

19. R. K., Maikhuri, S. Nautiyal, K. S. Rao & K. G. Saxena.1998. Role of medicinal plants in the traditional health care system: a case study from Nanda Devi Biosphere Reserve. *Current Science,* 75(2): 152-157.

20. P. C Pande,., D. S. Pokharia & J. C. Bhatt (Eds.). 1999. *Ethnobotany of Kumaun Himalaya.* Scientific Publishers, Jodhpur.

Miscellaneous References

1. Anonymous, *Survey of Tibetan Medicine,* Chinese Journal of Ethnomedicine and Ethnopharmacy, 1992; (1): 40-41.

2. Guo Jiening, *et al., Tibetan medicine: historical development and theoretical system,* Chinese Journal of Ethnomedicine and Ethnopharmacy, 1995; (14): 1-5.

3. Clark B (translator), *The Quintessence Tantras of Tibetan Medicine,* 1995 Snow Lion Press, Ithica, New York.

4. Jinhui Wang, *The characteristics of the Jingzhu Bencao,* Chinese *Journal of Ethnomedicine and Ethnopharmacy,* 1995; (13): 4-5.

5. LD Khangkar, *Lectures on Tibetan Medicine,* 1986 Library of Tibetan Works and Archives, Dharamsala.

6. Brekhman II and Dardymov IV, *New substances of plant origin which increase non-specific resistance, Annual Review of Pharmacology,* 1969; 9: 419-430.

7. Minyi Chang, *Anticancer Medicinal Herbs,* 1992 Hunan Science and Technology Publishing House, Changsha.

8. FP Smith and Stuart GA, *Chinese Medicinal Herbs,* 1973 Georgetown Press, San Francisco, CA.

9. Li Yingcun, *The characteristics of Tibetan medicine preparation in Sibu Yidian*, Chinese Journal of Ethnomedicine and Ethnopharmacy, 1995 (14): 16-19.

10. Pharmacopoeia Commission of the Ministry of Public Health, *Colored Atlas of the Chinese Materia Medica*, 1995 Guangdong Science and Technology Press, Guangzhou.

11. Hson-Mou Chang and Paul Pui-Hay But (eds.), *Pharmacology and Applications of Chinese Materia Medica*, (2 vols.), 1986 World Scientific, Singapore.

12. Li TSC and Schroeder WR, *Sea buckthorn (Hippophae rhamnoides): A multipurpose plant*, Horticultural Technology 1996; 6(4): 370-378.

13. Ji Lanju, *Free amino acids and vitamin C in the fruits of Hippophae rhamnoides, Nitraria tangutorum, and Berberis dasystachya*, ACTA Botanica Sinica 1989; 31(6): 487-488.

14. Zhong Fei, et al., *Effects of the total flavonoid of Hippophae rhamnoides on nonspecific immunity in animals*, Shanxi Medical Journal 1989; 18(1): 9-10.

15. Li Yong and Liu Huang, *Blocking effect of the juice of Hippophae rhamnoides on synthesis of nitrosodimethylamine in rat*, ACTA Nutrmenta Sinica, 1989; 11(1): 47-53.

16. Zhang Maoshun, et al., *Treatment of ischemic heart diseases with flavonoids of Hippophae rhamnoides, Chinese Journal of Cardiology*, 1987; 15(2): 97-99.

17. AK Nadkarni, *Indian Materia Medica*, 1908 (revised 1954), Popular Prakashan Private LTD, Bombay.

18. Huang Bingshan and Wang Yuxia, *Thousand Formulas and Thousand Herbs of Traditional Chinese Medicine*, 1993 Heilongjiang Education Press, Harbin, China.

19. TJ Tsarong, *Handbook of Traditional Tibetan Drugs*, 1986 Tibetan Medical Publications, Kalimpong.

20. Zhang Weiyun, *Recent development on application of Rhodiola spp. and its preparations*, Journal of the Gansu College of Traditional Chinese Medicine 1997; 14(4); 41-42.

21. Wang Liang, *Progress of research on the pharmacology of rhodiola*, Li Shizhen Medicine and Materia Medica Research 1999; 10(4): 295-296.

22. Qian Yancong, *et al.*, *Survey of research on Rhodiola kirilowii*, Acta Chinese Medicine and Pharmacology 1999; (5): 34-35.

23. Diao Jingli, et al., *Pharmacological actions of Hippophae rhamnoides*, Li Shizhen Medicine and Materia Medica Research 1999; 10(12): 956-957. *May 2001.*

24. Lama Tashi Namgyal (ed.), Thirangpu Rinpoche 'Medicine Buddha Sadhana', & 'Medicine Buddha Sutra' *Shenpen Osel*, Vol. 4, No. 1and 2.

25. Pasang Arya's article titled *Buddhism and Medicine* on *tibetanmedicine.edu.org*

26. James Hughes, Mclean Centre for Clinical Medical Ethics and Damien Keown, Goldsmiths, *Buddhism and Medical Ethics: A Bibliographic Introduction*, University of London, *Journal Of Buddhist Ethics*, Vol. II, 1995.

27. C. Pierce Salguero, Article on "Indian Influence on Chinese Medicine through Buddhism," in World History Encyclopedia, Oxford: ABC-CLIO, forthcoming in 2009. Johns Hopkins University, Institute of the History of Medicine, USA.

28. S. S. Begley,J Holist Nurs, *Tibetan Buddhist Medicine: A Transcultural Nursing experience*, Vol. 12, No. 3, Sep.1994.

29. Pankaj Goyal, *Medicine in Buddhist and Jaina Traditions*, Lok Vigyan Kendra, Almora 263601 India

30. D. P. Agrawal, and J. Kharakwal. 1998. *Central Himalayas: an Archaeological, Linguistic and Cultural Synthesis.* Delhi: Aryan Books International.

Separate Bibliography on Indian Traditional Medicine

Anticancer Herbal Drugs of India: With Special Reference to Ayurveda / Gyanendra Pandey. Delhi, Sri Satguru, 2002.

Astanga-Hrdaya of Vagbhata : The Book of Eight Branches of Ayurveda / translated by A Board of Scholars. 1999, 3, Vol.

Ayurved and Hepatic Disorders/edited by P.H. Kulkarni. Reprint. Delhi, Satguru, 2001.

Ayurveda Aahar (Food/Diet)/P.H. Kulkarni. Delhi, Satguru, 2000.

Ayurveda Chikitsa/P. H. Kulkarni. Reprint. Delhi, Sri Satguru, 2000.

The Ayurveda Encyclopedia : Natural Secrets to Healing, Prevention and Longevity/Swami Sada Shiva Tirtha. 1998.

Darsanodaya: Early Indian Thought/S.K. Ramachandra Rao. Bangalore, Kalpatharu Research Academy, 1999.

Database on Medicinal Plants Used in Ayurveda : Vol. I/P. C. Sharma, M. B. Yelne and T.J. Dennis. New Delhi, Central Council for Research in Ayurveda & Siddha, 2000.

Database on Medicinal Plants Used in Ayurveda, Vol. 2/P. C. Sharma, M. B. Yelne and T. J. Dennis. New Delhi, Central Council for Research in Ayurveda & Siddha, 2001.

Database on Medicinal Plants Used in Ayurveda : Vol. III/P.C. Sharma, M.B. Yelne and T. J. Dennis. New Delhi, Central Council for Research in Ayurveda & Siddha, 2001.

A Descriptive Glossary of Diseases in Ayurveda/S. R. Sudarshan. Delhi, Sri Satguru, 2002.

Diagnosis and Treatment of Diseases in Ayurveda : Based on Ayurveda Saukhyam of Todarananda/Vaidya Bhagwan Dash and Vaidya Lalitesh Kashyap. Reprint. New Delhi, Concept, 2000.

Diseases of Respiratory Tract : Ayurvedic Concept /V. B. Athavale and K. V. Athavale. Delhi, Chaukhamba Sanskrit Pratishthan, 2001.

Doctrines of Pathology in Ayurveda/K. R. Srikantha Murthy. 1998.

Dravyagunakosah : Dictionary of Ayurvedic Terms Relating to Names, Synonyms, Properties and Actions of Medicinal Plants (Sanskrit-Hindi-English)/Acharya Priya Vrat Sharma. 1997.

Eating Right the Natural Way : Ayurvedic Recipes for a Healthy Life/ Vinod Verma. New Delhi, Penguin, 2001.

Energetic Bodywork : Practical Techniques/Rita J. McNamara. Delhi, Motilal Banarsidass, 2002.

The Green Pharmacy : New Discoveries in Herbal Remedies for Common Diseases and Conditions from the World's Foremost Authority on Healing Herbs/James A. Duke. Reprint. Jodhpur, Scientific, 2002.

Handbook of Clinical Ayurveda Practice/P.H. Kulkarni. Reprint, Delhi, Sri Satguru, 2001.

The Healer's Wisdom : Fundamentals of Whole Body Healing/Jennifer Fraser. New Delhi, Health Harmony, 2002.

The Holistic Principles of Ayurvedic Medicine/R. H. Singh. 1998.

Home Doctor : Natural Healing Herbs, Condiments and Spices/P.S. Phadke. New Delhi, Roli Books, 2001.

Rasa-Dhatu-Kosha : Metallic and Mineral Drugs in Ayurveda/S.R. Sudarshan. Bangalore, Kalpatharu, 1999, 304.

Researches in Ayurveda : Past and Present (Felicitation Volume in Honour of Vaidya Pandit Gulraj Sharma Mishra)/edited by Vaidya Banwari Lal Gaur and Vaidya Santosh Kumar Sharma. Jaipur, Publication Scheme, 2000, 434.

Religious Therapeutics : Body and Health in Yoga, Ayurveda, and Tantra/ Gregory P. Fields. Delhi, Motilal Banarsidass, 2002, viii, 222.

Secrets of Marma : The Lost Secrets of Ayurveda (A Comprehensive Text Book of Ayurvedic Vital Points)/Avinash Lele, Subhash Ranade and David Frawley. Pune, International Academy of Ayurveda, 1999.

Sex Herbs : Nature's Sexual Enhancers for Men and Women/Beth Ann Petro Roybal and Gayle Skowronski. Reprint. New Delhi, Health Harmony, 2002, 326.

Traditional Knowledge on the Medicinal Plants of Ayurveda/Sandhya Singh, Preeti Pandey and Sushil Kumar. Lucknow, Central Institute of Medicinal and Aromatic Plants, 2000.

A Treatise on Ayurveda : Pharmaceutics and Therapies Being an English Translation of Sarngadhara Samhita. Delhi, 1999, vii, 387.

The Yoga of Herbs: An Ayurvedic Guide to Herbal Medicine/David Frawley and Vasant Lad. 1994.

Uncommon Plant Drugs of Ayurveda/Gyanendra Pandey. 1994, xxv, 359.

Understanding Rheumatoid Arthritis/Sanjeev Rastogi. Delhi, Pratibha, 2001.

The Vital Force in Health and Disease/S.K. Ramchandra Rao. Delhi, Sri Satguru, 2002, vi, 106 p., ISBN 81-7030-741-4.

Vrksayurveda of Parasara : A Treatise on Plant Science (Sanskrit Text, English Translation and Notes with Comparative References to Modern Botany)/edited by N. N. Sircar and Roma Sarkar. Delhi, Satguru, 1996.

Yoga and Ayurveda : Self Healing and Self-Realization/David Frawley. Delhi, Motilal Banarsidass, 2000, 333.

Secondary Buddhist Source Material

(1984) *Tibetan Buddhist Medicine: the Diamond Healing*. York Beach, Maine: Samuel Weiser.

Demieville, P. (1985), *Buddhism and Healing: Demieville's article 'Byoo' from Hooboogirin,* translated by Mark Tatz. Lanhan, Md:University Press of America.

Dhonden, Dr. Yeshe (1986), *Health Through Balance: An Introduction to Tibetan Medicine*. Ithaca: Snow Lion.

Duncan, A. S., G. R. Dunstan, and R. B. Welbourn (1981), "Buddhism", *Dictionary of Medical Ethics*. London: Darton, Longman and Todd.

Fenner, Edward Todd (1982), *Rasayana Siddhi: Medicine and Alchemy in the Buddhist Tantras*. Ann Arbor, Mich: University Microfilms International.

Haldar, J. R. (1977), *Medical Science in Pali Literature*. Indian Museum Monographs, 10. Calcutta: Indian Museum.

—— (1992), *Development of Public Health in Buddhism*. Varanasi: Indological Book House.

Jaqqi, Q. P. (1987), "India" (Medical Ethics of). In *Encyclopedia of Bioethics*, ed. W. Reich, London: Macmillan, 906-11.

Majupu, Trilok Chandra (1989), *Religious and useful plants of Nepal and India: medicinal plants and flowers as mentioned in religious myths and legends of Hinduism and Buddhism*. Lashkar (Gwalior): M. Gupta.

Massin, Christopher (1982), *La medicine Tibetaine*. Paris: Editions de la Maisnie.

Meulendbeld, G. Jan (ed.). (1991), *Medical Literature from India, Sri Lanka and Tibet*. Leiden: E.J. Brill.

Mitra, J. (1985), *A Critical Appraisal of Ayurvedic Materials in Buddhist Literature (with special reference to Tripitaka)*. Varanasi: The Jyotirlok Prakashan.

Ohnuki-Tierney, Emiko (1984), *Illness and Culture in Contemporary Japan*. Cambridge: Cambridge University Press.

Rechung Rinpoche, Ven. (1976), *Tibetan Medicine: Illustrated in Original Texts*. Berkeley: University of California Press.

Redmond, Geoffrey P. (1992), "Concepts of Disease in Buddhism," in *Buddhist Studies Present and Future*, ed. Ananda W.P. Guruge, Paris: The Permanent Delegation of Sri Lanka to Unesco, 143-159.

Soni, R. L. (1976), "Buddhism in Relation to the Profession of Medicine" in *Religion and Medicine*, ed. D. W. Millard, Vol.3. London: SCM Press, 135-51.

Unschuld, P. U. (1979), *Medical Ethics in Imperial China. A Study in Historical Anthropology*. Berkeley: University of California Press.

——(1987), "General Historical Survey" (of Asian Medical Ethics) in *Encyclopedia of Bioethics*, ed. W.Reich, London: Macmillan, 901-6.

Umezawa, K. (1988), "Medical Ethics in Japan," *Biomedicine and Pharmacotherapy* 42: 169-172.

Zysk, K. G. (1991), *Asceticism and Healing in Ancient India: Medicine in the Buddhist Monastery*. Oxford: Oxford University Press.

Buddhism and Bioethics

Beauchamp, Tom L. and James F. Childress (1989), *Principles of Biomedical Ethics,* Third ed. Oxford: Oxford University Press.

Epstein, Mark (1993), "Awakening with Prozac: Pharmaceuticals and Practice." *Tricycle* Fall: 30-34.

Florida, R. E. (1994), "Buddhism and the Four Principles". In *Principles of Health Care Ethics,* ed. R. Gillon and A. Lloyd, Chichester: John Wiley & Sons, 105-16.

Jones, Ken (1989), *The Social Face of Buddhism: An Approach to Political Activism.* Boston: Wisdom Publications.

Kabat-Zinn, Jon (1990), *Full Catastrophe Living: Using the Wisdom of Your Body and Mind to Face Stress, Pain and Illness.* New York: Dell.

——(1994), *Wherever You Go, There You Are: Mindfulness Meditation in Everyday Life.* Westport, Conn.: Hyperion.

Keown, Damien (1995), *Buddhism & Bioethics.* London and New York: Macmillan/St. Martins Press.

Kitagawa, J. (1987), "Medical Ethics of Japan through the Nineteenth Century," in *Encyclopedia of Bioethics,* ed. W.Reich, London: Macmillan, 922-924.

Leland, Charmiere (1995), "Bear Bile and Musk," *International Journal of Alternative and Complementary Medicine* 13: 16-17.

Lindbeck, Violette (1984), "Thailand: Buddhism meets the Western Model," *The Hastings Center Report* 14: 24-26.

Mettanando, Bhikkhu (1991), "Buddhist Ethics in the Practice of Medicine" in *Buddhist Ethics and Modern Society: An International Symposium,* ed.C.Wei-hsun Fu and S. A. Wawrytko, New York, etc: Greenwood Press, 195-213.

Nakasone, R. Y. (1990), *Ethics of Enlightenment.* Fremont, Ca: Dharma Cloud Publishers.

——(1994), "Buddhism". *Encyclopedia of Bioethics.* London: Macmillan.

Ratanakul, P. (1986), *Bioethics, an introduction to the ethics of medicine and life sciences*. Bangkok: Mahidol University.

——(1988), "Bioethics in Thailand: The Struggle for Buddhist Solutions," *Journal of Medicine and Philosophy* 13: 301-12.

——(1990), "Thailand: Refining Cultural Values." *The Hastings Center Report* 20: 25-27.

Sizemore, Russell and Donald Swearer, eds. (1990), *Ethics, Wealth and Salvation: A Study of Buddhist Social Ethics*. Columbia SC: University of South Carolina Press.

Taniguchi, S. (1987a), "A Study of Biomedical Ethics from a Buddhist Perspective". MA Thesis, Berkeley: Graduate Theological Union and the Institute of Buddhist Studies.

——(1987b), "Biomedical Ethics from a Buddhist Perspective". *Pacific World* New Series 3 Fall: 75-83.

Umezawa, K. (1988), "Medical Ethics in Japan," *Biomedicine and Pharmacotherapy* 42: 169-172.

Buddhist Approaches to Personhood

Chaube, D. B. (1991), *Mind-Body Relation in Indian Philosophy*. Varanasi: Tara Book Agency.

Collins, Steven (1982), *Selfless Persons: Imagery and Thought in Theravada Buddhism*. Cambridge: Cambridge University Press.

Harvey, P. (1987a), "The Buddhist Perspective on Respect for Persons". *Buddhist Studies Review* 4: 31-46.

—— (1987b), "A Note and Response to 'The Buddhist Perspective on Respect for Persons'". *Buddhist Studies Review* 4: 97-103.

Klein, A. (1987), "Finding a Self: Buddhist and Feminist Perspectives" in *Shaping New Vision: Gender and Values in American Culture*, ed. C. Atkinson, C. Buchana, and M. Miles, Ann Arbor: UMI Research Press.

Koyeli, G. D. (1987), "Individual Autonomy in Traditional Indian Thought," *Journal of Indian Philosophy* 15: 99-107.

MEDICAL ETHICISTS ON PERSONHOOD

Fletcher, Joseph (1979), *Humanhood: Essays in Biomedical Ethics.* Buffalo: Prometheus Books.

Gervais, Karen (1986), *Redefining Death.* New Haven: Yale University Press.

Lizza, John P. (1993), "Persons and Death: What's Metaphysically Wrong with our Current Statutory Definition of Death?" *Journal of Medicine & Philosophy* 18: 351-74.

More, Max. (1993), "The Diachronic Self: Identity, Continuity, Transformation" (Unpublished dissertation thesis, available at *gopher://gopher.etext.org:70/00/Politics/ Extropy.Institute/ more.03049**

Nelkin, Dorothy (1983), "The Politics of Personhood," *Milbank Quarterly* 61(1): 101-12.

Tooley, Michael (1984), *Abortion and Infanticide.* Oxford: Oxford University Press.

Parfit's Deconstruction of Personhood

Gruzalski, B. (1986a), "Parfit's impact on utilitarianism," *Ethics* 96: 760-83.

——(1986b), Symposium on Reasons and Persons. *Ethics* 96:832-72.

Kuczewski, Mark G. (1994), "Whose Will Is It Anyway? A Discussion of Advance Directives, Personal Identity and Consensus in Medical Ethics," *Bioethics*, 8(1): 27-48.

Parfit, Derek (1984), *Reasons and Persons.* Oxford: Oxford University Press.

Buddhism and Abortion

Florida, R. (1991), "Buddhist Approaches to Abortion," *Asian Philosophy* 1: 39-50.

Imamura, Ryo. (1984), "The Shin Buddhist Stance on Abortion." *Buddhist Peace Fellowship Newsletter* 6: 6-7.

Jones, K. (1989), *The Social Face of Buddhism*. London: Wisdom Publications.

Lecso, P. A. (1987), "A Buddhist View of Abortion," *Journal of Religion and Health* 26: 214-18.

Stott, D. (1985), *A Circle of Protection for the Unborn*. Bristol: Ganesha Press.

Tworkov, H. (1992), "Anti-abortion/Pro-choice: Taking Both Sides," *Tricycle* Spring: 60-69.

Key Western Writings on Abortion

Bennett, Michael (1989), "Personhood from a Neuroscientific Perspective" in *Abortion Rights and Fetal Personhood*, eds. Edd Doer and James Prescott. Long Beach, California: Centerline Press, 83-86.

Flower, Michael J. (1985), "Neuromaturation of the Human Fetus," *Journal of Medicine and Philosophy* 10: 237-251.

Luker, K. (1984), *Abortion and the Politics of Motherhood*. Berkeley: University of California Press.

Tooley, Michael (1984), *Abortion and Infanticide*. Oxford: Oxford University Press.

Writings on embryology, rebirth and Karma

"Abortion" in *Encyclopaedia of Buddhism*. Batchelor, Stephen (1992), "Rebirth: A Case for Buddhist Agnosticism," *Tricycle* Fall: 16-23.

Dhonden, Y. (1980), "Embryology in Tibetan Medicine" in *Tibetan Medicine*. Dharamsala: Library of Tibetan Works and Archives.

King, Winston (1994), "A Buddhist Ethics Without Karmic Rebirth?" *Journal of Buddhist Ethics* 1: 33-44.

Lipner, J. J. (1989), "The Classical Hindu View on Abortion and the Moral Status of the Unborn." In *Hindu Ethics*, ed. H. G. Coward, J. J. Lipner, and K. K. Young, Albany, New York: State University of New York Press, 41-69.

McDermott, James Paul (1984), *Development in the Early Buddhist Concept of Kamma/Karma.* New Delhi: Munshiram Manoharlal.

O'Flaherty, W. D., ed. (1980), *Karma and Rebirth in Classical Indian Traditions.* Berkeley: University of California Press.

Saksena, B. (1935), "Pali Bhuunahan," *Bulletin of the School of Oriental and African Studies* 8: 713-14.

Japan and Abortion

Brooks, Anne Page (1981), "*Mizuko Kuyoo* and Japanese Buddhism," *Japanese Journal of Religious Studies* 8: 119-47.

Eiki, H., and T. Dosho (1987), "Indebtedness and Comfort: The Undercurrents of *Mizuko kuyoo* in Contemporary Japan," *Japanese Journal of Religious Studies* 14: 305-20.

LaFleur, W. A. (1990), "Contestation and Confrontation: The Morality of Abortion in Japan," *Philosophy East and West* 40: 529-42.

——(1992), *Liquid Life: Abortion and Buddhism in Japan.* Princeton: Princeton University Press.

——(1995a), "The Cult of Jizo: Abortion Practices in Japan and What They Can Teach the West," *Tricycle* Summer: 41-44.

——(1995b), "Silences and Censures: Abortion, History, and Buddhism in Japan. A Rejoinder to George Tanabe," *Japanese Journal of Religious Studies* 22/1-2:185-196.

Miura, D. (1983), *The Forgotten Child.* Henley-on-Thames, England: Aidan Ellis.

Rand, Yvonne, Sensei (1994), "The Buddha's Way and Abortion - Loss, Grief and Resolution." *Mind Moon Circle* Autumn: 5-8 (Also Available Electronically, Filename jizo.zip, original site coombs.anu.edu.au).

Smith, B. (1988), "Buddhism and Abortion in Contemporary Japan: *Mizuko Kuyoo* and the Confrontation with Death," *Japanese Journal of Religious Studies* 15: 3-24.

Werblowsky, Z. (1984), "*Mizuko Kuyoo*; Notulae on the Most Important 'New Religion' of Japan," *Japanese Journal of Religious Studies* 18: 295-354.

Young, R. F. (1989), "Abortion, Grief and Consolation: Prolegomenon to a Christian Response to *Mizuko Kuyoo*," *Japanese Christian Quarterly* (Tokyo) 55: 31-39.

Buddhism on Sexuality and Contraception

Ling, T. (1969), "Buddhist Factors in Population Growth and Control," *Population Studies* 23: 53-60.

——(1980), "Buddhist Values and Development Problems: A Case Study of Sri Lanka," *World Development* 8: 577-586.

Genetics and Reproductive Technology

Kimura, R. (1990), "Religious Aspects of Human Genetic Information" in *Science, Law and Ethics*, Ciba Foundation Symposium. Chichester: Wiley.

Schenker, J. G. (1992), "Religious Views Regarding Treatment of Infertility by Assisted Reproductive Technologies," *Journal of Assisted Reproduction & Genetics* 9: 3-8.

Death Dying and Euthanasia

Amore, R. C. (1974), "The Heterodox Philosophical Systems" in *Death and Eastern Thought*, ed. Frederick H. Holck. Nashville, Tennessee: Abingdon, 114-163.

Becker, C. B. (1990), "Buddhist Views of Suicide and Euthanasia," *Philosophy East and West* 40: 543-56.

——(1993), *Breaking the Circle: Death and the Afterlife in Buddhism*. Carbondale, Illinois: Southern Illinois University Press.

Bilimoria, P. (1992), "The Jaina Ethic of Voluntary Death," *Bioethics* 6: 330-55.

Bowker, John (1991), *The Meaning of Death*. Cambridge: Cambridge University Press.

Feldman, E. (1988), "Defining Death: Organ Transplants, Tradition and Technology in Japan," *Social Science and Medicine* 27: 339-43.

Florida, Robert (1993), "Buddhist Approaches to Euthanasia," *Studies in Religion/Sciences Religieuses* 22(1): 35-47.

Green, J. (1989), "Death with Dignity: Buddhism," *Nursing Times* 85: 40-41.

Hardacre, Helen (1994), "Response of Buddhism and Shinto to the Issue of Brain Death and Organ Transplant," *Cambridge Quarterly of Healthcare Ethics* 3: 585-601.

Kapleau, P. (1989), *The Wheel of Life and Death*. New York: Doubleday.

——(1972), *The Wheel of Death*. London: George, Allen and Unwin.

Keown, D. and Keown, J. "Killing, Karma and Caring: Euthanasia in Buddhism and Christianity," *Journal of Medical Ethics* (forthcoming, October 1995).

LaFleur, W. R. (1974), "Japan" in *Death and Eastern Thought*, ed. Frederick H. Holck. Nashville, Tennessee: Abingdon Press, 226-256.

Lamotte, E. (1987), "Religious Suicide in Early Buddhism," *Buddhist Studies Review* 4: 105-26.

Lecso, P. A. (1986), "Euthanasia: A Buddhist Perspective," *Journal of Religion and Health* 25: 51-57.

Levine, S. (1982), *Who Dies? An Investigation of Conscious Living and Conscious Dying*. New York: Doubleday.

Lock, M. and C. Honde (1990), "Reaching Consensus about Death: Heart Transplants and Cultural Identity in Japan," in *Social Science Perspectives on Medical Ethics*, ed. G. Weisz, New York: Kluwer, 99-119.

Miura, D. (1983), *The Forgotten Child*. Henley-on-Thames, England: Aidan Ellis.

Mullin, Glenn H. (1986), *Death and Dying in Tibetan Tradition*. London: Routledge and Kegan Paul.

Nakasone, R. Y. (1994), "Buddhism," in *Encyclopedia of Bioethics*, London: Macmillan, 312-318.

Neuberger, J. (1987), *Caring for Dying People of Different Faiths*. The Lisa Sainsbury Foundation Series, ed. V. Darling and P. Clench. London: Austen Cornish Publishers.

Nudeshima, J. (1991), "Obstacles to Brain Death and Organ Transplantation in Japan," *Lancet* 338 (8774): 1063-64.

Picken, S. (1977), "The Understanding of Death in Japanese Religion," *Japanese Religion* (July) 9, 4, 48.

Powers, John (1995), *Introduction to Tibetan Buddhism*. Ithaca: Snow Lion.

Raft (1989), "Euthanasia." *Raft, the Journal of the Buddhist Hospice Trust* 2 Winter: 1-16.

Ratanakul, P. (1986), *Bioethics, an Introduction to the Ethics of Medicine and Life Sciences*. Bangkok: Mahidol University.

Sharma, A. (1987), "Emile Durkheim on Suicide in Buddhism," *Buddhist Studies Review* 4: 119-26.

Smart, N. (1968), "Attitudes Towards Death in Eastern Religions," in *Man's concern with Death*, ed. Arnold *et al.* Toynbee, Kent: Hodder and Stoughton, 95-115.

Sogyal Rinpoche (1992), *The Tibetan Book of Living and Dying*. San Francisco and London: Harper/Rider.

Sugunasiri, S. H. (1990), "The Buddhist view Concerning the Dead Body," *Transplantation Proceedings* 22: 947-49.

Thakur, U. (1963), *The History of Suicide in India*. New Delhi: Munshiram Manoharlal.

Tsomo, K. L. (1993), "Opportunity or Obstacle: Buddhist views of Organ Donation," *Tricycle* Summer: 30-35.

Van Loon, L. H. (1978), "A Buddhist Viewpoint." In *Euthanasia*. Human Sciences Research Council, Publication No.65, ed. Oosthuizen. G. C., H. A. Shapiro, and S. A. Strauss, Cape Town: Oxford University Press, 56-79.

——(1983), "Some Buddhist Reflections on Suicide," *Religion in Southern Africa* 4: 3-12.

Whitehill, James (1974), "Mystological Death: Some Buddhist Lessons on Dying and Selfhood," *The Drew Gateway*: 82-99.

Wiltshire, M. G. (1983), "The 'Suicide' Problem in the Pali Canon," *Journal of the International Association of Buddhist Studies* 6: 124-40.

Key Western Writings on Euthanasia

Grisez, Germain and Joseph M. Boyle (1979), *Life and Death with Liberty and Justice*. Notre Dame and London: University of Notre Dame Press.

Gormally, Luke, ed. (1994), *Euthanasia, Clinical Practice and the Law*. London: The Linacre Centre for Health Care Ethics.

Horan, Dennis J. and David Mall, eds. (1980), *Death, Dying and Euthanasia*. Frederick, Maryland: Aletheia Books, University Publications of America Inc.

Humphry, Derek and Ann Wickett (1986), *The Right to Die*. London: The Bodley Head.

Keown, John, ed. (1995), *Euthanasia Examined: Ethical, Clinical and Legal Perspectives*. Cambridge: Cambridge University Press.

Rachels, James (1986), *The End of Life*. Oxford: Oxford University Press.

APPENDICES

Appendix I

STATUE OF MEDICINE BUDDHA

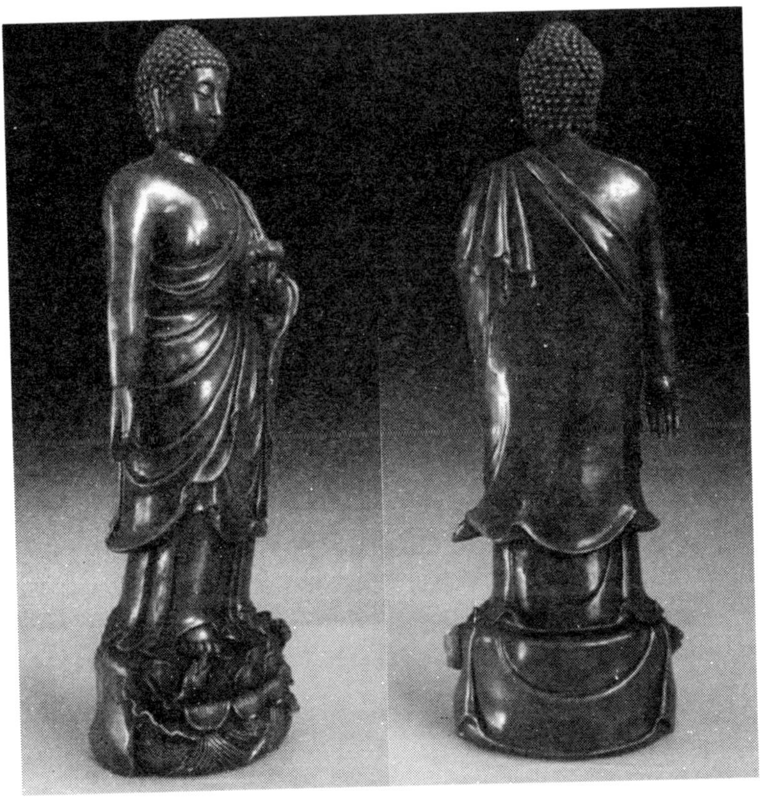

Antique Chinese Bronze

Medicine Buddha

With Lotus Medicine Bowl

Early 20th century

H 19" (48cm.), W 7" (18cm.), D 5" (15cm.)

Condition : Excellent

Standing in samapada on a circular plinth endorsed with double lotus, half opened lotus stems and leaves above interwoven patterns of wave forms. The Buddha is wearing a Tibetan style monk robes, with left shoulder bare, a **swastika** is embossed on his chest, his left hand is holding a medicine bowl in the form of a lotus, his right is pendent in the gesture of charity (Varada Mudra), his face with a serene expression, incised half moon shaped arch eyebrows, finely casted snail-curl hair, delicately modeled fingers. The statue has a rich deep bronze patina, it is meticulously rendered with no defects of any kind.

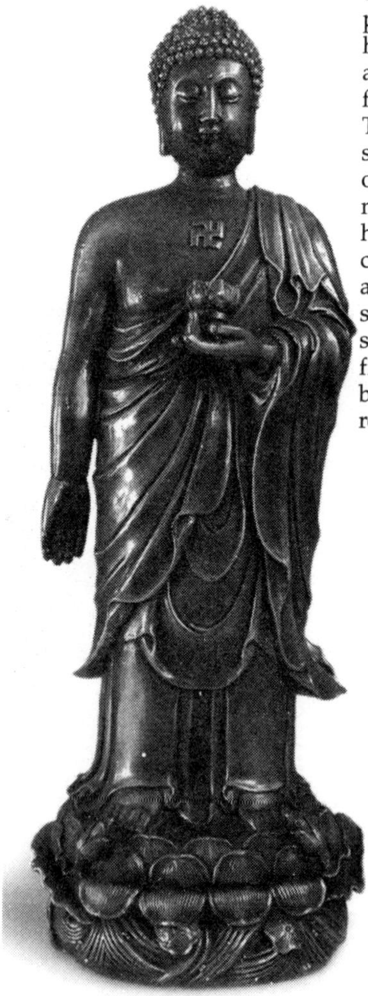

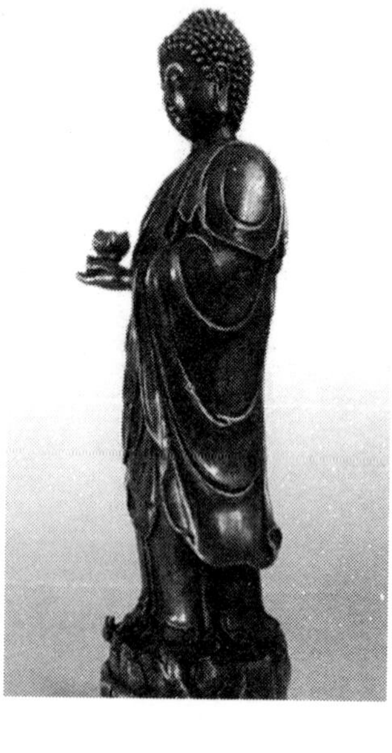

APPENDIX II

MEDICINAL PLANTS

The Tibetan Plateau region is estimated to contain 10,000 species of plants, of which more than 1,000 have any medicinal value.

Below we are giving you a few examples of medicinal plants from Ladakh. We display these plants here for various reasons. Either they are important in the Tibetan medical systems. Or they can serve as an example to explain about the specific problems and views of Tibetan medicine in Ladakh. Finally, some of these plants or their close relatives are known in the west as well and they can serve as a bridge between the two traditions, to show similarities and differences.

The descriptions of the plants which we present here are basically just a few field notes which we took during our excursions while herbarzing these plants. These plants have been selected from a collection of about 200 plants which we herbarized from '92 to '94.

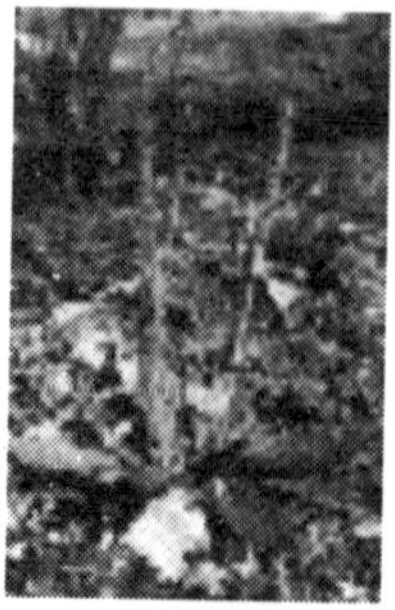

Plantago aff. depressa
Fam.: Plantaginaceae
Tibetan: tha ram

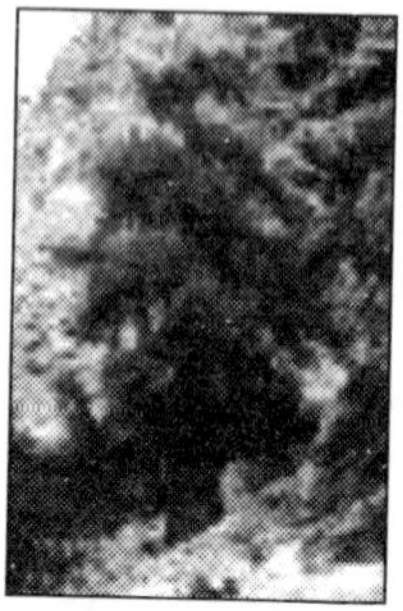

Juniperus macropoda Boiss. (J.excelsa M.B.)
Fam.: Cupressaceae
Tibetan: shug pa

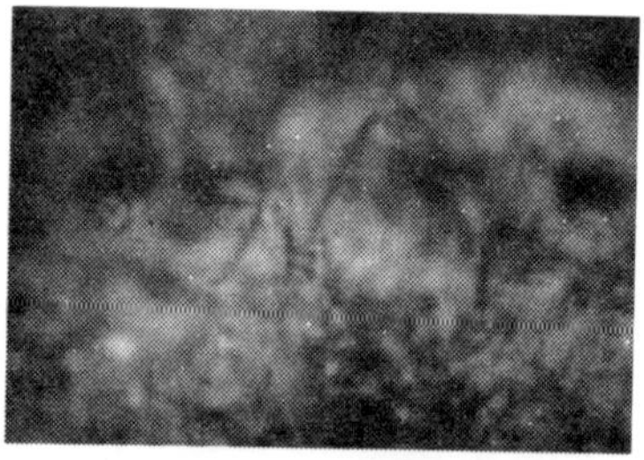

Koelpinia linearis Pallas
Fam.: Asteraceae (Compositae)
Tibetan: sngo chu srin sder ma ?
sngo lcags skyu

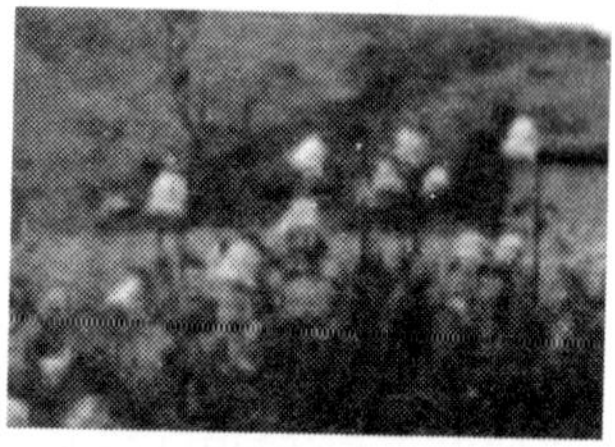

Codonopsis clematidea (Schrenk) Clarke
Fam.: Campanulaceae
Tibetan: klu bdud rdo rje

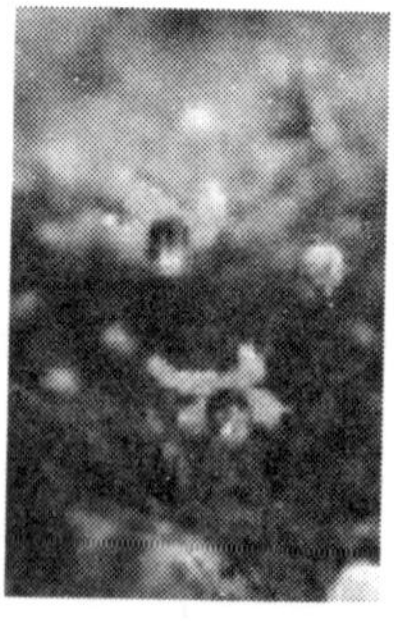

Clematis ladakhiana Grey-Wilson
Fam.: Ranunculaceae
Tibetan: dbyi mong rigs, dbyi mong dkar po

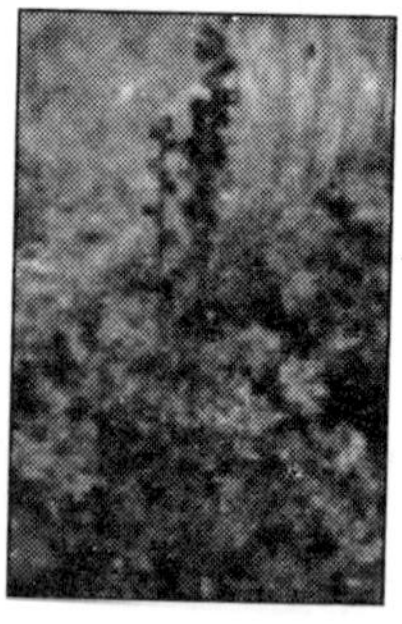

Aconitum aff. violaceum
Fam.: Ranunculaceae
Tibetan: bdud rtsi lo ma, bong nga nag po

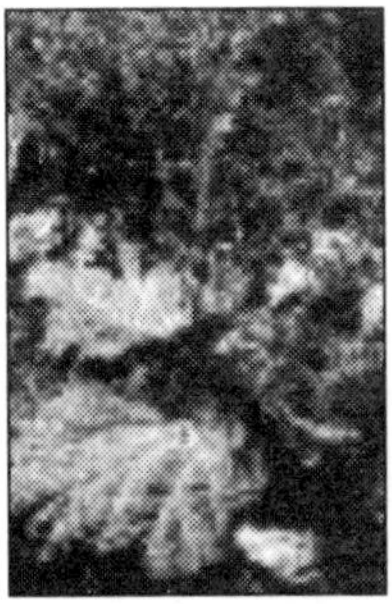

Rheum aff. webbianum
Fam.: Polygonaceae
Tibetan: chu rtsa

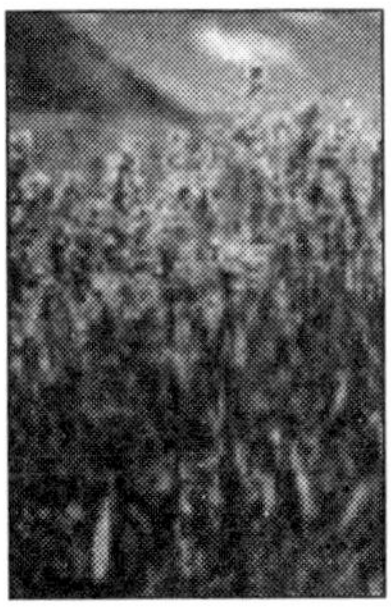

Bistorta affinis (D.Don) Greene (Polygonum affine)
Fam.: Polygonaceae Tibetan: li ga dur (gong li)

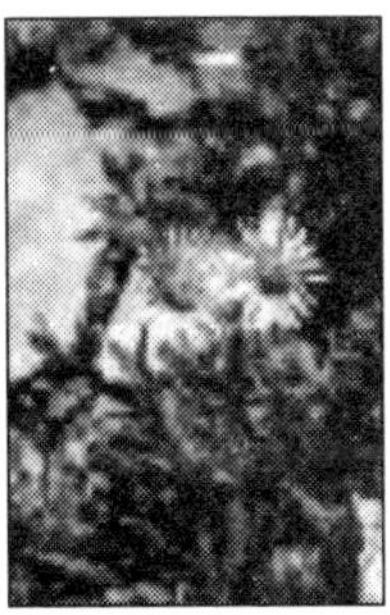

Aster sp.
Fam.: Asteraceae (Compositae)
Tibetan: lug mig

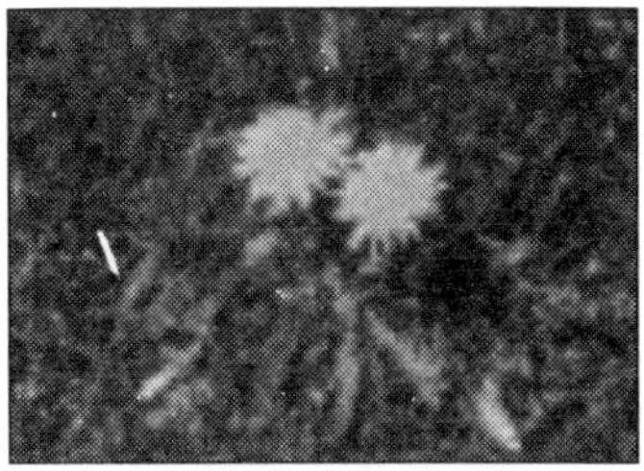

Taraxacum spp. agg.
Fam.: Asteraceae (Compositae)
Tibetan: khur mang

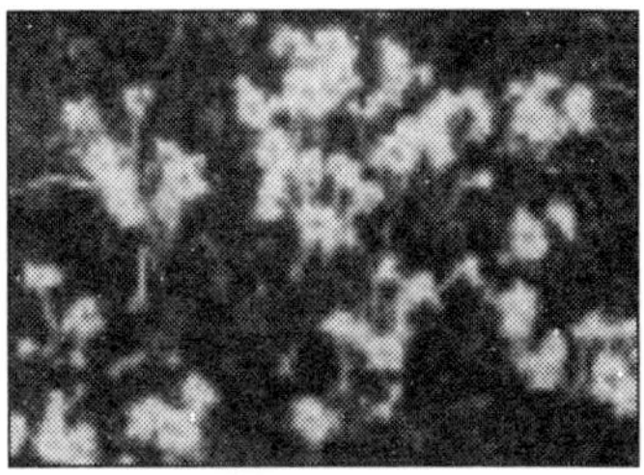

Pedicularis longiflora var. tubiformis
Fam.: Scrophulariaceae
Tibetan: lug ru ser po

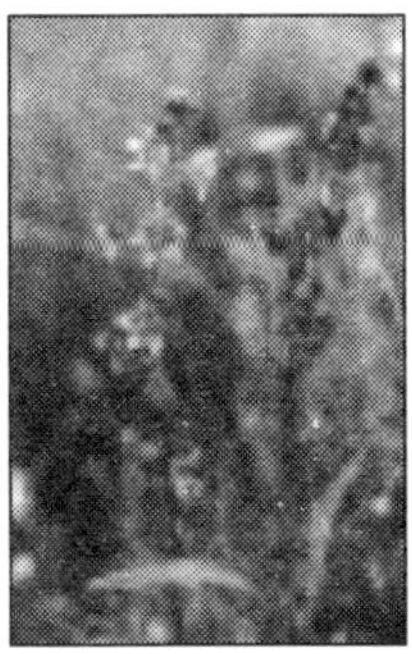

Swertia thomsonii Clarke
Fam.: Gentianaceae
Tibetan: tig ta rigs, lcag tig dkar po

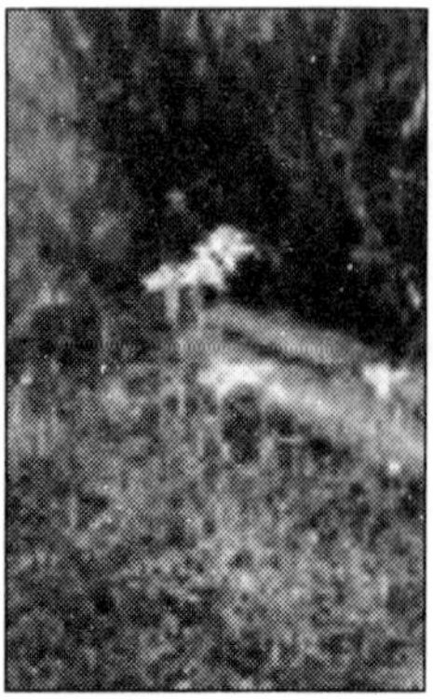

Leontopodium brachyactis
Fam.: Asteraceae (Compositae)
Tibetan: spra thog

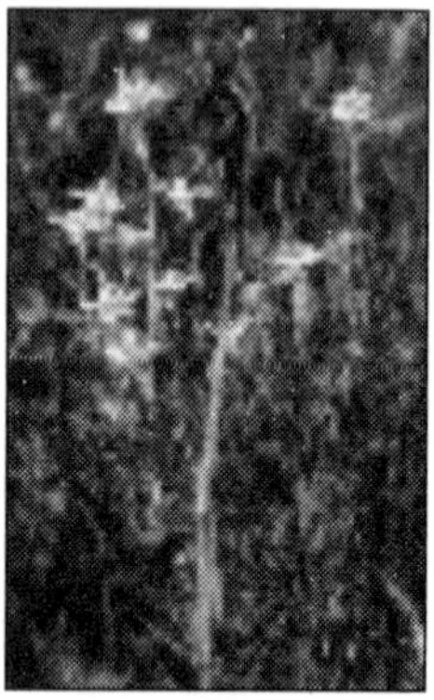

Dactylorhiza hatagirea (D.Don) Soo
Fam.: Orchidaceae
Tibetan: dbang lags

Appendix III

SUTRAS OF THE MERIT AND VIRTUE OF THE PAST VOWS OF MASTER VAIDURYA LGHT TATHAGATHA[1]

SAKYAMUNI BUDDHA came to the Saha world in order to help living beings resolve the problem of birth and death. He was born into a royal family, but he renounced the wealth of the kingdom and left his home in order to pursue the Truth. After he attained Buddhahood beneath the Bodhi Tree, he contemplated the living beings in the Saha world and discovered that we have the deepest affinities with two Buddhas-Medicine Master Vaidurya Light Tathagata in the East and Amitabha Tathagata in the West.

Medicine Master Vaidurya Light Tathagata is the Buddha of the Land of Vaidurya Light in the East. This Buddha bestows blessings and long life on people and helps them in times of disaster and difficulty. Amitabha Buddha of the Land of Ultimate Bliss in the West made a vow that whoever recites his name single-mindedly will be able to take his or her karma along and be reborn from a lotus in his Buddhaland, and that when his or her lotus opens he or she will see the Buddha and awaken to the patience of non-production.

The "Mantra of the Two Buddhas" says,
Two Buddhas proclaim and transform
in the Saha world-
Aksobhya in the East, Amitabha in the West.

Although Aksobhya (Medicine Master) Buddha is in the Vaidurya Land and Amitabha Buddha is in the Land of Ultimate Bliss, both of these Buddhas teach and transform the living beings of the Saha world. They have deep affinities with each and every one of us. Medicine Master Tathagata is also known as "Medicine Master Buddha Who Quells Disasters and Lengthens Life;" Amitabha Tathagata is known as both the "Buddha of Limitless Life" (Amitayus) and the "Buddha of Limitless Light" (Amitabha).

If you are mindful of Medicine Master Buddha, he will bestow blessings and long life upon you and save you from disasters, illnesses, and offenses. He fulfills the wishes of all living beings. Amitabha Buddha enables beings to be reborn in the Land of Ultimate Bliss. If you wish to be reborn in that land, simply recite Amitabha Buddha's name. If you wish to be born in the Vaidurya Land, then recite the name of Medicine Master Vaidurya Light Tathagata.

During their lives, people would like to avert disasters and live to a ripe old age. At death, they hope to be reborn in the Land of Ultimate Bliss. Therefore, in Buddhism, there are red plaques for extending life, which are associated with Medicine Master Buddha Who Quells Disasters and Lengthens Life. This Buddha's light shines upon your life-source. If you wish to be reborn in the Land of Ultimate Bliss when you die, then you can recite "Namo Amitabha Buddha." You can see that we are basically inseparable from these two Buddhas.

Yet we don't recognize or know very much about these two Buddhas. We might want to be mindful of them, but we don't even know their names. That's why Sakyamuni Buddha introduced them to us, telling us about their names, their vows, and their merit and virtue. Hence the name of this Sutra is the *Sutra of the Merit and Virtue of the Past Vows of Medicine Master Vaidurya Light Tathagata.*

"Medicine Master Vaidurya Light" is the name of this Buddha. Tathagata is one of the ten titles of all Buddhas. "Past Vows" refers to the vows to achieve Bodhi that Medicine Master Buddha made before he became a Buddha. If we sincerely make vows, we will

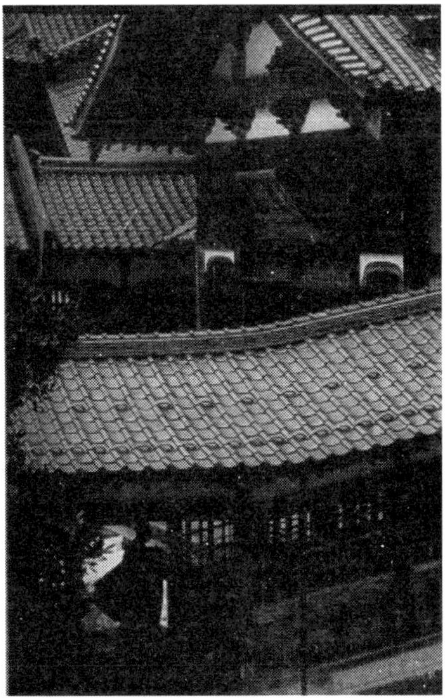

certainly reap the fruits of those vows. They won't be in vain. Vows are also a form of karma. If we make good vows, we will reap good results; bad vows bring bad results. Each person must make his own vows of his own initiative. Once we have made vows, there will be a driving force pushing us to accomplish those vows. Medicine Master Buddha made wholesome vows in his past lives, so he accomplished wholesome karma and reaped wholesome results.

His vows are wholesome because he made them for all living beings. He didn't vow, "When I become a Buddha, I'll enjoy my blessings and forget about other living beings." Having attained the greatest happiness, the Buddha wants to share it with all beings. He perfected his wholesome karma by practicing the Bodhisattva path in life after life. He made a great Bodhi resolve to benefit, enlighten, and rescue all beings. Forgetting themselves and thinking only of living beings, Bodhisattvas make wholesome vows, create wholesome karma, and reap the wholesome result of Buddhahood. When they become Buddhas, they are not arrogant. A Buddha is just the same as the other living beings, except that he has wisdom. He has truly left confusion behind and returned to enlightenment.

We create karma in our every word and deed, and many of them are bad. We might have an occasional good thought, but it is too weak to overcome our bad thoughts. If we were to tally up all our karma on the computer, we would find more bad karma than good. That's why quite often, our lives can get worse and worse. In each life, due to the impure karma we have created, we meet hard times and end up lost and lonely. Unlike the Buddha, we haven't always made wholesome vows, cultivated wholesome karma, and reaped wholesome results. Since the evil in our minds outweighs the goodness, we fall lower and lower in each successive life. When we try to make wholesome vows, our selfishness gets in the way. Sometimes we do good deeds, but our real motive is just to present a good image. Thus, the karma we create is very often not wholly good. Since our good intentions are usually polluted by selfish thoughts, quite often, we would experience more suffering than happiness in our lives.

Our happiness is not real. It is not the genuine happiness that arises from the virtues of "permanence, bliss, true self, and purity" of our inherent natures. The things we find happiness in are not genuine or lasting. When we dance, drink wine, or go to the theater, quite often, we"turn our backs on enlightenment and unite with the dust," deluding ourselves into thinking that we are happy.

"Is there no happiness in the world, then?" you ask. Think it over. Many forms of worldly happiness are indirect causes of suffering. Take clothing, food, and shelter, for instance. People like to dress up in style. But when you put on fancy and expensive clothes, they turn into a yoke around your neck. You can't move around freely, or stand naturally, or sit or lie down comfortably either. Why not? It is because you want to protect your fancy, expensive outfit. Just think about it: A human being, the highest of all creatures, becomes a slave to his clothes!

People like to eat good food, but even the most delicious food decomposes once it is ingested. If you ask people to regurgitate their food and eat it again, no one would do it.

As for shelter, there's a saying:

One may have ten thousand mansions,

But one doesn't need more than eight feet

of space to sleep in at night.

One may have ten thousand acres of fertile fields,

But one can only eat three meals a day.

Why should you work so frantically all day long, without a moment's rest, just for the sake of clothing, food, and shelter? When death arrives, you say to the Ghost of Impermanence, "Wait, I haven't finished taking care of my affairs. Can't you let me have a little more time?" The Ghost of Impermanence shakes his head and says, "Sorry, I can't let you live even a minute longer." And so off you go to die. What's the point at all? Failing to see things the way they really are, we spend our lives madly pursuing fame and fortune. This is where we differ from the Buddhas.

The Buddha has a clear view of everything. He has seen through everything and put it down, and so he has attained comfort and ease. When he saw through everything, he vowed to benefit living beings and practice the Bodhisattva Way.

Merit and virtue: Merit is created externally, while virtue is accumulated internally. One creates merit by building temples, repairing bridges or roads, or doing other work to benefit others. Virtue exists within one's self and doesn't rely on anything external. A virtuous person doesn't have a bad conscience. He has no reason to feel ashamed before the heavens or before other people. He doesn't cheat others or himself. In everything he does, he creates outer merit and amasses inner virtue. A saying about virtue goes,

Good done in the hope that others will notice

is not genuine good.

Evil done in the fear that others will find out

is truly great evil.

Don't boast about yourself, saying, "I've done good deeds. I've received the five precepts, the eight precepts, and the Bodhisattva precepts!" Virtuous deeds are done without others knowing. If you want others to notice your good deeds, you are not virtuous. If you try to cover up your bad deeds, then your offenses are great indeed.

Buddhists should not be boastful or competitive, saying, "I've done many good deeds and made lots of donations! I really do a lot to support Buddhism!" People with such an attitude are not fit to be Dharma-protectors. Therefore, in studying the teachings, we should remember this point: we should value genuine practice, not false publicity. This is very important. As Buddhists, we must be models for the world. If we have integrity and hold to our principles, other people will respect us and be influenced by us. That is merit and virtue.

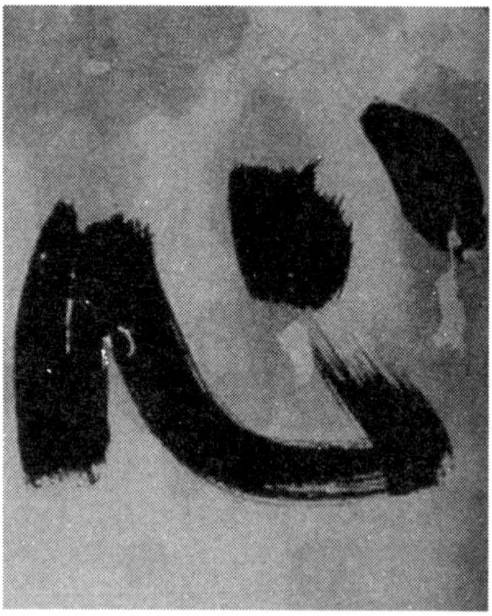

"Sutra" refers to the eternal Dharma, to teachings that are not subject to change. Since the Sutras are the teachings of sages, we should never delete or add even a single word to them. The word "Sutra" has many meanings, but in general, they do not go beyond the four meanings: "stringing together", "attracting", being "constant", and being "a standard".

The Four Meanings of Sutra

1. "Stringing together": The principles and meanings spoken by the Buddha are strung together from the beginning to the end.
2. "Attracting" means gathering all living beings.
3. Being "constant" means never changing from the ancient times to the present. Whether the Sutras are spoken by the Buddhas of the past, present, or future, they are the same.
4. Being "a standard:" A Sutra is a standard followed by all Buddhas and all living beings of the past, present, and future. By definition, a "standard" is honored by all throughout time.

The word Sutra has the meaning of "a chalk-line," for it is like the marking line that carpenters used in ancient times for making straight lines. Sutra also means "a bubbling spring", for it is like water gushing forth from a spring.

Now let us continue to explain the words of the title, "Sutra of the Meritand Virtue of the Past Vows of Medicine Master Vaidurya Light Tathagata." "Master" refers to the Buddha, who is a great king of physicians, one who can heal the sicknesses of all people. No matter what sort of incurable disease you have, the Buddha can certainly cure you. Even if you are supposed to die, he can bring you back to life. Therefore, he is the "Medicine Master."

"Vaidurya " is a translucent substance. It is also the name of Medicine Master Buddha's land of reward, where he is the teaching host. His body, which is made of *Vaidurya*, is pure and lustrous both inside and out. This Buddha thoroughly understands all the various kinds of medicines. In ancient China, the Emperor Shennong [c.2838 B.C.] was said to have tasted all the various medicinal herbs. His body was also as if transparent. When he ingested a medicine, he could observe its effects in his stomach and see what channels the medicine travelled to. He tasted all the medicinal herbs and classified them as sour, sweet, bitter, pungent, or salty; as cold, hot, warm, or neutral in nature; and as poisonous or nontoxic. "Light": this Buddha's body has an inner and outer radiance and is a pure, bright storehouse of light.

"Tathagata" is one of the ten titles of a Buddha. The ten titles are: Tathagata (Thus Come One), One Worthy of Offerings, One of Proper and Universal Knowledge, One Whose Understanding and Practice are Complete, Well Gone One Who Understands the World, Supreme Lord, Regulating Hero, Teacher of Gods and Humans, Buddha, and World Honored One. Originally, every Buddha had 100,000 titles, but that was too many for people to remember, so they were later condensed to 10,000. That was still too many, so they were reduced to 1000. But 1000 was still too numerous, so they were decreased to 100. One hundred titles were still too many, so they were reduced to only ten titles. These ten titles do not belong exclusively to any particular Buddha; every Buddha has them. All Buddhists should know these ten general, designations for the Buddhas. Some people who know nothing about Buddhism think "Tathagata Buddha" is the name of a Buddha, but actually, every Buddha can be called Tathagata. Tathagata ("Thus Come One") means: "Following the Way which is: 'Thus, he comes to realize right enlightenmen' ".

"Past Vows" refers to vows that the Buddha made in past lives, not to vows made in the present life.

Medicine Master Vaidurya Light Tathagata of the Eastern Land is also known as "Aksobhya Buddha." Medicine Master Buddha

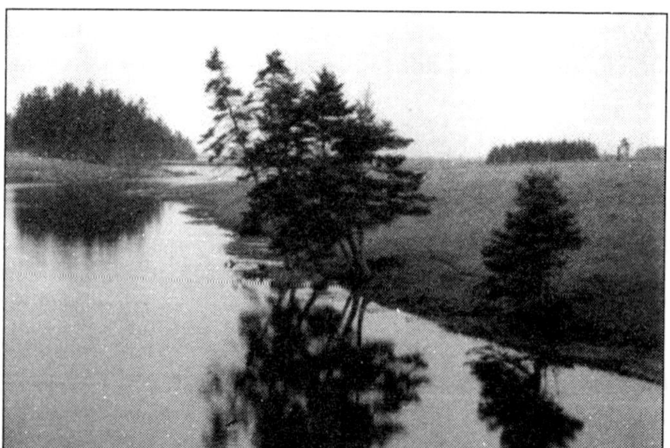

belongs to the Vajra Division in the East. The Vajra Division emphasizes the Dharmas of Subduing, which can overcome the heavenly demons and those of external sects. The demons and externalists become subdued as soon as they see the Vajra Dharma-protectors of the Vajra Division. If you sincerely recite the Surangama Mantra, which contains Dharmas of Subduing, you will have the constant protection of 84,000 Vajra Treasury Bodhisattvas.

Sutra: (in Chinese)

Thus I have heard. At one time the Bhagavan was travelling through various lands to teach living beings. He arrived at Vaisali ["City of Extensive Adornments"] and stayed beneath a tree from which music resounded. With him were eight thousand great Bhikshus and thirty-six thousand Bodhisattvas Mahasattvas; also kings, ministers, Brahmans, lay disciples; gods, dragons, and the rest of the eightfold division; beings both human and non-human. The immeasurable great multitude respectfully surrounded him, and he spoke Dharma for them.

Commentary

Thus I have heard. The word "thus" means, "The Dharma which is 'thus' can be believed, studied, and practiced. You should make vows to practice according to the Dharma which is 'thus.'" Ananda [who recited the Sutra after the Buddha's Nirvana] is saying, "The Dharma spoken in this Sutra is what I, Ananda, personally heard the Buddha speak with his golden mouth. It is not hearsay. I myself heard it."

The Four Matters

There were four reasons for saying "Thus I have heard," which the Buddha gave when Ananda asked about the Four Matters. When the Buddha was about to enter Nirvana, Ananda was so overcome with grief that he could only cry! Although Ananda was a Third Stage Arhat he was still emotional. He couldn't bear to think that the Buddha was going to enter Nirvana, so he wept piteously, forgetting about everything else.

Then another Bhikshu *[Venerable Aniruddha]* reminded him, "You're in charge of remembering the Dharma spoken by the Buddha. The Buddha is about to enter Nirvana, so you'd better think things over clearly! There are some important matters you should ask the Buddha about before he enters Nirvana. All you know how to do is cry! What will become of us in the future?"

Hearing the Venerable One's words, Ananda collected his wits and said, "Yes, you're right, but I've been crying so hard that I can't think straight. What should we ask the Buddha?"

The Venerable One said, "First of all, when we compile the Sutras in the future, how should they begin?" Ananda replied, "Right! That's very important!" "Second, when the Buddha is in the world, we take the Buddha as our teacher. After the Buddha enters Nirvana, whom should we take as our teacher?"

Ananda said, "Yes, that's also an important question!" "Third, when the Buddha is in the world, all the Bhikshus dwell with the Buddha. After the Buddha enters Nirvana, with whom should we dwell?"

"That's certainly a good question!" said Ananda.

"Fourth, when the Buddha is in the world, he can subdue the evil-natured Bhikshus. After the Buddha enters Nirvana, who should discipline them?"

"These four questions are all extremely important," said Ananda. "Now I will go and ask the Buddha."

Then he went before the Buddha, knelt, placed his palms together, and said, "World Honored One, since you are about to enter Nirvana, there are some important questions I would like to ask. I hope the Buddha will compassionately answer them."

The Buddha replied, "What are your questions? You may ask them now."

"Buddha, you have spoken the Dharma for forty-nine years

and expounded the Sutras in over three hundred assemblies," said Ananda, "In the future, when we compile the Sutras, how should they begin?"

The Buddha told Ananda, "Our Sutras are different from the scriptures of other religions, which begin by speaking of either existence or non-existence. You should begin the Buddhist Sutras with the four words, 'Thus I have heard,' which means, 'I, Ananda, personally heard this Dharma, which is thus; it is not hearsay.'"

Ananda said, "Okay, I will use the four words, 'Thus I have heard.' My second question is, when the Buddha is in the world, we Bhikshus take the Buddha as our teacher. Whom should we take as our teacher after the Buddha enters Nirvana?"The Buddha said, " After I enter Nirvana, you Bhikshus should take the precepts as your teacher. The Pratimoksa is your great teacher. If you uphold the precepts, it will be the same as when I am in the world. You should avoid all evil and practice all good deeds."In the beginning of the Buddha's teaching career, there were no precepts, but as the Sangha continued to grow, complications inevitably arose. Not everyone was well-behaved. The Buddha established the precepts one by one in response to the needs of the situation. In the final compilation of the precepts, there were 250 precepts for Bhikshus, 348 precepts for Bhikshunis, ten major and forty-eight minor precepts for Bodhisattvas, ten precepts for Shramaneras (novices), and eight precepts and five precepts for laypeople. All these various categories of precepts are aimed at helping people to behave well. People who are well-behaved will be good citizens who can help others and benefit the society. Thus, the moral precepts are the basis for world peace. Therefore, Bhikshus should take the precepts as their teacher."Now I'll ask the third question," continued Ananda. "When the Buddha is in the world, we dwell with the Buddha. We always live and study with the Buddha. After the Buddha enters Nirvana, with whom should the Bhikshus dwell?"

The Buddha answered, "After I enter Nirvana, all the Bhikshus should dwell in the Four Applications of Mindfulness."

The Four Applications of Mindfulness:

1. Contemplating the body as impure.
2. Contemplating feelings as suffering.
3. Contemplating thoughts as impermanent.
4. Contemplating dharmas as being without self.

The first application of mindfulness is to contemplate the body as impure. "But," you say, "I take a bath and keep my body clean every day, and I put on make-up and jewelry to make it beautiful." You may adorn your body with expensive jewelry and designer clothes, but it's just like decorating a toilet; no matter how beautiful the toilet looks, it will still stink!

The nine orifices of our bodies constantly discharge impurities. There is unclean matter from the eyes, wax from the ears, mucus in the nose, and saliva and phlegm in the mouth. Together with the anus and urethra, they make up the nine orifices that discharge impurities. If you don't bathe for several days, your body begins to stink. If you eat onions and garlic, your body will smell of onions and garlic. When you drink milk, it smells of milk. If you eat beef, veal, or pork, then you'll have those odors about you. If you eat dog meat, you'll smell like dog meat. You smell of whatever you eat.

"The flavor is in my mouth," you might say, "and all I have to do is brush my teeth and the flavor will be gone." Wrong! When you eat something, its flavor not only stays in your mouth, it permeates your whole body. You don't believe it? Drink a lot of milk, and you'll notice that your sweat has a milky smell to it. Since impurities are always coming from the nine orifices, what's so good about your body? Thus, you should contemplate the body as being impure. The origin of the body is unclean. It is composed of the four elements (earth, water, fire, and air) and is not real.

Second, contemplate feelings as suffering. Feelings refer to sensations. No matter how enjoyable the sensation is, it is basically suffering! Happiness is the cause of suffering. Third, contemplate thoughts as impermanent. Thoughts arise in continuous succession, one after another; they don't last. Fourth, contemplate dharmas as being without self. All dharmas (phenomena) are free of the notion of "me and mine." These are the Four Applications of Mindfulness.

Contemplate the body as impure; feelings, thoughts, and dharmas are also impure. Contemplate feelings as suffering; the body, thoughts, and dharmas are also suffering. Thoughts are impermanent, and so are the other three. Dharmas are without self, and the other three are also without self. The Four Applications of Mindfulness apply to each of body, feelings, thoughts, and dharmas. Since the time of the Buddha's Nirvana, the Bhikshus have "dwelt" in the Four Applications of Mindfulness as the Buddha instructed.

"Here is my fourth question," said Ananda. "When the Buddha is in the world, the Buddha can subdue the evil-natured Bhikshus. After the Buddha enters Nirvana, how should we deal with them?

The Buddha said, "When you encounter an evil-natured Bhikshu, just ignore him – don't talk to him." To ignore him is a passive way of expelling him. If no one pays attention to him or argues with him, he will soon grow bored of making trouble. If you pay attention to him or try to fight with him, he will think that he is getting somewhere. But if you ignore him, he won't be able to do anything! An "evil-natured Bhikshu" is a monk who doesn't practice. Not every left-home person wants to practice.

In the past, there were all kinds of left-home people in the great monasteries of China, including former murderers, arsonists, and robbers. Some of them reformed after they left the home-life. Others assumed the guise of monks in order to escape the authorities. There were both good and bad people in the Sangha in China, and I believe that this will be the case in other places as well.

Speaking of criminals, in China, vagrants are nick-named "naughty monkeys" and also "Thousand-handed Guanyins," because they have so many hands. They'll steal whatever catches

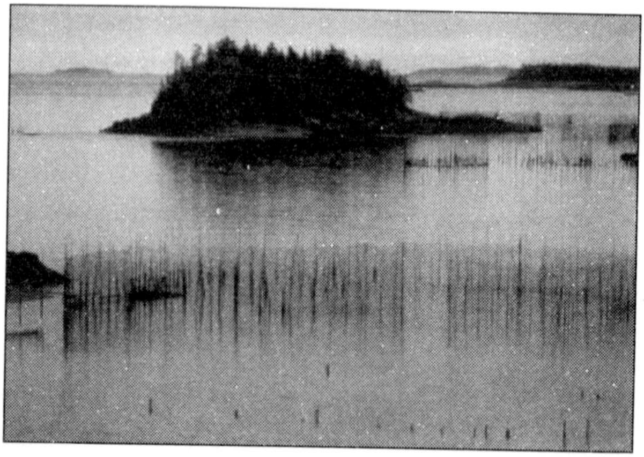

their fancy, and then sell it and use the money to buy alcohol or drugs. Don't be naive and think that all left-home people are good. Left-home people – and that includes myself-are not necessarily good people. However, I'm trying to be good. I don't know what bad deeds I did in the past, but now I want to become a better person.

Evil-natured Bhikshus are perverse and unreasonable. The more you argue with them, the more they enjoy it. That's why the Buddha instructed us to ignore them.

The Three Doubts of the Assembly

When Ananda first ascended the Dharma-seat – the seat where the Buddha spoke the Dharma – to begin the compilation of Sutras, there were many auspicious portents. For instance, Ananda became endowed with the thirty-two features and eighty subsidiary characteristics of a Buddha. Seeing those portents, the members of the assembly immediately had three kinds of doubts:

1. They thought that Ananda was their teacher, Sakyamuni Buddha, who had come back to life.
2. They thought that Ananda was a Buddha from another world. "Is this a Buddha who has come from another world to speak the Dharma in the Saha world? Otherwise, why would he look like that?"

3. They thought Ananda himself had become a Buddha. The entire assembly was startled and at a loss, but once Ananda said, "Thus I have heard," the three doubts were dispelled. He was in effect stating, "This is the Dharma that I, Ananda, personally heard Sakyamuni Buddha speak."

Even the Arhats had three doubts when they saw Ananda leading the compilation of the Sutras. As we listen to this Sutra, we may have a thousand or even ten thousand doubts! "Is this Sutra true? Did the Buddha really say this? What proof is there?" Our human brain starts plugging away, generating millions of doubts! So, you see, studying the Buddhadharma is not that easy. Why haven't we had any attainment? Too many doubts, that's why!

A cultivator should take care not to doubt.

Once you doubt, you go astray.

You shouldn't be so skeptical. You refuse to believe the truth, but you accept a false teaching right away. That's why you are utterly deluded. Once you have a doubt, you are sure to take the wrong road.

You should study the Dharma day after day and learn from the Buddha at all times. Don't be lax. If you really want to study Buddhism, you should memorize the *Surangama Sutra*. Everyone should master this Sutra, know it inside out. If you can recite the *Surangama Sutra* from memory, then your study of Buddhism will have been worth it. The *Surangama Sutra* is the Buddha's most genuine and penetrating teaching. It exposes all the short-comings and weaknesses of the heterodox sects. If you understand the *Surangama Sutra*, you will frighten the demons from the heavens and their followers in heterodox sects so much that their hair stands on end. Therefore, if you really want to support the Triple Jewel and propagate Buddhism, then you should start by studying, reciting, and explaining the *Surangama Sutra*.

Studying Sutras and listening to lectures requires patience. Just as plants and people grow and mature day by day, just as children study in school each day, we should set aside some time each day to study the Dharma. Studying Buddhism is worth more than any amount of money you save up in the bank! In terms of your Dharma body and wisdom life, the Dharma is far more important than money. Don't take worldly wealth so seriously. When you study the Dharma, you earn a transcendental kind of wealth, which can be used in the world and which is indispensable if you want to transcend the world. So, don't look lightly upon the wealth of Dharma and of merit and virtue.

Don't take this casually! It would be best if you could find some time in your busy schedule to come listen to the Sutra lecture and investigate Buddhism every day. "But the lecture is always about the same thing," you say, "It's boring. Why do I have to listen to it every day?" No matter how busy you are, you still have to eat, dress, and sleep every day, don't you? If only you would consider listening to the Sutra as important as dressing, eating, and sleeping!

The Six Requirements

There are Six Requirements found at the beginning of each Sutra. The first is the Requirement of Faith, indicated by the word "Thus." We should have faith in Dharma which is thus, cultivate it, and attain Buddhahood by means of it. Only by means of faith can you attain realization and derive benefit. It's like eating. If you don't believe that food can satisfy your hunger, you won't eat it and get full. Similarly, although the Dharma can lead you to Buddhahood, if you don't believe in it and cultivate it, then it's of no use. Talking about cultivation is not enough. "The Dharma is spoken; the Way is walked." You can benefit from the Dharma only if you believe in and practice it.

The second requirement, the Requirement of Hearing, is indicated by the words "1 have heard." Ananda refers to himself as "I," but this "I" is selfless and unattached, perfectly fused and unimpeded. It is the true self of the inherent nature, which has seen through all things and put them down. This "I" is spoken not to others, but rather, to oneself. This "I" is wise and not deluded, and is endowed with Dharma-selecting vision, so it can deeply enter the treasury of Sutras and have wisdom like the sea. How can one obtain Dharma-selecting vision? It develops through possessing the requirements of faith and hearing. "I have faith, and I would like to listen to the Sutra," you would say.

That's fine, but there must be a time – a time for listening to the lecture on the Medicine Master Sutra. This also refers to the time when Ananda compiled the Sutras. The words "**At one time**" fulfill the Requirement of Time. You may have faith and may wish to hear the Sutra, but if the lecture is scheduled at an inconvenient time, you still won't get to hear the Sutra.

The Bhagavan is another name for the Buddha. If you don't know what "Bhagavan" means, just remember that it's another Sanskrit name for the Buddha. In the text, the word "Bhagavan" fulfills the Requirement of a Host. The requirements of faith, hearing, and time may be satisfied, but if no one lectures on the Sutra, then what are you going to listen to? There's nothing to listen to and nothing to believe, and the time is irrelevant as well!

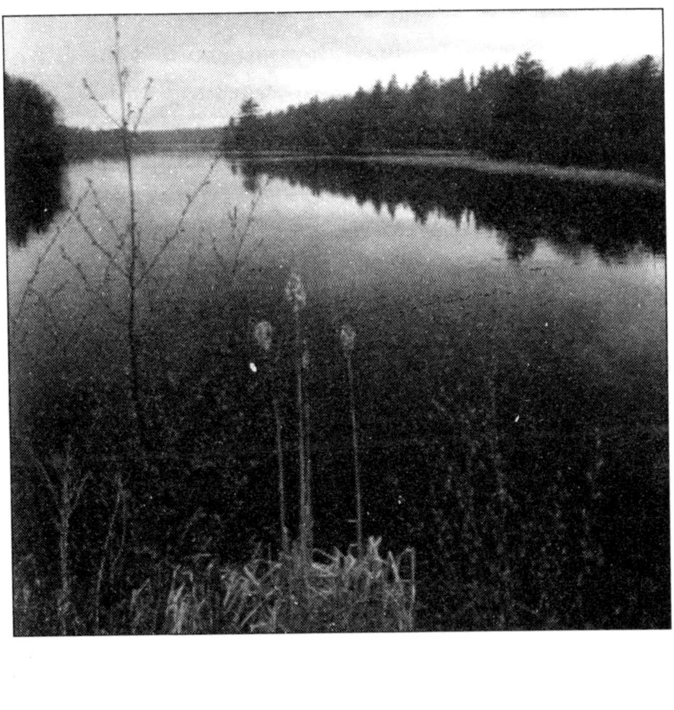

And so a "host," a person who explains the Sutra and speaks the Dharma, is necessary.

The word "Bhagavan," when translated, has six meanings:

1. Comfortable
2. Renowned
3. Adorned
4. Resplendent
5. Auspicious
6. Honored

"Auspicious:" Chinese people like auspiciousness, especially the Cantonese. At New Year's, they always say, "Good luck! May your wishes come true!" Although they like to have good luck, they spend their time playing mahjong and dancing. If you want things to be lucky and according to your wishes, you have to recite the Buddha's name. You also have to be good and follow the rules. If you play mahjong, you might even lose the shirt off your back! Now, would you call that lucky?

"Honored": The Buddha is the most honored one. If we wish to be honored, we should learn from the Buddha, the most venerable and perfect being, who is free of bad habits, faults, delusions, and scattered thoughts. The Buddha's state is much higher than that of an Arhat. *The Dharma Flower Sutra* begins, "Thus have I heard. At one time the Buddha dwelt on Mount Grdhrakuta, near the city of Rajagrha *["House of Kings"]* together with a gathering of great Bhikshus, twelve thousand in all. All were Arhats..." Why were they Arhats? They "had exhausted all outflows." One who attains the state of an Arhat no longer has any faults, bad habits, or idle thoughts. He has put an end to birth and death. They "had done what they had to do." They had done everything they were supposed to do. When the One is attained, all things are finished. They had attained the One, so they didn't seek outside anymore. Since they didn't seek outside, they had no more outflows. If you like to talk, that's an outflow, as is liking to look at things or to listen to sounds.

"But I can't keep my eyes from seeing and my ears from hearing," you say.

That's why you haven't become a Buddha yet. You're always running outside and forgetting to return. You aren't able to turn the light around and shine it within. Exhausting all outflows means having no faults whatsoever – you aren't greedy, you don't contend, you don't seek anything, you aren't selfish, and you don't pursue personal advantages. Affection and love are also faults, and thoughts of desire are the worst faults of all. To have exhausted all outflows means to have no thoughts of desire, thoughts of lust, or wild and deluded thoughts.

"And had no further afflictions": The Arhats no longer had any afflictions. "Having attained self-benefit": They had truly regained their inherent wisdom and gained the advantages of the Buddha's teaching. As I have said to you, "Who is the Buddha? The Buddha is a person of great wisdom. Whoever has true wisdom and is not deluded can become a Buddha." If you are still deluded and insatiably greedy, always seeking for more, fighting with everyone, being selfish and pursuing personal gain, then you haven't gained any benefit from the Dharma. Those who have attained genuine benefit do not crave external things. Gold, silver, and riches mean nothing to them. They do not know what forms, sounds, smells, tastes, and objects of touch are. Nothing can distract them. That is what is meant by "having attained self-benefit."

"They had exhausted the bonds of all existence." They had eradicated all residual habits and had escaped from all the entanglements that used to bind them. They were truly free. "And their hearts had attained self-mastery." Their hearts were carefree and at ease. However, the Buddha's state is much more advanced. That's why the Buddha is considered the most honored and venerable.

If we want to be like the Buddha, first we should learn not to contend, not to be greedy, not to seek, not to be selfish, and not to pursue personal advantage. But it doesn't mean that you won't do these things, while at the same time planning to commit a robbery. Then you're only cheating yourself and others! Genuine non-contention means letting things follow their natural course. If you are not greedy, you will also let things happen naturally. As for seeking nothing, it is said, "When one reaches the state of seeking nothing, one has no worries." Worries come from seeking things. You should also be unselfish. All the troubles in the world come from selfishness and desire. Being unselfish means seeking nothing and having no emotional attachments. Not pursuing personal advantage means not thinking about your own benefit, pleasure, or comfort. Cast out all these faults, and then you can become a Buddha!

The six meanings of "Bhagavan" are very important, and Buddhists should remember them. If you don't, you won't even recognize the Buddha. It's like knowing a person. If you can recognize someone by his appearance or his voice, you can say you know him. Knowing the Buddha is the same way. If you don't even know what the Buddha's title "Bhagavan" means, you are certainly a muddled Buddhist! So, you should memorize them and be prepared to say what they are next time. I have spent so much time and energy explaining the Sutra to you; it'd be a shame if you forgot everything once the lecture was over. If you aren't able to answer my questions, then I'll know that you've been sleeping!

The Buddha was travelling through various lands to teach living beings. He arrived at Vaisali (*"City of Extensive Adornments"*) and stayed beneath a tree from which music resounded. The Buddha teaches and transforms living beings not only in one country, but in all the countries where he has affinities.

As the Buddha was travelling around to teach living beings, he carne to the large city of Vaisali, where he seated himself in full-lotus posture at the base of a tree which put forth music, and spoke Dharma for the multitudes. "At Vaisali" and "beneath a tree from which music resounded" fulfill the Requirement of a Place. Above, we had the requirements of faith, hearing, time, and host. With the requirement of a host, there is a person to speak the Sutra, but if there is no place, how can he speak? For example, if we didn't have a lecture hall, how could we hold a lecture on the

Medicine Master Sutra? And so it is necessary to have a place. The tree from which music resounded is the location where the Medicine Master Sutra was spoken.

The Bhikshus and Bodhisattvas mentioned in the next passage of text fulfill the Requirement of an Audience. Once there is a lecturer and a place for the lecture, people have to go and listen. If no one went to listen to the Buddha when he spoke, his speaking would have been rather pointless. The Dharma is spoken for living beings. Each Dharma assembly has living beings who have affinities with it. For instance, you have come to this Sutra lecture because you have affinities with it. Those without affinities cannot come even if they want to. You have the chance to come listen every day now because you planted good roots during many past lives and many eons. It's not as simple as you think!

Since you don't realize how difficult it is to take part in a Dharma assembly, sometimes you become lazy, thinking, "The Master isn't here yet, so I think I'll just steal away for some fun." And so you go to watch a play or see a movie, or you go to a dance or a party. You waste your energy doing these things, which are of no benefit. When you come to the Sutra lecture, you hear the sound of the Dharma and it lightens your worldly defilements and deluded thoughts. You study the *prajna*-wisdom found in the Sutras. Every time you listen, you understand a little bit more.

"I already understand a lot!" you say. What's wrong with understanding a little bit more? Why do you think it's too much? I never hear you complain about having too much money! No matter how rich you are, you never think you have too much. "The more the better!" is your attitude. So why, when you study wisdom, when you study the true Dharma, are you afraid of learning too much? Isn't this delusion? Since you've never really thought about it, you simply forget what's fundamental so as to pursue the superficial; you look for what is far away and fail to notice what's right beside you. Instead of seriously investigating the Buddhadharma, you just waste your time!

With him were eight thousand great Bhikshus. Bhikshus are men who have left the home-life. They were called "great

Bhikshus" because they were virtuous and wise elders who had left home for at least twenty or thirty years. "Bhikshu" is Sanskrit and has three meanings:

1. Mendicant
2. Frightener of demons
3. Destroyer of evil

Although a mendicant is one who collects alms from others, he is not a common beggar. Common beggars sometimes obtain their food in unscrupulous ways, and they lack the spirit of equanimity. If they don't get enough food, they become afflicted. A mendicant, on the other hand, doesn't notice whether the food tastes good or not. Nor does he care whether you give him a lot or a little. He simply wants to give people the opportunity to "plant" blessings. The donor's blessings will be as bountiful as the seeds he or she sows.

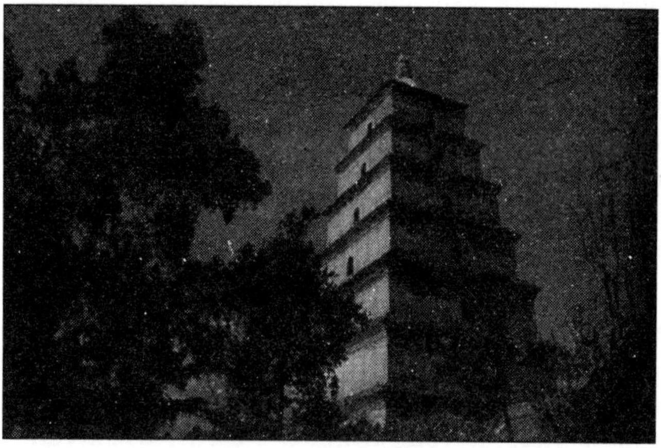

A mendicant monk is free of affliction and ignorance. He carries himself with dignity and obtains food in the proper manner. When Bhikshus walk on the road, they do not stare around at random. Instead, their eyes contemplate their noses, their noses contemplate their mouths, and their mouths contemplate their hearts. They do not look at, listen to, speak about, or do anything that does not accord with propriety. Bhikshus seek alms in silence, unlike common beggars, who may stand at people's doors and say flattering things, such as, "Sir! Madam! May blessings, wealth, and good fortune be yours!" When Bhikshus seek alms, they stand silently and accept whatever offerings are given. If none are offered, they simply leave, without becoming upset. That's how mendicant monks differ from ordinary beggars.

The second meaning of "Bhikshu" is "frightener of demons." Because a Bhikshu is very proper and upright, the demons from the heavens and the externalists are afraid of him. The demons and ghosts stay far away from him. His proper energy overcomes all deviant beings.

The third meaning is "destroyer of evil." Ordinary people find it difficult to give up their bad habits. Bhikshus who cultivate the Way, however, concentrate on giving up bad habits and reforming themselves. They are able to make a new start, changing their faults and becoming good. That's why they are called destroyers of evil.

Present in the assembly were eight thousand great Bhikshus **and thirty-six thousand Bodhisattvas Mahasattvas.** Bodhisattva is a Sanskrit word, but it has become a very popular term in China. Although many people use it, most don't know what it really means. "A Bodhisattva is just a Bodhisattva!" they say.

A "Bodhisattva" is a sage of the Great Vehicle. The full Chinese transliteration of the Sanskrit term is *putisaduo,* but the Chinese use the abbreviated form *pusa.* "Bodhisattva" means "one who enlightens sentient beings." Bodhisattvas are one of the nine Dharma Realms of living beings and also one of the Four Dharma Realms of Sages. A Bodhisattva uses his enlightened wisdom to rescue and liberate all sentient beings, beings with blood and breath. Although beings without blood and breath, such as plants, are considered insentient, they do have natures, and they are born and grow within the Buddhas' great, bright, light treasury.

A Bodhisattva is also defined as "an enlightened sentient being." The Bodhisattva is the same as other living beings, except that he is enlightened. Being enlightened, he "does no evil and practices all good deeds." He has no bad habits or faults. Having attained supreme wisdom, he is not confused anymore, so he does not act out of ignorance.

Ordinary living beings always bungle things up in their ignorance. They don't have any real wisdom. When confronted with a problem, they don't know how to handle it, because they are unenlightened. Those of the Two Vehicles are self-enlightened: they have come to such understanding and are no longer confused. However, they have not tried to teach other people the method by which they themselves became enlightened. Bodhisattvas are enlightened themselves, and they also share their enlightened wisdom with other living beings, teaching those beings to become enlightened through the method they themselves used. Bodhisattvas enlighten themselves and also enlighten others, but their enlightenment is not complete. A Buddha is one who has enlightened himself, enlightens others, and perfected his enlightened practice. Since he is perfect in the three enlightenments and replete with the myriad virtues he is called a Buddha.

When Bodhisattvas continue to advance, they can attain Buddhahood. There are many different levels of Bodhisattvahood; for example, there are Bodhisattvas of the First, Second, Third, Fourth, Fifth, Sixth, Seventh, Eighth, Ninth, and Tenth Grounds. When Tenth Ground Bodhisattvas reach the level of Equal Enlightenment, their enlightenment is virtually equal to that of the Buddhas – they are only one step away from Buddhahood.

"Mahasattvas" are great Bodhisattvas endowed with great vows, great wisdom, and great skill and accomplishment in cultivation. There were thirty-six thousand of such Bodhisattvas in the assembly of Medicine Master Buddha, which was as vast as the ocean.

Also kings, ministers. Various kings were also present. Kings rule the country in order to bring blessings and prosperity to the people, and they are assisted by ministers.

Brahmans. The Brahmans [the priestly class] were one of the two noble classes in ancient India. While practicing, Brahmans, like Buddhists, may observe certain ascetic practices and be vegetarian, their goal is to be born in the heavens. Although they cultivate purity and asceticism, they do not work on subduing greed, anger, and delusion. Their equivalent in China is the Taoists.

Despite their external differences, Brahmans and Taoists share similar practices and beliefs. There are quite a few skilled cultivators among the Brahmans.

Lay disciples. While others may address you by the title of "Upasaka" or "Upasika" [titles for a Buddhist layman and laywoman, respectively] it is not permissible to use these titles to refer to yourself. Some laypeople print business cards giving their names as "Upasaka So-and-so," and they also speak of themselves as Upasakas. Such people do not know the proper etiquette. Maybe you don't understand what I mean, so let me talk about "Mr." instead. In China, *xiansheng* ("Mr.") is the most common form of addressing the others. Other people may address you as "Mr. So-and-so" out of respect, but you certainly wouldn't introduce yourself as "Mr. Smith" or "Mr. Jones." If you shamelessly call yourself *xiansheng*, you simply don't understand the Chinese language. This is something everyone should know. Remember not to call yourself "Mr. Smith" or "Upasaka Smith." "Mr." is a title reserved for learned, virtuous elders, and "Upasaka" is used for a layman who has ten kinds of virtue.

"Dharma Master" is also a title used by others to address you. If you call yourself a Dharma Master, you are praising yourself. It's like calling yourself the emperor. Others can hail the emperor, "Long live your Majesty!" but the emperor does not say that to himself. That's common sense. The same goes for the title "Upasaka" and "Dharma Master." These are respectful forms of address. You use them to respect others, not yourself. Of course you should respect yourself, but you don't need to make a show of it. The lore and knowledge of Chinese culture is boundless and inexhaustible. If you miss one small point, you may end up making a big blunder. These rules of etiquette are commonly overlooked.

There were also **gods, dragons, and the rest of the eightfold division.** Our temple is protected by the gods, dragons, and the rest of the eightfold division of ghosts and spirits. You may all remember that when we first moved into Gold Wheel Monastery and began renovating it, some people saw a vision of Guanyin Bodhisattva sitting in mid-air with his foot resting on a tortoise.

On the eastern comer of thc property, there used to be a bar where drug dealers, winos, strippers, and other disreputable people would hang out. Then, just before our opening ceremony, the bar was closed down for good. It used to be a bad neighborhood, but now it's much cleaner. This is a response from the gods, dragons, and the rest of the eightfold division, who protect the monastery.

When this place was a church, some rather messy people came and left food allover the ground, attracting a lot of mice. We are now propagating the Buddhadharma here, so the gods, dragons, and the rest of the eightfold division should protect this temple and quickly chase the mice away. Actually, I wouldn't really mind the rats, except that they give people the impression that our place is very unsanitary. So now we request the Dharma-protecting spirits to do their job and protect this monastery. Chase away the mice and any other beings that should not be here. Don't be polite with them.

The eightfold division is comprised of the gods, dragons, *yaksas, gandharvas, asuras, garucjas, kinnaras, and mahoragas.*

The gods in the heavens made vows in the past to protect the Buddhas' temples.

Dragons are magical beings. When they cultivated in past lives, they were "fast with the Vehicle and slow with the precepts." They practiced Great Vehicle (Mahayana) Buddhism with tremendous vigor. Seeking a shortcut to obtaining spiritual powers, they practiced esoteric dharmas with intensity, but neglected to hold the precepts. They weren't careful to abstain from evil and practice good. For their esoteric practices, sometimes they would steal skulls from corpses and recite mantras over them. They would also steal the plaques that people put up to honor their ancestors, and then they would command ghosts and spirits using those ancestors as mediums.

Dragons were cultivators who advanced at a rocket-like speed, but who didn't pay much attention to the precepts. They casually broke the precepts against sexual misconduct, lying, killing, and stealing. They stole human skulls and ancestral plaques, and even the trees growing by people's graves, in order to carry out their practices. They approached the Dharma with crooked, greedy minds. That's how they were "fast with the Vehicle and slow with the precepts." Because they were fast with the Vehicle, they have spiritual powers when they become dragons. Because they were slow with the precepts, they fell into the animal realm.

Dragons are animals, but they are also spiritual creatures. Through its spiritual powers, a dragon has the ability to change size at will from the very small to the very large and can also suddenly vanish and just as suddenly reappear. However, dragons have a great fear of the sun because when they bake in the sun, it's as painful as being scorched by fire. They have to send down some rain to soak themselves-just like taking a shower. These are the dragons that dwell in the heavens.

Yaksas are called "speedy ghosts" because they travel very quickly. There are space-travelling *yaksa*, ground-travelling *yaksas*, and water-travelling *yaksas*. They travel faster than cars, airplanes, and even rockets. They can travel ten thousand miles in a single thought. There are a great variety of *yaksas*, just as there are great varieties of dragons: golden dragons, fire dragons, green dragons, white dragons, black dragons, and so on. There are also many ethnic groups in the human race, and within each ethnic group or nationality, there are further distinctions of southerners, northerners, easterners, and westerners. All these different groups of people have their own languages and writing systems. In general, countless species of living beings populate the world, and each species contains infinite variations within it. That's the wonder of the world.

People will never completely understand the secrets of the world. Now with people going to the moon, it seems we are about to experience a breakthrough and everything will be understood. However, when everything is understood, the world will come to an end. When everything has been discovered, it will all disappear. The play will be over! Once people on earth can communicate with and travel to other planets, the world's population will be wiped out by nuclear weapons, or by natural disasters such as earthquakes and volcanic eruptions. No matter how flourishing the world becomes, when it reaches the height of its glory, it will become dark again, just as day turns into night. We rise in the morning and begin the day; and when the day is over, we go to sleep. As soon as we close our eyes, we become muddled and unclear. All things, great and small, in the world, go through cycles.

Gandharvas are spirits that make delightful music. When they play their music in the heavens, the immortals sit there totally enraptured, oblivious to the passing of time. However, *gandharvas* won't play their music for just anyone. The Jade Emperor can enjoy their music, because he knows their weakness. He knows that once they get a whiff of incense, they immediately come wanting to sniff it, no matter how many tens of thousands of miles away they might be. The Jade Emperor has a special kind of incense that he uses to attract them. When they arrive at his palace and smell the incense, they start dancing and singing. That is why *gandharvas* are called "incense-inhaling spirits." There are eight dragon kings, and four *gandharva* kings.

There are four kinds of *asuras*. *Asuras* have huge tempers. They are always getting angry. People who have big tempers are controlled by *asuras*. In the heavens, *asuras* are called "those without wine" since they have no wine to drink. They are also known as "non-gods" because their status in the heavens is like that of illegal aliens in America, who live in America and can enjoy American bread and butter, but who cannot vote or run for office. The *asuras* in the heavens are constantly at war with Lord Shakra's heavenly troops, hoping to overthrow Shakra *[the Jade Emperor]* and usurp his throne. They can live in the heavens and enjoy the blessings of the gods, but they do not have any authority there.

Garudas are the great golden-winged Peng birds. They also have the ability to grow large or small, and to appear and disappear at will. Their wingspan is 330 *yojanas*. One *yojana* is 40 miles long, so you can see how long 330 *yojanas* must be! With one flap of its wings, a Peng bird dries up the waters of the sea so that it can gobble up all the exposed dragons-big, little, young, and old! With another flap of its wings, it can level the mountains by moving them into the ocean.

Garudas have very great spiritual penetrations, and dragons used to fear them more than anything. But since the garudas have taken refuge with the Buddha, they live in peace with the dragons and don't eat them anymore. Chapter One of the Wonderful Dharma Lotus Flower Sutra explains the four kinds of garudas.

Kinnaras are called "doubtful spirits," because they look like humans, except that they have a single horn growing on top of their heads. They also make extremely fine music.

Mahoragas are spirits of huge pythons. The gods, dragons, and the rest of the eightfold division include former demons, ghosts, and goblins who reformed and became Dharma-protectors of Buddhism. So you see, bad people sometimes turn around and become good. As it is said, "The sea of suffering is boundless; a turn of the head is the other shore." Those who committed the ten evil deeds or the five rebellious acts can still start anew and become good. Since the ghosts and spirits of the eightfold division felt bad about the harm they had done to Buddhism before, they vowed to protect Buddhism.

Note

1. Explained by the Venerable Master Hua in 1983 at Gold Wheel Monastery in Los Angeles.

Appendix IV

"TIBETAN MEDICINE IN AMERICA": THE 2008 SYMPOSIUM OF TIBETAN MEDICINE

By Adam Okerblom

This June 13th through 15th, the American Tibetan Medical Association(ATMA) presented its first major public event, "Tibetan Medicine in America": 2008 Symposium of Tibetan Medicine. The symposium was co-sponsored by the Shang Shung International Institute for Tibetan Studies, USA, and the local university of Amherst College. This unique event was held in two of the stately lecture halls of Amherst College, in Amherst Massachusetts. The symposium was made possible largely due to the inspiration of Dr. Phuntsog Wangmo, president of the board of ATMA and director of the Shang Shung Institute School of Traditional Tibetan Medicine; also by the invaluable efforts of Paola Zamperini, President of the board of the Shang Shung International Institute for Tibetan Studies, USA, and professor of Asian Languages and Civilizations at Amherst College. After much hard work, the circumstances for the symposium arose very favorably; the auspiciousness of the event greatly increased when our precious master Chögyal Namkhai Norbu graciously accepted to personally inaugurate the event.

The symposium participants consisted of numerous Tibetan physicians, including the guest keynote presenters as well as physicians residing in the local region, Tibetan medical students of the Shang Shung Institute, interested members of the academic community from across the country, and also interested people of the local community.

Chogyal Namkhai Norbu inaugurated the symposium with an opening keynote address. He described the ancient roots of Tibetan culture in the kingdom of Shang Shung, and the necessity to protect Tibetan knowledge and culture today. He encouraged the participants to utilize the opportunity to learn from traditional Tibetan physicians, who carry the valuable ancient knowledge of the Tibetan Healing Science.

In the following two days the keynote speakers delivered presentations on topics of traditional Tibetan Medicine, and its current situation throughout the world. The guest speakers consisted of Tibetan physicians trained in the traditional Tibetan Healing Science both in Tibet and India. All of the presenters had extensive experience with their specialized practice of medicine, as well as with teaching and practicing abroad in countries beyond their homeland.

Dr. Yang ga, professor at the Tibetan Medicine Institute of Lhasa and board member of ATMA, presented from his current PHD research on the historical precedent of the traditional texts of the Tibetan Healing Science Lineage. Dr. Kunchok Gyaltsen, doctoral student at the UCLA School of Public Health and current board member of ATMA, demonstrated the fundamental theory of the Tibetan Medicine system for the public audience. He also shared his broad experience in teaching and applying Tibetan Medicine among diverse groups of patients and medical professionals, from the far East to the far West.

The presentations continued with Dr. Phuntsog Wangmo, graduate of the Tibetan Medicine Institute of Lhasa. Citing the classic Tibetan Healing Science Text, "Remaining Free from Disease", Dr. Wangmo lectured on vital themes such as seasonal and dietary considerations for maintaining health and wellness. These topics were further expounded by Dr. Yangdron Kalsang, graduate of the Tibetan Medicine Institute of Lhasa, the Five

Branches Acupuncture Institute in Santa Cruz California, and current board member of ATMA. Dr. Kalsang offered health tips and lifestyle guidelines for modern living, from the Tibetan medical perspective.

Dr. Tenzin Dakpa, current instructor at the Shang Shung School of Traditional Tibetan Medicine, provided a thorough account of the current situation of Tibetan medicine in India, and described in detail the curriculum for contemporary students at Men Tsi Khang University in Dharamsala, the largest school of Tibetan medicine and astrology outside of Tibet. Dr. Yangbum Gyal described the current condition of Tibetan Medicine inside Tibet, presenting the successes and the challenges facing modern practitioners. Dr. Tashi Rabten lectured on the opportunities and challenges of practicing Tibetan medicine in the United States, insightfully recounting his experience in the context of modern urban communities in America.

The keynote presentations of the symposium provided clear insight into the world-wide Diaspora of the Tibetan Healing Science, its burgeoning roots across the modern world, and its value in modern society. Tibetan medicine has endured for so many centuries as a highly regarded science of healing. However today Tibetan medicine faces modern challenges. Through the works of the American Tibetan Medical Association(ATMA), and other groups, Tibetan physicians world-wide are beginning to collaborate to continue the authentic lineage of the Tibetan Healing Science, and secure its legal protection and precedence in the United States.

For the guest Tibetan physicians the symposium was a rare occasion to network and collaborate with other practitioners living here in the U.S.. For the fortunate medical students of the Shang Shung Institute it was an unprecedented privilege to learn from these eminent physicians of renowned lineage. The physicians shared with the students moving accounts of their personal experience. They described their reverence for their teachers above them, their exhaustive studies and intensive training. They shared their individual work, innovative research, as well as their experience within the United States. These laudable senior physicians reiterated the pivotal role of the students in perpetuating the authentic Tibetan Healing Science practice, and their continuing support in that work. Thus the Shang Shung Institute Tibetan medical students, representative of many different nations, developed their global perspective on the contemporary situation of the Tibetan Healing Science, and were greatly inspired in their pursuit of this dynamic medical lineage.

Thanks to the dedicated work and generous contributions of the sponsors, organizers, symposium volunteers, and of course the continual support and blessings of Chogyal Namkhai Norbu, "Tibetan Medicine in America" was a complete success. The Tibetan Healing Science Lineage is rooted in thousands of years of history. Compared to this root, its seeds here in the West are tiny young sprouts. But as one keynote guest observed, America is the Land of Opportunity. In this fertile soil, Tibetan medicine is free to develop, to continue its ancient lineage for the benefit of people today, and for all beings.

APPENDIX V

THE TZU CHI FOUNDATION

Tzu-Chi temple and hospital, Hualien, Taiwan

At 4 am each day, a 70-year-old Buddhist nun rises from her sleep and leads 150 nuns in prayer in a modest wooden temple on the east coast of Taipei, nestled between a mountain range and the Pacific Ocean.

This unlikely setting is the home of the biggest non-government organization (NGO) in the Chinese-speaking world, with 10 million members in more than 30 countries around the world and annual donations of US$300 million.

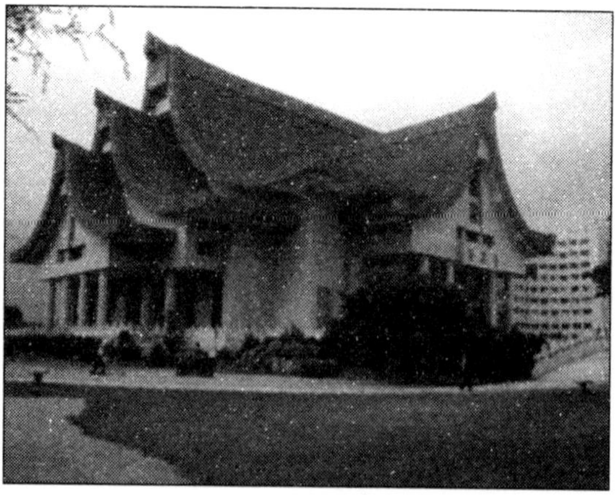

Founded in 1966 by Master Cheng Yen, as she is now known, the Tzu Chi Foundation runs seven hospitals, a university, a recycling programme with 57,000 volunteers, more than 60 schools, Asia's largest bone marrow bank, a global television station and has delivered medical and humanitarian aid to more than 60 countries.

Inspired by the teachings of Buddha and the work of Albert Schweitzer and Mother Theresa, its volunteers seek to follow a creed of 'Buddhism in action,' implementing love and good works all over the world. The core are its 1 million volunteers, of whom 10 percent work full-time for no pay. It is a Buddhist organization in which lay people are the key players.

This year Tzu Chi has delivered food, clothes and medicine to victims of disasters in countries across the world, including China, Indonesia, Malaysia, Philippines, South Africa, Lesotho, Bolivia, Argentina, Mexico, and the United States, as well as Taiwan. No other charity in the Chinese world provides aid on this scale and to people of all races and religions. The bone marrow bank, established in 1993, has provided bone marrow to more than 1,400 people from 23 countries.

"Traditionally, Chinese only helped their own family or their own community," said Richard Madsen, head of the sociology department at the University of California at San Diego and a Maryknoll father for three years in Taiwan.

"Tzu Chi helps the whole world. This is a global vision, suitable to the cosmopolitan and middle-class Taiwanese. Cheng Yen has given a vision to this. This is a major contribution to the Chinese world."

The charity's biggest program of aid outside Taiwan is to mainland China, where it has built 38 schools, 4,100 homes for the poor, 10 nursing homes for old people, 13 day care centres, dug 5,000 wells for farmers in arid Gansu province and provided scholarships for 7,000 students.

This aid has provoked fierce controversy in Taiwan, where many opposed giving aid to what they see as 'the enemy', especially during times of tension, such as the 1996 missile crisis and the Qiandao Lake incident of March 1994, when 24 Taiwanese were murdered on a tourist boat and the was investigation handled ineptly by the police. But Cheng Yen has insisted on continuing the aid, which she sees as a 'bridge of love' between the two sides.

"The people in the mainland and Taiwan are innocent," said Kao Ming-san, a volunteer from Taiwan working in the mainland since 1997. "The tensions between the two sides are the result of politicians. Love can ease the tensions and avoid war. The people there are very polite to us. We do not talk of politics or religion."

Cheng Yen was born into a modest family in Chingshui, west Taiwan on May 14, 1937, when Taiwan was a Japanese colony. When she was 11 months old, her parents gave her to the brother of her father and his wife, who brought her up. She was traumatized by the sudden death of her adopted father, a cinema manager, of a brain hemorrhage in June 1960 at the age of 51 and turned to Buddhism. She left home and established her own community of nuns in Hualien, a port city on the east coast and one of the poorest regions of Taiwan.

Their early work was to provide cash, food and clothes to the poor and victims of natural disasters in the Hualien area. Its first major project was construction of a hospital in the town, which opened in August 1986. It was the first Buddhist hospital offering western medicine in the Chinese world.

The foundation grew rapidly after the lifting of martial law in July 1987, when civil society blossomed in Taiwan, and it opened its first overseas branch in the United States in December 1989. Its membership rose from 80,000 members in 1986 to 1 million in 1990 and 3 million in 1994.

In October 1999, the foundation launched a global channel, Da Ai Tai (Great Love Television), to reach members abroad and help it expand beyond the Taiwanese community, who account for a majority of its members. It was also out of disgust at the sensationalism and tabloid journalism of the Taiwan media.

Cheng Yen gives her disciples 10 interdictions, which include chewing betel nut, because it causes cancer, and taking part in politics. She has succeeded in keeping her foundation neutral in the intense political climate of Taiwan.

INDEX